Movement and Allied Disorders in Childhood

Movement and Allied Disorders in Childhood

Edited by
MARY M. ROBERTSON
University College London Medical School, London, UK
VALSAMMA EAPEN
United Arab Emirates University, Al Ain, United Arab Emirates
& University College London Medical School, London, UK

JOHN WILEY & SONS
Chichester · New York · Brisbane · Toronto · Singapore

Telephone National 01243 779777
International (+44) 1243 779777

Other Wiley Editorial Offices

John Wiley & Sons, Inc., 605 Third Avenue,
New York, NY 10158-0012, USA

Jacaranda Wiley Ltd, 33 Park Road, Milton,
Queensland 4064, Australia

John Wiley & Sons (Canada) Ltd, 22 Worcester Road,
Rexdale, Ontario M9W 1L1, Canada

John Wiley & Sons (SEA) Pte Ltd, 37 Jalan Pemimpin #05-04,
Block B, Union Industrial Building, Singapore 2057

Library of Congress Cataloging-in-Publication Data

Movement and allied disorders in childhood / edited by Mary M. Robertson and Valsamma Eapen.
p. cm.
Includes bibliographical references and index.
ISBN 0-471-95324-5 (alk. paper)
1. Movement disorders in children. I. Robertson, Mary M.
II. Eapen, Valsamma.
[DNLM]: 1. Movement Disorders—in infancy & childhood. WS 340
M935 1995]
RJ496.M68M68 1995
618.92'8—dc20
DNLM/DLC
for Library of Congress 95–9400
CIP

British Library Cataloguing in Publication Data

A catalogue record for this book is available from the British Library

ISBN 0-471-95324-5

Typeset in 10/12 pt Palatino by Mackreth Media Services, Hemel Hempstead
Printed and bound in Great Britain by Biddles Ltd, Guildford
This book is printed on acid-free paper responsibly manufactured from sustainable forestation, for which at least two trees are planted for each one used for paper production.

To the
MEMORY OF OUR PARENTS

Contents

List of Contributors ix

Preface xiii
Mary M. Robertson and Valsamma Eapen

1 **Gilles de la Tourette Syndrome** 1
Mary M. Robertson and Valsamma Eapen

2 **The Genetics of Tics and Related Disorders** 13
David L. Pauls and Ben J. M. van de Wetering

3 **Inner Lives of Individuals and Families Living with Tourette Syndrome** 31
Donald J. Cohen, Sharon I. Ort and James F. Leckman

4 **Obsessive–Compulsive Disorder in Children and Adolescents** 43
Robert A. King and Lawrence Scahill

5 **Attention Deficit Disorder** 57
Gerald S. Golden

6 **Juvenile Wilson's Disease: The Neurological Syndrome** 69
John M. Walshe

7 **Phenylketonuria: An Unfolding Story** 83
Alan J. Thompson

8 **Chorea, Athetosis, Dystonia, Tremor and Parkinsonism** 105
Kimberly S. Trinidad and Roger Kurlan

9 **Myoclonus and Infantile Spasms** 149
Frank M. C. Besag

10 **Rare Movement Disorders Associated with Metabolic and Neurodegenerative Diseases** 177
Mark Stacy and Joseph Jankovic

11 **Drug-related Movement Disorders** 199
David G. Cunningham-Owens

12 Genetics of Movement Disorders: Dystonia, Dopa-responsive Dystonia and Huntington's Disease 237
Susan B. Bressman and Neil J. Risch

13 Functional Neuroanatomy of the Basal Ganglia 257
Garrett E. Alexander

14 Structural Neuroimaging: Magnetic Resonance 279
Alina Greco

15 Radionuclide Neuroimaging 293
Durval Campos Costa

16 Developmental Dysexecutive Syndrome: Does it Exist? A Neuropsychological Perspective 305
Simon Baron-Cohen and John Moriarty

Index 317

List of Contributors

Garrett E. Alexander
Department of Neurology, Emory University School of Medicine, WMB-6000, 1639 Pierce Drive, Post Office Drawer V, Atlanta, GA 30322, USA

Simon Baron-Cohen
Departments of Experimental Psychology and Psychiatry, University of Cambridge, Downing Street, Cambridge CB2 3EB, UK

Frank M.C. Besag
Honorary Consultant, St Piers Lingfield, St Piers Lane, Lingfield, Surrey RH7 6PW, UK

Susan B. Bressman
Dystonia Clinical Research Center, Neurological Institute, Columbia-Presbyterian Medical Center, New York, NY 10032, USA

Donald J. Cohen
Yale Child Study Center, Yale University School of Medicine, 230 South Frontage Road, PO Box 3333, New Haven, CT 06510-8009, USA

Durval Campos Costa
Senior Lecturer in Nuclear Medicine, Institute of Nuclear Medicine, University College London Medical School, Middlesex Hospital, Mortimer Street, London W1N 8AA, UK

David G. Cunningham-Owens
Department of Psychiatry, University of Edinburgh, Kennedy Tower, Royal Edinburgh Hospital, Morningside Park, Edinburgh EH10 5HF, UK

Valsamma Eapen
Assistant Professor in Child Psychiatry, UAE University, Faculty of Medicine and Health Science, PO Box 17666, Al Ain, UAE
& Honorary Lecturer, UCL Medical School, London, UK

Gerald S. Golden
Vice President, Medical School Liaison, National Board of Medical Examiners, Adjunct Professor of Neurology, University of Pennsylvania School of Medicine, 3750 Market Street, Philadelphia, PA 19104, USA

Alina Greco
Department of Magnetic Resonance Imaging, Centre Hospitalier Princesse Grace, Principality of Monaco. Address for Correspondence: c/o Dr Durval Campos Costa, Department of Nuclear Medicine, Middlesex Hospital, Mortimer Street, London W1N 8AA, UK

Joseph Jankovic
Department of Neurology, Baylor College of Medicine, Houston, TX 77030, USA

Robert A. King
Yale Child Study Center, Yale University School of Medicine, 230 South Frontage Road, PO Box 3333, New Haven, CT 06510-8009, USA

Roger Kurlan
Department of Neurology, University of Rochester, Strong Memorial Hospital, 601 Elmwood Avenue, Rochester, NY 14642, USA

James F. Leckman
Yale Child Study Center, Yale University School of Medicine, 230 South Frontage Road, PO Box 3333, New Haven, CT 06510-8009, USA

John Moriarty
Department of Neuropsychiatry, Raymond Way Suite, Institute of Neurology, University of London, Queen Square, London WC1N 3BG, UK

Sharon I. Ort
Yale Child Study Center, Yale University School of Medicine, 230 South Frontage Road, PO Box 3333, New Haven, CT 06510-8009, USA

David L. Pauls
Yale Child Study Centre, Yale University School of Medicine, 230 South Frontage Road, PO Box 3333, New Haven, CT 06510-8009, USA

Neil I. Risch
Department of Epidemiology, Yale University School of Medicine, 60 College Street, PO Box 3333, New Haven, CT 06510, USA

Mary M. Robertson
Senior Lecturer in Psychiatry and Consultant Neuropsychiatrist, Department of Psychiatry, Middlesex Hospital, Wolfson Building, Riding House Street, London W1N 8AA, UK

Lawrence Scahill
Yale Child Study Center, Yale University School of Medicine, 230 South Frontage Road, PO Box 3333, New Haven, CT 06510-8009, USA

Mark Stacy
Assistant Professor of Neurology, Columbia School of Medicine, University of Missouri, Columbia, MO 65212, USA

Alan J. Thompson
Consultant Neurologist, The National Hospital for Neurology and Neurosurgery, Queen Square, London WC1N 3BG, UK

Kimberly S. Trinidad
Assistant Professor of Neurology, Buffalo General Hospital, Department of Neurology, School of Medicine and Biomedical Services, 100 High Street, Buffalo, NY 14203, USA

Ben J. M. van de Wetering
Department of Psychiatry, University Hospital Rotterdam-Dijkzigt and Erasmus University, Postbus 1738, Dr Molewaterplein 50, 3015 CN Rotterdam, The Netherlands

John M. Walshe
Consultant Neurologist, The Department of Neurology, Faculty of Clinical Sciences, University College London School of Medicine, London WC1E 6BT, UK

Preface

Movement disorders serve as a paradigm for understanding both neurological and psychiatric disorders, and bridge the narrowing gap between the two disciplines. In many of these conditions, there is a familial neurobiological basis, and yet environmental influences may modify both the nature and course of these disorders. A developmental perspective is particularly crucial when the onset is in childhood.

This volume documents recent advances in the understanding of movement disorders and allied conditions. It is not intended to be exhaustive, but rather, to provide an update on research developments in a wide range of childhood movement disorders. For readers with a background in clinical medicine, the special emphasis on management issues will offer practical guidance in the management of children with a range of movement disorders. For researchers, the contributors have attempted to provide sufficient information to achieve a critical assessment of the state of the art and identify directions for future research.

We hope that this book will aid interdisciplinary communication in an area where an increasing range of researchers are involved in clinical management and research. There is a worldwide range of contributors from the various clinical specialities, as well as the basic sciences. The former include neurology, paediatrics, psychiatry and psychology, while examples for the latter are genetics, neuroimaging and neuroanatomy. Linking them is the acknowledgement that childhood movement disorders result from a basic disturbance in specific areas of the brain, the effects of which include not only involuntary movements, but also a variety of neurobehavioural manifestations.

We begin with three chapters on Gilles de la Tourette syndrome (GTS), covering the clinical syndrome itself (Robertson and Eapen), the genetics (Pauls and van de Wetering), and psychosocial aspects (Cohen, Ort and Leckman). This is because we regard GTS as a paradigm of neuropsychiatric disorders, which is a particularly useful model for the application of the full range of neuroscience and behavioural methodologies, and as one that could provide insights into other developmental and neurobehavioural conditions. For example, advances in understanding the genetics of GTS have profoundly influenced both the conceptualization and research, not only pertaining to this disorder, but also to a variety of associated disorders such as obsessive–compulsive disorder (OCD) and attention deficit hyperactivity disorder (ADHD). Thus, Pauls and van de Wetering in their chapter on the genetics of tics and related disorders highlight directions for future research, including studies to illuminate the physiological and biochemical aetiology of a disorder by examination of the gene product and its impact on the manifestation of the syndrome. From a slightly different perspective, Cohen, Ort and Leckman in their chapter on living with Tourette syndrome illuminate the 'inner worlds' of afflicted children, and the struggle for both themselves and their families. This is true for any young person suffering from movement disorders, irrespective of the type, and the authors go on to consider the role of the clinician in aiding afflicted children and their families. Due to their links with GTS and other movement disorders, OCD and ADHD have merited inclusion in the volume as chapters in their own right. King and Scahill give a comprehensive account of childhood OCD, highlighting the relationship between this and movement disorders such as Sydenham's chorea and GTS. Golden highlights the complexities involved in the diagnosis and management of children with comorbid ADHD and movement disorders.

The following chapters deal directly with other individual disorders, providing information on the epidemiology, aetiology, pathogenesis and clinical and management issues. For example, Trinidad and Kurlan provide comprehensive clinical descriptions of the commonly occurring movement disorders such as chorea, athetosis, dystonia, tremor and parkinsonism. Besag provides a comprehensive account of myoclonus and infantile spasms, and describes how to distinguish these from other involuntary movements. Clinicians will undoubtedly find this information valuable, since distinguishing one involuntary movement from another is the key not only to correct diagnosis but also to optimal subsequent management. The chapter on juvenile Wilson's disease by Walshe gives special emphasis to treatment issues. Thompson begins with the history of phenylketonuria (PKU), then brings the reader up to date with all aspects of the disorder. The chapter on rare childhood movement disorders by Stacy and Jankovic gives an overview of the metabolic and neurodegenerative diseases that may present to the clinician as a movement disorder, highlighting the differentiating features between different involuntary movements. The chapter on drug related movement disorders by Cunningham-Owens is extensive in its review of research literature on the topic, and provides a brief overview of some standardized techniques for recording symptomatology in these disorders.

We have chosen to conclude the book with chapters providing comprehensive information about the genetics as well as the functional neuroanatomical models in the understanding of some of these disorders. The functional and structural neuroimaging chapters are complementary to these, bringing together the basic sciences and their clinical applications. The underlying importance of developmental issues in these disorders is highlighted by the fact that the chapter by Bressman and Risch covers the genetics of movement disorders, illustrating the varying strategies that are now being applied to localize disease genes. In addition, the ability to utilize genetic linkage and other aspects of genetic analysis to study non-genetic aetiological factors in illnesses is a significant methodological advancement that has not been possible before. Although we acknowledge a slight overlap between this chapter and the one by Trinidad and Kurlan, we felt that it is appropriate as the chapters are very different and rounded in their own right. Alexander describes the functional organization of the basal ganglia, the motor circuitry central to the production of involuntary movements, and the neurotransmitters (particularly dopamine) that are involved in the operational control of these circuits. There is also emphasis on how movement parameters are encoded in the discharge patterns of basal ganglia neurons, how the basal ganglia communicate with other brain regions that are involved in movement control, and how therapeutic manipulations of these areas can ameliorate symptoms in certain movement disorders. Natural sequels to the functional neuroanatomy of the brain include brain imaging techniques, which have increased our understanding of the neuroanatomical substrates and have brought together structural, functional and neurochemical concepts in the pathogenesis of movement disorders. In this regard the chapters by Greco and Campos Costa on structural and functional neuroimaging are noteworthy. They describe the findings and implications of currently available techniques such as magnetic resonance imaging (MRI), positron emission tomography (PET) and single photon emission tomography (SPET), all of which have revolutionized the understanding of the pathophysiology in a wide range of movement disorders.

Furthermore, throughout the book, there is emphasis on the interaction between brain and behaviour, including information about the site, range and characteristics of brain involvement which have behavioural and psychological implications. In this regard, the frontal lobe–basal ganglia circuits are particularly important. Baron-Cohen and Moriarty provide a neuropsychological perspective to the arguments for the existence of a developmental dysexecutive syndrome, examining the specific links between cognitive architecture as shown by neuropsychological tests, brain and behaviour. They focus on several disorders included in this volume such as GTS, ADHD, OCD and PKU as well as autism, highlighting the similarities and differences between them.

In both basic science and clinical medicine the search continues for a better understanding of the precise mechanisms of how disturbances in neuronal circuits result in behavioural manifestations. There is no doubt that movement disorders will continue to be an important testing ground for exploring the brain behaviour relationships for years to come. We hope that this volume helps give some insight into the complexities of the disorders and the challenges that they offer to scientists and clinicians alike.

Mary M. Robertson
Valsamma Eapen

1 Gilles de la Tourette Syndrome

MARY M. ROBERTSON
University College London (UCL) Medical School, London, UK
and
The National Hospital for Neurology and Neurosurgery, London, UK
and
VALSAMMA EAPEN
UAE University, Al Ain, UAE
and
University College London (UCL) Medical School, London, UK

INTRODUCTION

Gilles de la Tourette Syndrome (GTS) is a movement disorder characterized by both multiple motor and one or more vocal (phonic) tics (noises) of more than a year's duration[1,2] and, in many cases, a variety of associated behaviours and psychopathology.

GTS was first described in the medical literature by Itard in 1825[3], and subsequently by Georges Gilles de la Tourette in 1885[4], who documented nine cases of the syndrome, emphasizing the triad of multiple tics, coprolalia and echolalia, which gained him eponymous fame. GTS was once thought to be rare and a bizarre curiosity and only around 50 isolated case reports were found in the medical literature during the 80 years after its description; moreover in an International Registry published in 1973, only 174 GTS cases were documented in the USA and 53 in the UK[5]. However, in the last three decades there has been a growing interest and substantial research into the condition[6–8]. Today GTS is regarded as a paradigm for scientists and clinicians interested in the relationship between brain and behaviour.

The disorder is complex and fascinating, and has thus attracted much attention in both the popular and scientific press. It has been convincingly speculated that Dr Samuel Johnson, the famous 18th century literary figure had GTS[9,10], while others including Mozart[11–13] have been suggested to have GTS. While we agree that Dr Johnson almost certainly did have GTS, we feel that the evidence for Mozart is insufficient.

EPIDEMIOLOGY AND DEMOGRAPHY

The exact prevalence of GTS is unknown and depends, at least in part, on the definition of GTS, the type of ascertainment and epidemiological

Movement and Allied Disorders. Edited by M. M. Robertson and V. Eapen

methods used[7,14]. Eight epidemiological studies in GTS have been undertaken with the majority being in the USA ($N = 4$), others being in France ($N = 2$), England ($N = 1$) and Israel ($N = 1$)[14]. The generally accepted figure has been 0.5/1 000 (5/10 000) (approximately 110 000 patients in the USA and 25 000 in the UK)[15]. The only population-based study performed in Israel[16] reported a prevalence estimate of 4.28/10 000 (sex specific prevalences were 4.90/10 000 for boys and 3.10/10 000 for girls).

GTS is found in all social classes, cultures and racial groups. There have been cohorts with substantial numbers reported from the USA, Europe (UK, The Netherlands, Denmark), the Soviet Union, the Far East and Australasia. In addition there have been numerous case reports highlighting the worldwide distribution of the disorder. It is generally agreed that GTS occurs three to four times more commonly in males than in females[7,8,17].

CLINICAL CHARACTERISTICS

Phenomenologically, GTS patients share a similar clinical profile irrespective of culture, underlining the biological nature of the condition. The age of onset of symptoms ranges from 2–15 years, with a mean of 7 years. The first commonly reported motor tic is eyeblinking ('squinting') and the most common initial vocal tics are sniffing and throat clearing. Complex movements are common in GTS and include touching, licking, spitting, hitting, jumping, smelling, squatting, abnormalities of gait, and forced touching. Vocal tics, by and large, have a later age of onset with a mean of 11 years[7,17]. Many GTS patients describe premonitory 'sensory' experiences[18] and stimulus-induced tic behaviours[19].

Coprolalia (the involuntary uttering of obscenities) occurs in roughly one-third of clinic patient populations, but has been reported to be less common in children, mild cases and in certain cultures (e.g. Japan). The mean age of onset is usually 13–15 years, disappearing later in up to one-third of patients[17]. Copropraxia (involuntary making of obscene gestures) is reported in up to 20% of clinic samples, with the palm-backed V sign being common in Europe[7].

Echolalia (the imitation of sounds or words of others) and echopraxia (the imitation of actions of others) occur in some 10–40% of patients. Palilalia (the repetition of the last word or phrase in a sentence or the last syllable of a word uttered by the patient) occurs in roughly 10% of patients. Symptoms such as mental coprolalia (the thinking of obscenities), coprographia (the writing of obscenities) and mental palilalia are usually unrecognized unless specifically asked about. Whilst these clinical features are not essential in making the diagnosis of GTS, their presence would increase one's diagnostic confidence[7,17].

Motor tics and vocalizations are made worse by stress, boredom, fatigue and excitement, while sleep, alcohol, orgasm, fever, relaxation or concentrating on an enjoyable task often reduce symptoms[7]. In addition it has been reported that premenstrual stress and stimulants such as caffeine, methylphenidate and amphetamines exacerbate tics[20,21].

Characteristically, the symptoms wax and wane, and the type and nature of tics change over time, with older tics being replaced by new ones[7]. Symptoms may increase during adolescence but once the person reaches early adulthood, the symptoms remit or significantly improve in about two-thirds of cases; the remaining third will continue to be symptomatic during adulthood[20].

PSYCHOPATHOLOGY, ASSOCIATED BEHAVIOURS AND COMORBID CONDITIONS

GTS and associated psychopathology has been an area of considerable controversy[7,17,23,24] and the conditions which have attracted most interest have been depression and anxiety disorders, obsessive–compulsive behaviours (OCB), attention deficit and hyperactivity disorder (ADHD) and self-injurious behaviours (SIB).

While some investigators (see Comings[22,24]) have suggested that GTS is associated with a wide variety of psychopathology (including learning difficulties, anxiety, phobias, panic attacks, manic depressive disorder, schizoid behaviours, alcoholism, drug abuse and pathological gambling), others[5,25] assert that no specific psychopathology is found in association with GTS.

Most investigators, however, regard the psychopathology in GTS to be somewhat specific. It has been found that GTS patients are more anxious and depressed when compared to controls[26–29] and that this is related to the duration of the GTS[30]. This is not surprising given the fact that GTS is a chronic and disabling condition with considerable social stigma[7,17].

There is now increasing evidence to suggest that OCB is clinically[30] and aetiologically[31] related to GTS. The evidence has come from phenomenological[32], family[33] and epidemiological investigations[7,17,34] (for full review see Eapen and Robertson[35]). However, recent studies[30,32,36] and Eapen, Pauls and Robertson's study (1995, in preparation) have shown that the obsessive–compulsive (OC) symptom profile is different in GTS when compared to primary obsessive–compulsive disorder (OCD) with sexual, violent, aggressive and symmetrical themes being significantly more common in GTS.

The precise relationship between GTS and ADHD is less clear[21] although this has been studied extensively[22,37,38]. Whilst symptoms suggestive of ADHD occur in a substantial proportion (40%) of GTS subjects, this may well be due to an overlap in symptoms, neurotransmitter involvement or common neuroanatomical substrates rather than a primary genetic relationship[39]. However, it is also possible that there is a subtype of GTS where ADHD is an integral part[40].

Clinical experience suggests an association between some types of SIB and GTS[41], although the exact nature of this is unclear (for reviews see Eapen and Robertson[35], and Robertson and Yakeley[42]). In this regard it is interesting to note that in epidemiological[34] and pedigree[43] studies even mild GTS cases have exhibited SIB.

Other associated behaviours, although occurring less frequently but often resulting in seeking medical attention, include exhibitionism, antisocial behaviours, aggression and discipline problems[7,17].

In reviews of neuropsychological studies[7,44] it has been noted that there are discrepancies between verbal and performance IQs (by about 15 points, with performance being the lower) as well as specific deficits in reading, writing and arithmetic. Dysfunction in the 'intention editor' (a mechanism that is triggered when there are several simultaneously activated intentions competing in parallel with one another) has been reported in GTS[45] as have deficits in attention and complex tasks (e.g. serial addition, block sequence span (forwards), the trail making test and letter cancellation vigilance tasks)[46].

AETIOLOGY

GENETICS

The hereditary nature of the condition has been recognized from the time of its original description[4]. However, the exact genetic mechanism underlying the disorder is still unknown. There is growing evidence to suggest the existence of a single major gene(s) and an autosomal dominant pattern of inheritance (for full review see chapter 2).

NEUROCHEMISTRY

It has been suggested that the neurochemical basis for GTS is an imbalance of central nervous system neurotransmitter agents. Dopamine has received most support mainly based on the fact that dopamine blockers are effective in relieving the symptoms in a large number of patients, while stimulants such as pemoline and methylphenidate exacerbate the symptoms[7,21,47]. Others such as the noradrenergic system, acetylcholine, γ-aminobutyric acid and endogenous opioids have all been implicated (for full review see chapter 13).

With no one transmitter convincingly implicated to date, the importance of animal models and further post-mortem (PM) studies are crucial. Recent exciting PM findings however, have suggested decreased 5-hydroxytryptamine and glutamate in many areas of the basal ganglia[48], a reduction in the second messenger cyclic AMP, an increased number of dopamine uptake carrier sites in the striatum[49], and a decrease in dynorphin-like immunoreactivity in the globus pallidus[50,51].

PATHOPHYSIOLOGY

Apart from non-specific changes in some cases there are no characteristic EEG findings in GTS[7,52]. Obeso and colleagues reported that there is no evidence of any paroxysmal activity time-locked to the tics[53], but an absence of a pre-movement, readiness or Bereitschafts-potential (probably representing the summed activity of changing firing patterns in cortical neurons in preparation for willed voluntary movement) before spontaneous simple tics in patients with GTS[53]. This may suggest therefore that the simple tics of GTS are not generated through the normal cortical motor pathways utilized for willed human movements.

Electromyelogram (EMG) patterns have been shown to vary according to the type and nature of tics[7]. No consistent findings have emerged from the visual and sensory evoked potential studies[7] except for minor abnormalities of the late components of the event-related auditory evoked potentials perhaps reflecting specific attention deficits occurring in the context of GTS[54].

NEUROIMAGING

Earlier structural neuroimaging using predominantly computed tomography (CT) scans have not demonstrated any specific abnormalities1[7,17,55–57]. More recent studies using magnetic resonance imaging (MRI) have demonstrated left/right asymmetries in the basal ganglia as well as reductions in basal ganglia volumes in GTS. Furthermore, functional imaging and, in particular, positron emission tomography (PET) and single photon emission tomography (SPET) have found perfusion abnormalities in the frontal lobe and basal ganglia areas[58–61]. For full details see chapters 14 and 15 of this volume.

GTS thus probably reflects the interaction between genetic, neurophysiological, behavioural and environmental factors[62,63]. From all the available evidence to date it seems highly likely that more than one monoamine and more than one area of the brain will be implicated in the aetiology and pathogenesis of GTS.

MANAGEMENT

Chemotherapy is the mainstay of treatment for the motor and vocal tics as well as some of the associated behaviours of GTS, and includes dopamine blockers such as haloperidol, pimozide[64,65] and sulpiride[66]. For comorbid GTS and ADHD, clonidine[67,68] may well be the treatment of choice since stimulants are known to worsen tics[21]. Specific serotonin reuptake inhibitors (SSRIs) (e.g. fluoxetine[69,70]) have been successfully used to treat the OCB aspects of GTS, and augmentation of the antiobsessional effects of SSRIs by neuroleptics has been reported in patients with OCD and GTS[71,72]. Other neuroleptics such as fluphenazine and penfluridol have also been used with some success, as have the antidepressant clomipramine, the anticonvulsant clonazepam, the calcium antagonists (verapamil and nifedipine), naloxone, lithium carbonate, tetrabenazine, progabide and physostigmine[7]. Our preliminary clinical experience with risperidone (with effects on both serotonin and dopamine) has not been as encouraging as was originally thought[73].

In addition to pharmacotherapy, psychosocial interventions are important both for the individual with GTS as well as for the family. Explanation about the nature, cause and course of the disorder is often sufficient for those with a mild form of the disorder. Parents are usually reassured by a diagnosis and explanation about the nature of the disorder, and often benefit from self-help groups. However, the management is far from simple in those with moderate to severe GTS, especially when the associated features of ADHD, SIB, and aggressive behaviour are present.

Many parents of GTS children suggest that certain food items affect their GTS symptomatology but few studies have been performed in the area. Symptom exacerbation associated with seasonal allergy responses, the ingestion of allergens in food as well as the drugs used to treat allergies have been reported by Bruun[15]. However, to date there is little scientific evidence for the involvement of allergy in GTS (Kalali, Brostoff and Robertson 1995, in preparation).

CONCLUSIONS

GTS is no longer considered uncommon, and the clinical characteristics and phenomenological features are well established. Whilst the core symptoms (motor and vocal tics) are probably genetically determined, the genesis and exact relationship of associated symptoms (SIB, ADHD) is unclear. This may well be the result of an interaction between genetic and environmental factors, or due to an overlap in the intermediate (neuroanatomy and neurochemistry) and final (symptoms) pathways of expression of these behaviours.

Whilst there are no demonstratable structural changes in GTS, functional abnormalities in the basal ganglia, cingulum and frontal areas, have been consistently reported. SPET and superimposed quantitative MRI studies might shed light on subtle structural and correlating functional changes.

With regard to the clinical phenotypes of GTS, there is increasing evidence that OCB is an alternative phenotypic expression of the putative GTS gene(s). Whilst more than 50% of the genome has already been excluded, it is difficult to be certain whether this is merely a reflection of imprecise definition of the phenotypes, or due to genetic heterogeneity. Clinically it is difficult to distinguish phenotypes (with links to the genotype) from phenocopies, and identification of an endophenotype, perhaps using a combination of genetic and neuroimaging techniques, may well be a way forward. Once genetic linkage is established, it may be possible to identify the actual gene and its causative mutations, followed by prenatal diagnosis and genetic counselling, as well as development of new treatments based on a knowledge of the disease pathways.

REFERENCES

1. American Psychiatric Association (1994) *Diagnostic and Statistical Manual of Mental Disorders* (4th revision) (DSM 1V) American Psychiatric Association, Washington, DC.
2. World Health Organisation (1992) *International Classification of Diseases and Health Related Problems* (10th revision), WHO, Geneva.
3. Itard, J. M. G. (1825) Memoire sur quelques fonctions involontaires des appareils de la locomotion de la prehension et de la voix. *Arch. Gen. Med.*, **8**, 385–407.
4. Gilles de la Tourette, G. (1885) Etude sur une affection nerveuse caracterisee par de l'incoordination motrice accompagnee d'echolalie et de copralalie. *Arch. Neurol.*, **9**, 19–42, 158–200.
5. Abuzzahab, D. E. and Anderson, F. O. (1973) Gilles de la Tourette's syndrome. *Minn. Med.*, **56**, 492–496.
6. Kurlan, R. (1989) Tourette's syndrome: current concepts. *Neurology*, **39**, 1625–1630.
7. Robertson, M. M. (1994) Annotation: Gilles de la Tourette Syndrome—an update. *J. Child Psychol. Psychiatry*, **35**, 597–611.
8. Shapiro, A. K., Shapiro, E. S., Young, J. F. and Feinberg, T. E. (1988) *Gilles de la Tourette Syndrome* (2nd edition). Raven Press, New York.
9. McHenry, L. C. Jr. (1967) Samuel Johnson's tics and gesticulations. *J. His. Med.*, **22**, 152–168.
10. Murray, T. J. (1979) Dr Samuel Johnson's movement disorders. *BMJ*, **i**, 1610–1614.
11. Fog, R. and Regeur, E. (1983) Did Mozart suffer from Tourette's syndrome? In *Abstracts of the Ninth World Congress of Psychiatry*, Vienna, F501.
12. Gunne, L. (1991) Hade Mozart Tourette's syndrom? *Lakartidningen*, **88**(50), 4325–4326.
13. Simkin, B. (1992) Mozart's scatological disorder. *BMJ*, **305**, 1563–1567.
14. Tanner, C. M. (1993) Epidemiology. In *Handbook of Tourette's Syndrome and Related Tic and Behavioural Disorders* (R. Kurlan, Ed). Marcel Dekker, New York, pp. 337–344.
15. Bruun, R. D. (1984) Gilles de la Tourette's syndrome: an overview of clinical experience. *J. Am. Acad. Child Psychiatry*, **23**, 126–133.
16. Apter, A., Pauls, D. L., Bleich, A., Zohar, A. H., Kron, S., Ratzoni, G., Dycian, A.,

Kotler, M., Weizman, A. and Cohen, D. J. (1992) A population based epidemiological study of Tourette Syndrome among adolescents in Israel. *Adv. Neurol.*, **58**, 61–65.

17. Robertson, M. M. (1989) The Gilles de la Tourette Syndrome: The current status. *Br. J. Psychiatry*, **154**, 147–169.
18. Lange, A. E. (1993) Premonitory ('sensory') experiences. In *Handbook of Tourette's Syndrome and Related Tic and Behavioral Disorders* (R. Kurlan, Ed). Marcel Dekker, New York, pp. 17–25.
19. Eapen, V., Moriarty, J. and Robertson, M. M. (1994) Stimulus induced behaviours in Gilles de la Tourette syndrome. *J. Neurol. Neurosurg. Psychiatry*, **57**, 853–855.
20. Leckman, J. F. and Scahill, L. (1990) Possible exacerbation of tics by androgenic steroids. *N. Engl. J. Med.*, **322**, 1674.
21. Robertson, M. M. and Eapen, V. (1992) Pharmacologic controversy of CNS stimulants in Gilles de la Tourette's Syndrome. *Clin. Neuropharmacol.*, **15**, 408–425.
22. Comings, D. E. and Comings, B. G. (1987) A controlled study of Tourette syndrome, I–VII. *Am. J. Hum. Genet.*, **41**, 701–866.
23. Pauls, D. L., Towbin, K. E., Leckman, J. F., Zahner, G. E. P. and Cohen, D. J. (1988) Gilles de la Tourette syndrome and obsessive compulsive disorder: evidence supporting an etiologic relationship. *Arch. Gen. Psychiatry*, **43**, 1180–1182.
24. Comings, D. E. (1990) *Tourette Syndrome and Human Behavior*. Hope Press, Duarte, California.
25. Shapiro, A. K. and Shapiro, E. S. (1992) Evaluation of the reported association of obsessive compulsive symptoms or disorder with Tourette's disorder. *Compr. Psychiatry*, **33**, 1–10.
26. Coffey, B., Frazier, J. and Chen, S. (1992) Comorbidity, Tourette syndrome, and anxiety disorders. *Adv. Neurol.*, **58**, 95–104.
27. Van de Wetering, B. J. M., Cohen, A. P., Minderaa, R. B. *et al.* (1988) Het syndroom van Gilles de la Tourette: klinische bevindigen. *Ned. Tijd. Geneeskd.*, **132**, 21–25.
28. Robertson, M. M., Channon, S., Baker, J. and Flynn, D. (1993) The psychopathology of Gilles de la Tourette Syndrome: a controlled study. *Br. J. Psychiatry*, **162**, 114–117.
29. Robertson, M. M., Trimble, M. R. and Lees, A. J. (1988) The psychopathology of the Gilles de la Tourette syndrome: a phenomenological analysis. *Br. J. Psychiatry*, **152**, 383–390.
30. Frankel, M., Cummings, J. L., Robertson, M. M., Trimble, M. R., Hill, M. A. and Benson, D. F. (1986) Obsessions and compulsions in Gilles de la Tourette's syndrome. *Neurology*, **36**, 378–382.
31. Eapen, V., Pauls, D. L. and Robertson, M. M. (1993) Evidence for autosomal dominant transmission in Gilles de la Tourette Syndrome—United Kingdom cohort study. *Br. J. Psychiatry*, **162**, 593–596.
32. George, M. S., Trimble, M. R., Ring, H. A., Sallee, F. R. and Robertson, M. M. (1993) Obsessions in obsessive–compulsive disorder (OCD) with and without Gilles de la Tourette Syndrome. *Am. J. Psychiatry*, **150**, 93–97.
33. Pauls, D. L., Leckman, J. F. and Towbin, K. E. (1986) A possible genetic relationship exists between Tourette's syndrome and obsessive–compulsive disorder. *Psychopharmacol. Bull.*, **22**, 730–733.
34. Robertson, M. M., Verrill, M., Mercer, M., James, B. and Pauls, D. L. (1994) Tourette syndrome in New Zealand; a postal survey. *Br. J. Psychiatry*, **164**, 263–266.
35. Eapen, V. and Robertson, M. M. (1994) Tourette's syndrome and

obsessive–compulsive behaviours. In *Psychiatry in Europe: Directions and Developments* (T. Sensky, C. Katona and S. Montgomery, Eds). Gaskell Press, London, pp. 48–57.
36. Pitman, R. K., Green, R. C., Jenike, M. A. and Mesulam, M. M. (1987) Clinical comparison of Tourette's disorder and obsessive–compulsive disorder. *Am. J. Psychiatry*, **144**, 1166–1171.
37. Pauls, D. L., Hurst, C. R., Kruger, S. D., Leckman, J. F., Kidd, K. K. and Cohen, D. J. (1986) Gilles de la Tourette's syndrome and attention deficit disorder with hyperactivity. *Arch. Gen. Psychiatry*, **43**, 1177–1179.
38. Erenberg, G., Cruse, R. P. and Rothner, A. D. (1986) Tourette Syndrome: an analysis of 200 pediatric and adolescent cases. *Cleve. Clin. Q.*, **53**, 127–131.
39. Eapen, V. and Robertson, M. M. (1994) *Gilles de la Tourette Syndrome and Attention Deficit Hyperactivity Disorder: Evidence against a Genetic Relationship.* Abstract presented to American Neuropsychiatry Association Meeting, Newport Rhode Island, July 1994.
40. Pauls, D. L., Leckman, J. F. and Cohen, D. J. (1993) Familial relationship between Gilles de la Tourette's syndrome, attention deficit disorder, learning disabilities, speech disorders, and stuttering. *J. Am. Acad. Child Adolesc. Psychiatry*, **32**, 1044–1050.
41. Robertson, M. M., Trimble, M. R. and Lees, A. J. (1989) Self-injurious behaviour and the Gilles de la Tourette Syndrome: a clinical study and review of the literature. *Psychol. Med.*, **19**, 611–625.
42. Robertson, M. M. and Yakeley, J. (1993) Obsessive–compulsive and self injurious behavior. In *Handbook of Tourette's Syndrome and Related Tic and Behavioral Disorders* (R. Kurlan, Ed). Marcel Dekker, New York, pp. 45–87.
43. Robertson, M. M. and Gourdie, A. (1990) Familial Tourette's syndrome in a large British pedigree: associated psychopathology, severity, and potential for linkage analysis. *Br. J. Psychiatry*, **156**, 515–521.
44. Como, P. G. (1993) Neuropsychological Testing. In *Handbook of Tourette's Syndrome and Related Tic and Behavioral Disorders* (R. Kurlan, Ed). Marcel Dekker, New York, pp. 221–239.
45. Baron Cohen, S., Cross, P., Crowson, M. and Robertson, M. M. (1994) Can children with Gilles de la Tourette Syndrome edit their intentions. *Psychol. Med.*, **24**, 29–40.
46. Channon, S., Flynn, D. and Robertson, M. M. (1992) Attentional deficits in Gilles de la Tourette Syndrome. *Neuropsychiat. Neuropsychol. Behav. Neurol.*, **5**, 170–177.
47. Rubowitz, R. and Klawans, H. L. (1972) Implications of amphetamine-induced stereotyped behaviour as a model for tardive dyskinesia. *Arch. Gen. Psychiatry*, **27**, 502–507.
48. Singer, H. S. (1992) Neurochemical analysis of postmortem cortical and striatal brain tissue in patients with Tourette Syndrome. *Adv. Neurol.*, **58**, 135–144.
49. Anderson, G. M., Pollack, E. S., Chatterjee, D., Leckman, J. F., Riddle, M. A. and Cohen, D. J. (1992) Postmortem analysis of subcortical monoamines and amino acids in Tourette syndrome. *Adv. Neurol.*, **58**, 123–133.
50. Haber, S. N., Kowall, N. W., Vonsattel, J. P., Bird, E. D. and Richardson, E. P. Jr. (1986) Gilles de la Tourette's syndrome. A postmortem neuropathological and immunohistochemical study. *J. Neurol. Sci.*, **75**, 225–241.
51. Haber, S. N. and Wolfer, D. (1992) Basal ganglia peptidergic staining in Tourette syndrome. *Adv. Neurol.*, **58**, 145–150.
52. Shapiro, A. K., Shapiro, E. S., Bruun, R. D. and Sweet, R. D. (1978) *Gilles de la Tourette Syndrome*. Raven Press, New York.
53. Obeso, J. A., Rothwell, J. C. and Marsden, C. D. (1982) The neurophysiology of Tourette syndrome. *Adv. Neurol.*, **35**, 105–114.

54. Van de Wetering, B. J. M., Martens, C. M. C., Fortgens, C. *et al.* (1985) Late components of the auditory evoked potentials in Gilles de la Tourette syndrome. *Clin. Neurol. Neurosurg.*, **87**, 181–186.
55. Baxter, L. R. and Guze, B. H. (1993) Neuroimaging. In *Handbook of Tourette's Syndrome and Related Tic and Behavioral Disorders* (R. Kurlan, Ed). Marcel Dekker, New York, pp. 289–304.
56. Peterson, B., Riddle, M. A., Cohen, D. J., Katz, L. D., Smith, J. C., Hardin, M. T. and Leckman, J. F. (1993) Reduced basal ganglia volumes in Tourette's syndrome using three-dimensional reconstruction techniques from magnetic resonance images. *Neurology*, **43**, 941–949.
57. Singer, H. S., Reiss, A. L. and Brown, J. E. (1993) Volumetric MRI changes in basal ganglia of children with Tourette's syndrome. *Neurology*, **43**(5), 950–956.
58. Chase, T. N., Foster, N. L., Fedio, P., Brooks, R., Mansi, L., Kessler, L. and Chiro, G. D. (1984) Gilles de la Tourette syndrome: studies with the fluorine-18-labelled fluorodeoxyglucose positron emission tomographic method. *Ann. Neurol.*, **15** (Suppl), S175.
59. Chase, T. N., Geoffrey, V., Gillespie, M. *et al.* (1986) Structural and functional studies of Gilles de la Tourette syndrome. *Rev. Neurol.* (Paris), **142**, 851–855.
60. George, M. S., Trimble, M. R., Costa, D. C., Robertson, M. M., Ring, H. A. and Ell, P. J. (1993) Elevated frontal cerebral blood flow in Gilles de la Tourette Syndrome: a Tc99HM-PAO SPECT study. *Psychiatry Res.—Neuroimaging*, **45**, 143–151.
61. Costa, D. C., George, M. S., Ell, P. J., Pilowsky, L., Verhoeff, N. P. G. L. and Robertson, M. M. (1992) Dopamine D_2 receptor availability in patients with Gilles de la Tourette syndrome studied with SPET. *Nucl. Med.* **(Suppl. 28)**, 414–417.
62. Leckman, J. F., Dolnansky, E. S. and Hardin, M. T. (1990) Perinatal factors in the expression of Tourette's syndrome: an exploratory study. *J. Am. Acad. Child Adolesc. Psychiatry*, **29**, 220–226.
63. Leckman, J. F., Pauls, D. L., Peterson, B. S., Riddle, M. A., Anderson, G. M. and Cohen, D. J. (1992) Pathogenesis of Tourette syndrome; clues from the clinical phenotype and natural history. *Adv. Neurol.*, **58**, 15–24.
64. Shapiro, A. K., Shapiro, E., Fulop, G., Hubbard, M., Mandeli, J., Nordie, J. and Phillips, R. A. (1989) Controlled study of haloperidol, pimozide, and placebo for the treatment of Gilles de la Tourette's syndrome. *Arch. Gen. Psychiatry*, **46**, 722–730.
65. Shapiro, A. K. and Shapiro, E. (1984) Controlled study of pimozide versus placebo in Tourette's syndrome. *J. Am. Acad. Child Psychiatry*, **23**, 161–173.
66. Robertson, M. M., Schnieden, V. and Lees, A. J. (1990) Management of Gilles de la Tourette syndrome using sulpiride. *Clin. Neuropharmacol.*, **13**(3), 229–235.
67. Comings, D. E., Comings, B. G., Tacket, T. and Li, S. (1990) The clonidine patch and behavior problems. *J. Am. Acad. Child Adolesc. Psychiatry*, **29**(4), 667–668.
68. Hunt, R. D., Minderaa, R. B. and Cohen, D. J. (1989) Clonidine benefits children with attention deficit disorder and hyperactivity: report of a double-blind placebo-crossover therapeutic trial. *J. Am. Acad. Child Psychiatry*, **24**, 583–586.
69. Riddle, M. A., Hardin, M. T., King, R. A., Scahill, L. and Woolston, J. L. (1990) Fluoxetine treatment of children and adolescents with Tourette's and obsessive–compulsive disorders: preliminary clinical experience. *J. Am. Acad. Child Adolesc. Psychiatry*, **29**, 45–48.
70. Kurlan, R., Como, P. G., Deeley, C., McDermot, M. and McDermot, M. P. (1993) A pilot controlled study of fluoxetine for obsessive–compulsive symptoms in children with Tourette's syndrome. *Clin. Neuropharmacol.*, **16**(2), 167–172.

71. George, M. S., Trimble, M. R. and Robertson, M. M. (1993) Serotonin and dopamine agents in comorbid obsessive–compulsive disorder and Gilles de la Tourette Syndrome. *Hum. Psychopharmacol.*, **8**, 327–334.
72. McDougle, C. J., Goodman, W. K., Price, L. H., Delgado, P. L., Krystal, J. H., Charney, D. S. and Heninger, G. R. (1990) Neuroleptic addition in fluvoxamine-refractory obsessive–compulsive disorder. *Am. J. Psychiatry*, **147**, 652–654.
73. Van der Linden, C., Bruggeman, R. and Van Woerkom, T. C. A. M. (1994) Serotonin–domamine antagonist and Gilles de la Tourette's syndrome: an open pilot dose-titration study with riseridone. *Mov. Disord.*, **9**(6), 687–688.

2 The Genetics of Tics and Related Disorders

DAVID L. PAULS
Yale University, New Haven, CT, USA
and
BEN J. M. VAN DE WETERING
University Hospital Rotterdam-Dijkzigt and Erasmus University, Rotterdam, The Netherlands

INTRODUCTION

Tics are recurrent, non-rhythmical, 'involuntary' motor acts that are usually short and explosive, but occasionally may have dystonic features[1]. Tics may vary in complexity from simple to complex. Examples of simple motor tics include increased eye blinking, facial twitches and jerks. Complex tics are characterized by rubbing, touching, dystonic postures and symmetry behaviours. Phonic or vocal tics are sounds that result from a motor tic that sets air in the pharynx into motion. Simple phonic tics are exemplified by throat clearing, yelping, squealing and snorting. Yelling words and phrases (including obscenities as seen in the Gilles de la Tourette's syndrome) are examples of complex vocal tics.

Tics have been reported incidentally as secondary to organic brain syndromes caused by intoxication, inflammation and trauma[2–12]. However, the majority of tics are idiopathic and occur frequently in children of school age. The estimated prevalence of tics in American and European school populations varies between 12 and 16%, although limited epidemiological data are available[13,14]. A prevalence of 3–5% seems to be a minimal estimate for the general population[15].

The vast majority of tics disappear within one year following their onset[1]. These transient tics (TT) are most frequently simple tics (eye-blinking or facial twitches). Tics that exist longer than one year are diagnosed as chronic motor tics (CMT) or chronic vocal tics (CVT)[16]. An individual having both CMT and CVT usually meets diagnostic criteria for Gilles de la Tourette syndrome (GTS).

According to the DSM-IV criteria, a diagnosis of GTS is made when multiple motor tics and at least one vocal tic have been present for a period of more than one year, with onset before the age of 18[16]. GTS is usually a more severe clinical condition than either CMT or CVT. Thus, GTS has been studied more extensively than the other tic syndromes. Most of the research

Movement and Allied Disorders. Edited by M. M. Robertson and V. Eapen

on CMT and/or CVT has been done to determine their possible relationship to GTS.

The initial prevalence estimates of GTS were obtained in heterogeneous clinical samples and ranged between 0.0008 and 0.00007[17,18]. Lucas and co-workers calculated an incidence rate of 4.6/1 000 000 based on data extrapolated from clinical data in an American urban area[19]. Burd and colleagues, using questionnaires sent to health professionals in North Dakota, reported prevalence rates of 1/10 000 girls and 9.3/10 000 boys at school age and a much lower prevalence in adults (males 0.77 and females 0.22/10 000)[20,21]. In a single Los Angeles school district, Comings and co-workers found prevalence rates of 1 in 95 for boys and 1 in 759 for girls[22].

All of these epidemiological data have been difficult to interpret and compare for several reasons. First, given that GTS is a relatively rare condition, large population samples need to be studied using proper diagnostic criteria to obtain reliable data. Second, the extent to which more or less severe cases have been included in previous studies has dramatically influenced the prevalence rates.

Caine and co-workers identified 41 GTS cases from approximately 140 000 school-age children in Monroe county (Rochester, NY, USA) using DSM-III criteria[23]. Of these cases, 24 had already been diagnosed as GTS and 17 new cases were identified during the study. Of the 24 earlier diagnosed cases, 19 (79%) had associated behavioural problems compared with only 1 (6%) of the new cases. This suggests that more severe and/or more complicated cases will more readily come to medical attention and be diagnosed as compared to mild cases. This observation emphasizes the need to use proper diagnostic criteria to estimate the true rate of tics and GTS. In another population-based study, Apter *et al.*[24] screened approximately 30 000 adolescent recruits in the Israeli army. These investigators found an overall prevalence for GTS of 4.28/10 000 and sex-specific prevalences of 4.90/10 000 for males and 3.10/10 000 for females[24]. These rates may be somewhat low since they were calculated in an adolescent population.

THE GENETICS OF TICS

Only a few studies have focused on the familial occurrence of tics. Zausmer and Torup, in their follow-up studies of children with tics, reported an increased positive family history for tics in a number of cases[25,26]. Using these data, Abe and Oda calculated the rate of tics to be 9.5 and 11 respectively among the parents of these children[27]. In a case report, Frost and co-workers described an extended pedigree of a GTS patient[28]. None of the 14 interviewed relatives had GTS, but six had tics (one first-degree, two second-degree and three third-degree relative(s)). Interestingly, one paternal cousin had a tic syndrome that went into full remission after 2 years.

Abe and Oda investigated the prevalence of tics in 76 children having at least one parent with childhood tics ('index group') and 177 children of parents without a history of tics ('control group')[27]. The rate of tics in the index group was significantly higher when compared to the control group—15/76 (20%) versus 17/177 (10%). For one of the index children with tics, both parents had had tics in their childhood. Of the remaining 14 children, 10 were boys and four were girls. Of the 10 boys with tics, seven had a ticking father and three a ticking mother. Of the four girls with tics, one had a father with tics and three had a mother with tics. There was also some indication of parent–child similarity in the type of tics (either motor or vocal), but no definite conclusion could be drawn due to the small size of the sample. In considering genetic explanations for their findings, the authors concluded that X-linked inheritance seemed unlikely because of the frequent occurrence of male-to-male transmission and the male-to-female ratio of the tics. They suggested that the most likely genetic explanation would be either polygenic inheritance or autosomal dominance with incomplete penetrance.

The familial character of tics was partially supported by Zausmer and Dewey in a re-analysis of their 1954 data[29]. They found a relative risk of 14% for parents of tickers. However, this risk was three times greater than for siblings of the index cases. These authors suggested that the hereditary pattern was not consistent with recessive transmission. A dominant model also seemed unlikely, as in only three of the 91 pedigrees was there direct transmission over three generations.

In summary, these studies suggest that tics are familial but transmission within families does not follow classic mendelian patterns. More work is needed with current assessment and analytical methodologies to understand more completely the familiality of tics.

THE GENETICS OF GTS

Georges Gilles de la Tourette, in his original description of the syndrome, suggested a genetic aetiology[30]. However, it was not until the 1960s and 1970s that research was initiated to examine genetic hypotheses[2,31–33]. However, anecdotal reports suggested that there was a positive family history in only about 10% of GTS cases. These early reports relied on incidental clinical samples of GTS and family histories obtained during clinical work-up. Additional cases were not systematically evaluated or personally seen by the investigator, neither were systematic studies performed on all first- and second-degree relatives. Nevertheless, the interpretation was that 'a family history of tics does not characterize patients with Tourette syndrome'[34].

The first report of multiple diagnosed GTS cases in a nuclear family concerned two sisters with childhood onset GTS[35]. These sisters had six children; four of them had definite and obvious multiple motor tics, only one of them had vocal tics. Other evidence at that time for the involvement of genetic mechanisms in the aetiology of GTS came from adoption and twin studies.

ADOPTION AND TWIN STUDIES

Adoption studies are helpful in establishing that genetic factors are important for the manifestation of some traits, since they provide a research paradigm that disentangles genetic factors from familial environmental factors. By comparing adopted-away offspring of affected individuals to offspring raised by affected individuals, it is possible to estimate the relative influence of genetic and non-genetic familial factors.

There is only one adoption study of GTS reported in the literature. Adoptive families of 22 adopted GTS patients were compared with the family histories of the biological families of 641 GTS patients using the family history method[2]. None of the adoptive relatives had a history of tics. Of the 641 GTS patients, 227 had a positive family history in at least one of their first-degree biological relatives. Adding second- and third-degree relatives raised this number to 302. A limitation of this study is that data on the biological parents and other relatives of the adopted-away patients were not available. Nevertheless, the differences observed between the adoptive parents and biological first-degree relatives support the hypothesis of a genetic diathesis underlying GTS and tics.

Twin studies can also provide evidence for the importance of genetic factors. Monozygotic (MZ) twins are genetically identical and share (nearly) the same prenatal environment. Dizygotic (DZ) twins share on average 50% of their genes and also the same prenatal environment. If a disorder is completely determined genetically, MZ twins should be 100% concordant for the disorder and DZ twins should show a concordance rate of 50% or less.

There are anecdotal and incidental observations on DZ and MZ twins with GTS, with a larger than expected proportion of MZ twins (probably caused by reporting bias), showing variation in age of onset, and type and severity of symptoms between co-twins[27,33,36–44]. Taken together, a pairwise concordance of 50–70% for GTS, and 75–90% for GTS and tics combined, can be calculated for MZ GTS twins[2,44]. For DZ GTS twins, the concordance rates in both conditions were around 10% and 20% respectively[2,44]. Non-genetic circumstances like perinatal and postnatal factors may influence the expression of the GTS genetic vulnerability in individuals at risk, explaining the absence of a 100% concordance rate for GTS and/or tics in MZ twins. All the affected discordant MZ co-twins in one of the series had a lower birth weight as compared to the unaffected co-twins[45,46]. Moreover, in a series of MZ twins concordant for GTS and tics, the co-twin with the lowest birth weight consistently had the most severe symptoms.

Twin studies may be relevant to study the phenotypic relationships between GTS, tics and associated behavioural problems. Anecdotal concordance in GTS twins has been reported for obsessional traits and for attention deficit disorder[31,38,41,42,44].

FAMILY STUDIES

The findings from the first family history studies in GTS families were criticized by Wilson and colleagues because, given the high population frequency of tics, the observed increase in positive family histories was not significantly different from that expected[47]. Furthermore, the early studies did not estimate rates of illness among relatives. The first study to do so was reported by Kidd and colleagues[48]. This study combined GTS and chronic tics (CT) into a single category and showed that the risk to relatives was significantly elevated over what would be expected by chance. In fact, all of the early studies combined GTS and CT into a single category. This was based on the assumption that CT represented a milder variant manifestation of GTS. In 1981, Pauls and colleagues[49] re-analysed the data collected by Kidd and colleagues[48] as well as family history data collected from a sample of consecutive GTS clinic patients to examine empirically this hypothesis of relationship between GTS and CT. The results of those analyses demonstrated the following:

1. CT appeared to represent a variant expression of GTS.
2. The increased risk for GTS and CT was consistent across the two samples.
3. The patterns of occurrence within families of GTS probands were consistent with a hypotheses of vertical transmission.

GENETIC ANALYSES OF FAMILY HISTORY DATA

Subsequently, five separate studies[50–54] used family history data to test specific genetic hypotheses regarding the inheritance of GTS and CT. All studies reported that the pattern of inheritance within families was consistent with a genetic hypothesis that postulated the existence of a single gene of major effect that conferred susceptibility to GTS and/or CT. However, this was not the only hypothesis supported. Kidd and Pauls were unable to reject a hypothesis of multifactorial–polygenic transmission[51]. This hypothesis posits that there are many genes, each with equal and additive effect, which contribute to the expression of the disorder. Although the single locus hypothesis provided the best fit to the data, the multifactorial–polygenic hypothesis could not be rejected statistically. Comings and colleagues also could not reject the multifactorial–polygenic hypothesis unless extended relatives were included, and the population prevalence for GTS and CT was restricted to be less than 0.0075[52]. Nevertheless, the consistent conclusion in all studies was that a two allele single-major-locus genetic model best explained the observed data.

While the results from all studies were consistent with a single locus hypothesis, not all studies supported an identical model of inheritance. Results from three of the studies were consistent with an autosomal dominant hypothesis[50,52,54]. Results from the remaining two studies were consistent with single gene inheritance in which the penetrance of the heterozygote was smaller than the penetrance of the homozygote with two susceptibility alleles[51,53]. The fact that the penetrance of the homozygote is greater than the penetrance of the 'normal homozygote' suggests some dominance. However, such a trait is not inherited as a classically dominant condition since the probability of being affected is dependent on the number of susceptibility alleles an individual has. This latter pattern is consistent with an additive model of inheritance. Nevertheless, while not all studies supported the same genetic model, all models predicted that males were more likely to develop GTS and/or CT if they inherited at least one susceptibility allele.

As indicated, all of the initial family studies relied on family history data. That is, the diagnosis of the relatives was based on information obtained from one or at most two informants; not all of the relatives were personally assessed. It has been demonstrated that family history data underestimate the 'true' rates of GTS and CT obtained with direct interviews[55]. Thus, the results from family history studies should be interpreted with caution. This is particularly true if the underestimation of rates does not occur equally in all classes of relatives. For example, if the rate of illness is consistently underestimated in the parents of the patients, then the pattern of illness will more closely resemble the pattern for a recessive or additive condition.

Results from analyses presented by Pauls and colleagues[55] suggested that there was a consistent underestimation of rates in the parents of GTS probands in the family history studies of Kidd, Pauls and colleagues[48,49]. If this is generally true for other family history studies of GTS, the model parameters resulting from genetic analyses of family history data are most likely inaccurate. Specifically, the penetrances for the heterozygotes would be expected to be underestimated since, in any single locus model, at least one of the parents would be heterozygous for the susceptibility allele. If parents were systematically being incorrectly identified as unaffected, the penetrance estimates for the heterozygotes would be too low. It is quite remarkable, however, that all studies supported a single gene hypothesis regarding the mode of inheritance.

Comings and colleagues, using family history data, have recently hypothesized that the mode of inheritance for GTS is not strictly dominant or recessive[56]. They suggest that the inheritance of GTS may be best described as 'semi-dominant, semi-recessive'. The model they are proposing is essentially the same as an additive model. That is, they are proposing a differential probability of manifesting GTS that is dependent on the number of alleles. This hypothesis is based on the assumption that a wide range of other behaviours are also a manifestation of the GTS gene. Family history data are presented that suggest that obsessive–compulsive behaviour, panic attacks, attention deficit hyperactivity disorder, alcohol and/or drug abuse and eating disorders including obesity are elevated among first-, second- and third-degree relatives of GTS probands. Since many of their families have relatives with these disorders on both maternal and paternal sides of the family, these authors suggest that a single dose of the GTS gene will be likely to result in these variant expressions and a double dose (i.e. homozygosity) will be more likely to result in GTS. No formal segregation analyses are presented to support their hypothesis.

To address the potential problem of reporting biases, family studies are needed in which all available first-degree relatives are personally assessed using structured clinical interviews. Several studies have been completed using this paradigm. Results from the first of these studies suggest that GTS is familial and that some chronic tics and some forms of obsessive–compulsive disorder are variant expressions of the syndrome[57]. The hypothesis that OCD is a variant manifestation of the syndrome grew out of a number of studies of GTS patients that documented the increased frequency of obsessive–compulsive symptomatology among GTS patients[58–69]. Others such as Robertson and Gourdie[70] have directly interviewed 85 members of a kindred containing 122 individuals. Complex segregation analysis supported the hypothesis that a single major gene inherited in autosomal dominant fashion but with incomplete penetrance contributed most of the variance in the liability to develop GTS and CMT[71]. Moreover, results suggested that obsessive–compulsive behaviour (OCB) can occur as a variant expression of the putative GTS gene[70,71].

THE GENETICS OF OTHER ASSOCIATED CONDITIONS

Early data from the Yale Family Study suggested that OCD alone (no current or past history of tics) could represent a variant expression of GTS[72]. Several more recent studies have supported these findings[68,73–75], as well as another series of families collected in the Yale Family Study[57]. The hypothesis that OCD is a variant expression of the syndrome is supported by family data that show that the rate of OCD is increased significantly in the families of GTS probands regardless of whether the proband has a concomitant diagnosis of OCD. That is, the rate of OCD is equally high in families of probands with both GTS and OCD, and families of probands with GTS only. Of interest is that OCD by itself occurs more frequently in female relatives of GTS probands suggesting some sex-related expression of the syndrome, with males being more likely to express GTS and tics, and females being more likely to express OCD in the absence of any tics[57].

The familial relationship between GTS and attention deficit disorder (ADD), learning problems, speech disorders and stuttering was also examined in a controlled study[76]. No evidence was found that the attentional and speech problems represent variant expressions of GTS. However, the data suggested that GTS and ADD may be aetiologically related in relatives with GTS, regardless of the ADD diagnosis of the GTS proband. There may be two types of individuals with GTS and ADD: ones in whom ADD is independent of GTS and others in whom ADD is secondary to the occurrence of GTS.

GENETIC ANALYSES OF FAMILY STUDY DATA

Family study data result in higher estimates of the rates of GTS and CT in the first-degree relatives of GTS probands when compared to the rates obtained in family history studies[55]. To examine whether the family study data would result in different genetic hypotheses being supported, segregation analyses were undertaken. Pauls and Leckman demonstrated that the pattern within families was consistent with autosomal dominant transmission[77]. This hypothesis was supported when:

1. only relatives with GTS were included as affected;
2. relatives with GTS or CT were included as affected; and
3. when relatives with GTS, CT or OCD were included as affected.

These findings have been replicated in an extension of the Yale sample and two independent samples[78–80]. Eapen and co-workers studied the families of 40 consecutive GTS probands seen in a London clinic and Van de Wetering and colleagues studied the families of approximately 45 GTS patients seen in Rotterdam[79,80]. All studies found strong statistical evidence that the pattern of transmission of GTS, CT with OCD, and OCD without tics, was consistent with autosomal dominant inheritance. In all analyses except the affected scheme of GTS or CT, all models except a mendelian dominant were rejected when compared with the mixed model. These findings from the total data set replicated those reported earlier[77]. While the earlier findings suggested a dominant model could explain the transmission patterns for all diagnostic schemes, goodness of fit tests suggested that the scheme that included GTS and CT could be rejected. Given that the population prevalence of chronic tics is estimated to be between 1 and 5%, it is likely that some of the individuals in these families could have tics genetically unrelated to the GTS spectrum and thus not be part of the mendelian transmission patterns observed for the other diagnoses in the spectrum. It has been suggested that relatives with CT and obsessive–

compulsive symptoms (CT + OCS) are more likely to be related to those with GTS. The family patterns obtained including CT + OCS individuals are consistent with mendelian inheritance[81]. Since all published reports of genetic analyses suggest that the GTS spectrum is inherited as a single gene, genetic linkage studies are warranted as the next step in our understanding of the inheritance of this syndrome.

LINKAGE ANALYSIS

Genetic linkage studies provide a powerful method for confirming the conclusions of segregation analysis studies. Linkage results can demonstrate the existence of a major locus and help clarify the pattern of inheritance even in the absence of a known association between a biological abnormality and a disorder. The objective of linkage analysis is to demonstrate that a distinct segment of DNA (i.e. a 'DNA-marker' with known chromosomal localization) co-segregates with a disease in a family.

Due to recent developments in molecular biology, a large number of disease genes have been cloned and analysed. In most cases disease genes could be cloned because information was available about the biochemical defect, i.e. the gene product or the function of the gene. The strategy of identifying a disease gene by its known abnormal gene product or function is referred to as 'functional cloning'. For genetic diseases with unknown aetiology, an alternative strategy, called 'positional cloning', is applied to identify the responsible genes. Positional cloning begins with the localization of a gene to a particular region of a chromosome. The next steps involve narrowing down the candidate region until the gene is identified. The genes for Huntington's disease, Duchenne muscular dystrophy, cystic fibrosis, neurofibromatosis type I and the fragile X syndrome have recently been identified by positional cloning.

Although there is some indication that specific brain structures are involved in GTS, the aetiology is still unknown. In addition, there are currently no biological markers available. In the absence of specific abnormal gene products and candidate brain regions, several strategies will have to be used to localize the GTS gene(s).

SEARCH FOR CHROMOSOMAL ABNORMALITIES IN GTS PATIENTS

While most GTS patients have normal karyotypes[82], there have been incidental reports describing chromosomal abnormalities in some. Each of these reports has been examined in more detail, since the site of a chromosomal rearrangement might provide a clue regarding the localization of a gene for GTS.

Comings and colleagues reported a 46,t(7:18)(q22;q22.1) balanced reciprocal translocation in six relatives with GTS[83]. This report suggested that a gene for GTS could be near the 18q22.1 breakpoint. Subsequently, Donnai reported a female patient with a mildly hypoplastic mid-face, tic-like movements, mild OCD, panic attacks and visual hallucinations, who carried a deletion of the long arm of chromosome 18 at 18q22.1[84]. Given the relationship between OCD and tics, this report provided additional support for the hypothesis that a gene for GTS might be located in this region. These two reports led to the tentative assignment of the GTS gene to chromosome 18q22.1 by the Chromosome 18 Committee at the Human Gene Mapping Conference IX. Unfortunately, linkage analyses using chromosome 18 probes on Dutch and Norwegian caucasian families did not confirm linkage of a gene for GTS to this region[85].

Another cytogenetic abnormality (a *de novo* deletion, del(9) (qter−>p2304:)) was reported in a Latin-American male GTS patient by Taylor and colleagues[86]. This patient was mildly dysmorphic with microcephaly, prominent supraorbital ridges and slight mid-facial hypoplasia. In addition, he exhibited a number of characteristics of the 9p deletion syndrome in the oral cavity and the fingers. Linkage analysis of chromosome 9p has been hampered by a lack of polymorphic DNA markers in this region. The available markers on chromosome 9p that have been tested have provided no evidence for linkage.

CANDIDATE GENE APPROACH

Genes coding for proteins (e.g. enzymes or receptors) possibly involved in the aetiology of a disease are referred to as 'candidate genes'. If the candidate gene is the same as the disease gene, it will co-segregate with the disease in the families studied. The DNA markers for a number of candidate genes, such as the dopamine receptors, dopamine β-hydroxylase, pro-dynorphin (PDYN), proopiomelanocortin (POMC), tyrosine hydroxylase and the gastrin releasing peptide (GRP) have been tested. All of these loci can be excluded as the gene conferring susceptibility for GTS[87,88].

Association studies form an alternative to test for candidate genes. In this approach, co-segregation of a specific allele of a locus and the disease is studied in patients and matched controls. The goal of these analyses is to determine whether the allele and the disease co-occur more frequently than can be expected by chance alone. Association can be caused by the marker being located at or in the near vicinity of the functional mutation in the gene, or it can occur because the marker is close to a gene that modifies the expression of the disease. When modifier genes are involved, the phenotype results from the interaction of alleles at two or more loci. Recently, possible associations of the Dopamine D_2 and D_3-receptor loci and GTS were reported[89,90]. These initial results have not been consistently replicated in well-defined, large groups of GTS patients[91,92].

SYSTEMATIC SEARCH FOR POLYMORPHIC MARKERS LINKED TO THE DISEASE LOCUS

Another approach is to screen the genome in a systematic way using highly polymorphic markers that have been mapped. Several groups have undertaken such a search[93]. At the present time, over 600 autosomal markers have been tested in an attempt to map the GTS gene. No definite linkage has been obtained, although several markers produced several non-significant positive lod scores in some families. Further work is under way in order to obtain more conclusive results.

An exact calculation of the proportion of the genome that has been excluded is not possible for several reasons. First, not all markers have been typed on all families being studied. If there is genetic heterogeneity, exclusion in one family does not imply exclusion in another. Second, the exact length of the human autosomal map is not known. Third, exclusion zones of markers that are not exactly mapped could overlap with well-localized markers. Finally, exclusions are dependent on the genetic model used in the linkage analyses. Since the precise genetic parameter values are not known, it is not possible to estimate precisely the extent of the current exclusion. The search continues. Given the likelihood that GTS is heterogeneous, additional strategies are being employed that are not as dependent on a specific genetic model for the analyses.

FUTURE DIRECTIONS

The localization of a gene or genes responsible for the expression of GTS will be a major step forward in our understanding of the genetic/biological risk factors important for the expression of this syndrome. In addition, this work will allow the potential identification of non-genetic factors associated with the manifestation or the amelioration of the symptoms of the disorders[94,95]. On the one hand, the identification of a linked marker will permit the design of much more incisive studies to illuminate the physiological/biochemical aetiology of GTS by examination of the gene product and its impact on the manifestation of the syndrome. On the other hand, by controlling for genetic factors it will be possible to document more carefully the environmental/non-genetic factors important for the expression of the GTS spectrum.

Once the location of a gene or genes has been verified, it will be possible to genotype unaffected children at risk, to determine with a high probability who is carrying a susceptibility gene. It will then be possible to examine in more detail the interaction between genotype and environment. Linked genetic markers can serve as the basis for defining an appropriate control group for a 'genetic case-control' design[96]. Closely linked genetic markers can identify quite accurately those children who are genetically identical with their affected sibs and/or parents for the relevant loci.

The ability to utilize genetic linkage and other aspects of genetic studies to design and carry out a study of non-genetic aetiological factors of a psychiatric illness is a significant methodological advancement that has not been possible up to now. Data from prospective studies of children at risk will make it possible to examine individuals with specific genotypes to determine which factors protect some from manifesting the syndrome[97]. It is important to begin data collection now, before genes are localized. After the genes are localized, it will be ethically unacceptable to withhold the test for identification of carriers from individuals at risk and knowledge of carrier status may change the care-giving environment.

REFERENCES

1. Lees, A. J. (1985) *Tics and related disorders*. Churchill Livingstone, Edinburgh.
2. Shapiro, A. K., Shapiro, E. S., Bruun, R. D. and Sweet, R. D. (1978) *Gilles de la Tourette's Syndrome*. Raven Press, New York.
3. Devaugh-Geiss, J. (1980) Tardive Tourette syndrome. *Neurology*, **30**, 562–563.
4. Klawans, H. L., Falk, A. K., Nausieda, P. A. and Weiner, W. J. (1978) Gilles de la Tourette syndrome after long-term chlorpromazine therapy. *Neurology*, **28**, 1064–1066.
5. Mueller, J. and Aminoff, M. J. (1982) Tourette-like syndrome after long-term neuroleptic drug treatment. *Br. J. Psychiatry*, **141**, 191–193.
6. Pulst, S.-M., Walshe, T. M. and Romero, J. A. (1983) Carbon monoxide poisoning with features of Gilles de la Tourette syndrome. *Arch. Neurol.* **40**, 443–444.
7. Koryani, E. K. (1977) Remarkable aetiology in Gilles de la Tourette's disease. *Psychiatr. J. Univ. Ott.*, **1**, 507.
8. Wohlfart, G., Ingvar, D. H. and Hellberg, A. M. (1961) Compulsory shouting (Benedek's 'Klazomania') associated with oculogyric spasms in chronic epidemic encephalitis. *Acta Psychiatr. Scand.*, **30**, 369–377.
9. Sacks, O. (1982) Acquired Tourettism in adult life. In *Gilles de la Tourette Syndrome* (A. J. Friedhoff and T. N. Chase, Eds). Raven Press, New York, pp. 88–92.
10. Northam, R. S. and Singer, H. S. (1991) Postencephalitic acquired Tourette-like syndrome in a child. *Neurology*, **41**, 592–593.
11. Fahn, S. (1982) A case of post-traumatic tic syndrome. In *Gilles de la Tourette Syndrome* (A. J. Friedhoff and T. N. Chase, Eds). Raven Press, New York, pp. 349–350.
12. Bleeker, H. E. (1978) Gilles de la Tourette's syndrome with direct evidence of organicity. *Psychiatr. Clin.*, **11**, 147–154.
13. La Pouse, E. and Monk, M. (1964) Behavior deviations in a representative sample of children: variation by sex, age, race, social class and family size. *Am. J. Orthopsychiatry*, **34**, 436–446.
14. Shapiro, E. and Shapiro, A. K. (1981) Tic disorders. *JAMA*, **245**, 1583–1558.

15. Kurlan, R. (1933) Preface. In *The Handbook of Tourette's Syndrome and Related Tic and Behavioral Disorders* (R. Kurlan, Ed). Marcel Dekker, New York, p. vii.
16. American Psychiatric Association (1995) *Diagnostic and Statistical Manual of Mental Disorders* (4th edition). American Psychiatric Association, Washington, in press.
17. Koester, G. (1899) Über die maladie des tics impulsifs (mimische Krampfneurose). *Deutsche Zeitschr Nervenheil*, **15**, 147–159.
18. Ascher, E. (1948) Psychodynamic considerations in Gilles de la Tourette's disease (maladie des tics). *Am. J. Psychiatry*, **105**, 267–276.
19. Lucas, A. R. (1973) Report of Gilles de la Tourette's disease in two succeeding generations. *Child Psychiatry Hum. Dev.*, **3**, 231–233.
20. Burd, L., Kerbeshian, J., Wikenheiser, M. and Fisher, W. (1986) A prevalence study of Gilles de la Tourette syndrome in North Dakota school-aged children. *J. Am. Acad. Child Psychiatry*, **25**, 552–553.
21. Burd, L., Kerbeshian, J., Wikenheiser, M. and Fisher, W. (1986) Prevalence of Gilles de la Tourette's syndrome in North Dakota adults. *Am. J. Psychiatry*, **143**, 787–788.
22. Comings, D. E., Himes, J. A. and Comings, B. G. (1990) An epidemiological study of Tourette's syndrome in a single school district. *J. Clin. Psychiatry*, **51**, 463–469.
23. Caine, E. D., McBride, M. C., Chiverton, P., Bamford, K. A., Rediess, S. and Shiao, J. (1988) Tourette's syndrome in Monroe County school children. *Neurology*, **38**, 472–474.
24. Apter, A., Pauls, D. L., Bleich, A., Zohar, A. H., Kron, S., Ratzoni, G., Dycian, A., Kotler, M., Weizman, A., Gadot, N. and Cohen, D. J. (1993) An epidemiological study of Gilles de la Tourette syndrome in Israel. *Arch. Gen. Psychiatry*, **50**, 734–738.
25. Zausmer, D. M. (1954) Treatment of tics in childhood. *Arch. Dis. Child.*, **29**, 537–542.
26. Torup, E. (1972) A follow-up study of children with tics. *Acta Paediatr.*, **51**, 261–268.
27. Abe, K. and Oda, N. (1980) Incidence of tics in the offspring of childhood tiiquers: a controlled follow-up study. *Dev. Med. Child Neurol.*, **22**, 649–653.
28. Frost, N., Feighner, J. and Schuckit, M. A. (1976) A family study of Gilles de la Tourette's syndrome. *Dis. Nerv. System*, **37**, 537–538.
29. Zausmer, D. M. and Dewey, M. E. (1987) Tics and heredity—a study of the relatives of child ticqueurs. *Br. J. Psychiatry*, **150**, 628–634.
30. Gilles de la Tourette, G. A. E. B. (1885) Etude sur une affection nerveuse caractérisée par l'incoordination motrice accompagnée d'écholalie et de coprolalie. *Arch. Neurol.*, **9**, 19–42, 158–200.
31. Kelman, D. H. (1965) Gilles de la Tourette's disease in children: a review of the literature. *J. Child Psychol. Psychiatry*, **6**, 219–226.
32. Fernando, S. J. M. (1967) Gilles de la Tourette's syndrome. A report on four cases and a review of published case reports. *Br. J. Psychiatry*, **113**, 607–617.
33. Eldridge, R., Sweet, R., Lake, C. R., Ziegler, M. and Shapiro, A. K. (1977) Gilles de la Tourette's syndrome: clinical, genetic, psychological and biochemical aspects in 21 selected families. *Neurology*, **27**, 115–124.
34. Shapiro, A. K., Shapiro, E. S. and Wayne, H. (1972) Birth, developmental and demographic information in Tourette's syndrome. *J. Nerv. Ment. Dis.*, **155**, 335–344.
35. Friel, P. B. (1973) Familial incidence of Gilles de la Tourette's disease, with observations on aetiology and treatment. *Br. J. Psychiatry*, **122**, 655–658.
36. Ellison, R. M. (1964) Gilles de la Tourette's syndrome. *Med. J. Aust.*, **1**, 153–155.

37. Escalar, G., Majeron, M. A., Finavera, L. and Zamberletti, P. (1972) Contributo alla conoscenza della sindrome di Gilles de la Tourette. *Minerva Med.*, **63**, 3517–3522.
38. Jenkins, R. L. and Ashby, H. B. (1983) Gilles de la Tourette's syndrome in identical twins. *Arch. Neurol.*, **40**, 249–251.
39. Waserman, J., Lal, S. and Gauthier, S. (1983) Gilles de la Tourette's syndrome in monozygotic twins. *J. Neurol. Neurosurg. Psychiatry*, **46**, 75–77.
40. Vieregge, P., Schäfer, C. and Jörg, J. (1988) Concordant Gilles de la Tourette's syndrome in monozygotic twins: a clinical, neurophysiological and CT-study. *J. Neurol.*, **235**, 366–367.
41. Walkup, J. T., Leckman, J. F., Price, R. A., Hardin, M., Ort, S. I. and Cohen, D. J. (1988) The relationship between obsessive–compulsive disorder and Tourette's syndrome: a twin study. *Psychopharmacol. Bull.*, **24**, 375–379.
42. Goetz, C. G. and Tanner, C. M. (1988) Gilles de la Tourette syndrome in twins: clinical and neurochemical data. *Ann. Neurol.*, **24**, 152.
43. Segal, N. L., Dysken, M. W., Bouchard, T. J., Pedersen, N. L., Eckert, E. D. and Heston, L. L. (1990) Tourette's disorder in a set of reared-apart triplets: genetic and environmental influences. *Am. J. Psychiatry*, **147**, 196–199.
44. Price, R. A., Kidd, K. K., Cohen, D. J., Pauls, D. L. and Leckman, J. F. (1985) A twin study of Tourette syndrome. *Arch. Gen. Psychiatry*, **42**, 815–820.
45. Leckman, J. F., Price, R. A., Walkup, J. T., Ort, S., Pauls, D. L. and Cohen, D. J. (1987) Birthweights of monozygotic twins discordant for Tourette's syndrome. *Arch. Gen. Psychiatry*, **44**, 100.
46. Hyde, T. M., Aaronson, B. A., Randolph, C., Rickler, K. C. and Weinberger, D. R. (1992) Relationship of birth weight to the phenotypic expression of Gilles de la Tourette's syndrome in monozygotic twins. *Neurology*, **42**, 652–658.
47. Wilson, R. S., Garron, D. C. and Klawans, H. L. (1978) Significance of genetic factors in Gilles de la Tourette syndrome: A review. *Behav. Genet.*, **8**, 503–510.
48. Kidd, K. K., Prusoff, B. A. and Cohen, D. J. (1980) The familial pattern of Tourette syndrome. *Arch. Gen. Psychiatry*, **37**, 1336–1339.
49. Pauls, D. L., Cohen, D. J., Heimbuch, R., Detlor, J. and Kidd, K. K. (1981) Familial pattern and transmission of Gilles de la Tourette syndrome and multiple tics. *Arch. Gen. Psychiatry*, **38**, 1091–1093.
50. Baron, M., Shapiro, E., Shapiro, A. and Ranier, J. D. (1981) Genetic analysis of Tourette syndrome suggesting a major gene. *Am. J. Hum. Genet.*, **33**, 767–775.
51. Kidd, K. K. and Pauls, D. L. (1982) Genetic hypotheses from Tourette syndrome. In *Gilles de la Tourette Syndrome* (A. J. Friedhoff and T. N. Chase, Eds). Raven Press, New York, pp.243–249.
52. Comings, D. E., Comings, B. G., Devor, E. J. and Cloninger, C. R. (1984) Detection of a major gene for Gilles de la Tourette syndrome. *Am. J. Hum. Genet.*, **36**, 586–600.
53. Devor, E. J. (1984) Complex segregation analysis of Gilles de la Tourette syndrome: further evidence for a major locus mode of transmission. *Am. J. Hum. Genet.*, **36**, 704–709.
54. Price, R. A., Pauls, D. L., Kruger, S. D. and Caine, E. D. (1988) Family data support a dominant major gene for Tourette syndrome. *Psychiatry Res.*, **24**, 251–261.
55. Pauls, D. L., Kruger, S. D., Leckman, J. F., Cohen, D. J. and Kidd, K. K. (1984) The risk of Tourette Syndrome (TS) and Chronic Multiple Tics (CMT) among relatives of TS patients obtained by direct interview. *J. Am. Acad. Child. Psychiatry*, **23**, 134–137.
56. Comings, D. E., Comings, B. G. and Knell, E. (1989) Hypothesis: homozygosity in Tourette syndrome. *Am. J. Med. Genet.*, **34**, 413–421.

57. Pauls, D. L., Raymond, C. L., Leckman, J. F. and Stevenson, J. M. (1991) A family study of Tourette's syndrome. *Am. J. Hum. Genet.*, **48**, 154–163.
58. Kelman, D. H. (1965) Gilles de la Tourette's disease in children: a review of the literature. *J. Child. Psychol. Psychiatry*, **6**, 219–226.
59. Fernando, S. J. M. (1967) Gilles de la Tourette's syndrome. *Br. J. Psychiatry*, **113**, 115–124.
60. Morphew, J. A. and Sim, M. (1969) Gilles de la Tourette's syndrome: a clinical and psychopathological study. *Br. J. Med. Psychol.*, **42**, 293–301.
61. Nee, L. E., Caine, E. D., Polinsky, R. J., Eldridge, R. and Ebert, M. H. (1980) Gilles de la Tourette syndrome: clinical and family study of 50 cases. *Ann. Neurol.*, **7**, 41–49.
62. Yaryura-Tobias, J. A., Neziroglu, F., Howard, S. and Fuller, B. (1981) Clinical aspects of Gilles de la Tourette syndrome. *Orthomol. Psychiatry*, **10**, 263–268.
63. Jagger, J., Prusoff, B. A., Cohen, D. J., Kidd, K. K., Carbonari, C. M. and John, K. (1982) The epidemiology of Tourette's syndrome: a pilot study. *Schizophr. Bull.*, **8**, 267–278.
64. Montgomery, M. A., Clayton, P. J. and Friedhoff, A. J. (1982) Psychiatric illness in Tourette syndrome patients and first-degree relatives. In *Gilles de la Tourette Syndrome* (A. J. Friedhoff and T. N. Chase, Eds). Raven Press, New York, pp. 335–339.
65. Nee, L. E., Polinsky, R. J. and Ebert, M. H. (1982) Tourette syndrome: clinical and family studies. In *Gilles de la Tourette Syndrome* (A. J. Friedhoff and T. N. Chase, Eds). Raven Press, New York, pp.291–295.
66. Stefl, M. E. (1984) Mental health needs associated with Tourette syndrome. *Am. J. Public Health*, **74**, 1310–1313.
67. Cummings, J. L. and Frankel, M. (1985) Gilles de la Tourette syndrome and the neurological basis of obsessions and compulsions. *Biol. Psychiatry*, **20**, 1117–1126.
68. Robertson, M. M., Trimble, M. R. and Lees, A. J. (1988) The psychopathology of the Gilles de la Tourette syndrome: a phenomenological analysis. *Br. J. Psychiatry*, **152**, 383–390.
69. Robertson, M. M. (1989) The Gilles de la Tourette syndrome: the current status. *Br. J. Psychiatry*, **154**, 147–169.
70. Robertson, M. M. and Gourdie, A. (1990) Familial Tourette's syndrome in a large British pedigree. Associated psychopathology, severity, and potential for linkage analysis. *Br. J. Psychiatry*, **156**, 515–521.
71. Curtis, D., Robertson, M. M. and Gurling, H. M. D. (1992) Autosomal dominant gene transmission in a large kindred with Gilles de la Tourette syndrome. *Br. J. Psychiatry*, **160**, 845–849.
72. Pauls, D. L., Towbin, K. E., Leckman, J. F., Zahner, G. E. P. and Cohen, D. J. (1986) Gilles de la Tourette syndrome and obsessive–compulsive disorder: Evidence supporting an etiological relationship. *Arch. Gen. Psychiatry*, **43**, 1180–1182.
73. Frankel, M., Cummings, J. L., Robertson, M. M., Trimble, M. R., Hill, M. A. and Benson, D. F. (1986) Obsessions and compulsions in the Gilles de la Tourette syndrome. *Neurology*, **36**, 379–382.
74. Pitman, R. K., Green, R. C., Jenike, M. A. and Mesulam, M. M. (1987) Clinical comparison of Tourette's disorder and obsessive–compulsive disorder. *Am. J. Psychiatry*, **144**, 1166–1171.
75. Walkup, J. T., Leckman, J. F., Price, R. A., Harden, M. T., Ort, S. and Cohen, D. J. (1988) The relationship between Tourette syndrome and obsessive–compulsive disorder: a twin study. *Psychopharmacol. Bull.*, **24**, 375–379.
76. Pauls, D. L., Leckman, J. F. and Cohen, D. J. (1990) Familial relationship between Gilles de la Tourette's syndrome, attention deficit disorder, learning disabilities,

speech disorders, and stuttering. *J. Am. Acad. Child Adolesc. Psychiatry*, **32**, 1044–1150.

77. Pauls, D. L. and Leckman, J. F. (1986) The inheritance of Gilles de la Tourette's syndrome and associated behaviours: Evidence for autosomal dominant transmission. *N. Engl. J. Med.*, **315**, 993–997.
78. Pauls, D. L., Pakstis, A. J., Kurlan, R., Kidd, K. K., Leckman, J. F., Cohen, D. J. and Kidd, J. R. (1990) Segregation and linkage analyses of Gilles de la Tourette's syndrome and related disorders. *J. Am. Acad. Child Adolesc. Psychiatry*, **29**, 195–203.
79. Eapen, V., Pauls, D. L. and Robertson, M. M. (1993) Evidence for autosomal dominant transmission in Gilles de la Tourette syndrome: United Kingdom Cohort Study. *Br. J. Psychiatry*, **162**, 593–596.
80. Wetering, B. J. M. van de (1993) *The Gilles de la Tourette Syndrome: A Psychiatric–Genetic Study*. PhD Thesis, Rotterdam.
81. Pauls, D. L. (1993) The inheritance pattern. In *Handbook of Tourette's Syndrome and Related Tic and Behavioral Disorders* (R. Kurlan, Ed). Marcel Dekker, New York, pp. 1–9.
82. Robertson, M. M. and Trimble, M. R. (1993) Normal chromosomal findings in Gilles de la Tourette syndrome. *Psychiatr. Genet.*, **3**, 95–99.
83. Comings, D. E., Comings, B. G., Dietz, G., Muhleman, D., Okada, T. A., Arinana, F., Simmer, R. and Stock, D. (1986) Evidence the Tourette syndrome gene is at 18q22.1. *Proc. VIIth International Congress of Hum. Genet.*, Berlin, p. 620.
84. Donnai, D. (1987) Gene location in Tourette syndrome. *Lancet*, **i**, 627.
85. Heutink, P., Wetering, B. J. M. van de, Breedveld, G. J., Weber, J., Sandkuyl, L. A., Devor, E. J., Heiberg, A., Niermeijer, M. F. and Oostra, B. A. (1990) No evidence for genetic linkage of Gilles de la Tourette syndrome on chromosome 7 and 18. *J. Med. Genet.*, **27**, 433–436.
86. Taylor, L. D., Krizman, D. B., Jankovic, J., Hayani, A., Steuber, P. C., Greenberg, F., Fenwick, R. G. and Caskey, C. T. (1991) 9p Monosomy in a patient with Tourette syndrome. *Neurology*, **41**, 1513–1515.
87. Devor, E. J., Grandy, D. K., Civelli, O., Litt, M., Burgess, A. K., Isenberg, K. E., Wetering, B. J. M. van de and Oostra, B. A. (1990) Genetic linkage is excluded for the D_2-dopamine receptor lambdaHD2G1 and flanking loci on chromosome 11q22-q23 in Tourette syndrome. *Hum. Hered.*, **40**, 105–108.
88. Gelernter, J., Pakstis, A. J., Pauls, D. L., Chapell, P., Kurlan, R., Grandy, D. K., Bunzow, J., Retief, A. E., Litt, M., Civelli, O. and Kidd, K. K. (1990) Tourette syndrome is not linked to D_2 dopamine receptor. *Arch. Gen. Psychiatry*, **47**, 1073–1077.
89. Comings, D. E., Comings, B. G., Muhleman, D., Dietz, G., Shahbahrami, B., Tast, D., Knell, E., Kocsis, B. W., Baumgarten, R., Kovacs, B. W., Levy, D. L., Smith, M., Borison, R. L., Evans, D. D., Klein, D. N., Macmurray, J., Tosk, J. M., Sverd, J., Gysin, R. and Flanagan, S. D. (1991) The dopamine D_2 receptor locus as a modifying gene in neuropsychiatric disorders. *JAMA*, **266**, 193–200.
90. Comings, D. E., Muhleman, D., Dietz, G., Dino, M., Legro, R. and Gade, R. (1993) Association between Tourette's syndrome and homozygosity at the dopamine D_3 receptor gene. *Lancet*, **341**, 906.
91. Hebebrand, J., Nothen, M. M., Lehmkuhl, G., Poustka, F., Schmidt, M., Propping, P. and Remschmidt, H. (1993) Tourette's syndrome and homozygosity for the Dopamine D_3 receptor gene. *Lancet*, **341**, 1483–1484.
92. Brett, P., Robertson, M. M., Gurling, H. and Curtis, D. (1993) Failure to find linkage and increased homozygosity for the Dopamine D_3 receptor. *Lancet*, **341**, 1225.
93. Pakstis, A. J., Heutink, P., Pauls, D. L., Kurlan, R., Wetering, B. J. M. van de,

Weber, J., Leckman, J. F., Sandkuyl, L. A., Kidd, J. R., Breedveld, G. J., Castiglione, C. M., Sparkes, R. S., Cohen, D. J., Kidd, K. K. and Oostra, B. A. (1991) Progress in the search for genetic linkage with Tourette syndrome: an exclusion map covering more than 50% of the autosomal genome. *Am. J. Hum. Genet.*, **48**, 281–294.

94. Pauls, D. L. (1990) Emerging genetic markers and their role in potential preventive intervention strategies. In *Conceptual Research Models for Preventing Mental Disorders* (P. Muehrer, Ed). NIMH, Rockville, MD, pp.184–195.
95. Leckman, J. F., Dolnansky, E. S., Hardin, M., Clubb, M., Walkup, J. T., Stevenson, J. and Pauls, D. L. (1990) The perinatal factors in the expression of Tourette's syndrome. *J. Am. Acad. Child Adolesc. Psychiatry*, **29**, 220–226.
96. Kidd, K. K. (1985) New genetic strategies for studying psychiatric disorders. In *Genetic Aspects of Human Behavior* (T. Sakai and T. Tsuboi, Eds). Igaku-Shoin Ltd, Tokyo, pp.325–346.
97. Carter, A. S., Pauls, D. L., Leckman, J. F. and Cohen, D. J. (1995) A prospective longitudinal study of Gilles de la Tourette's syndrome. *J. Am. Acad. Child Adolesc. Psychiatry*, **33**, 377–385.

3 Inner Lives of Individuals and Families Living with Tourette Syndrome

DONALD J. COHEN
SHARON I. ORT
and
JAMES F. LECKMAN
Yale University School of Medicine, New Haven, Connecticut, USA

A central struggle for many individuals and families afflicted with Gilles de la Tourette syndrome (GTS) and related conditions concerns issues of control and self-regulation that are at once intimate and all too public in their expression[1,2]. For the individual with GTS, internal questions such as, 'What do I have control over with respect to my bodily sensations and movements?' and 'What is "beyond" my control?' emerge over the course of development. Similar questions vex families, 'What of our son's behaviour does he have control over and where do we draw the line between his Tourette's and just bad behaviour?' This chapter attempts to envision these inner worlds and their vicissitudes and consider the role of the clinician in aiding afflicted children and families.

THE INNER WORLD OF GTS

GTS may erupt with volcanic force, literally within a few days, transforming a normal tic-free child into one tormented by dozens of tics every minute. Over the course of weeks, such a youngster may feel that he is being driven crazy and his parents, too, may feel their child has been possessed. More often, GTS has a more gradual onset, with one or several episodes of 'innocent' childhood tics being followed by more persistent motor and phonic tics which are severe enough to move the child's symptoms into the range of clinical disorder. In these more typical cases, the tics are initially experienced as 'meaningless' events, as isolated movements or sounds which simply and rapidly pop out of the body or throat. The child may be unaware of their occurrence, either before or after.

Yet, over the course of months or years, children do become aware of their tics and resent them, consciously and in other ways. They see them

Movement and Allied Disorders. Edited by M. M. Robertson and V. Eapen

reflected in their parents' eyes when their parents knowingly try to overlook them; they see them evoke tension, embarrassment and anger. And they are taught to be aware of their tics—'Why are you having so many tics today?'—and of their role in producing them—'Please try not to do your tics when grandma is visiting . . . they upset her so'.

By the age of 10 or 11, many children recognize and report premonitory experiences which precede the tics and to which they capitulate[3,4]. These sensory experiences, which may be intrinsic to the phenomenology of the tic, typically consist of a feeling of tightness, tension, increased sensitivity or a mounting discomfort/anxiety, located in a specific part of the body. The sensory prodrome, which is likened to the expectation which precedes a sneeze or an itch at some unreachable spot on the back, is felt as requiring some type of vigorous, quick, tic-like action for its attenuation. Sometimes the patient feels that an effective action must include a dangerous or aggressive quality, as an essential constituent (and not merely a secondary effect) of the tic experience. For example, a young man needed to scream in a way that would frighten others in order to feel his inner tension relieved. Another young adult felt the need to punch at someone with whom he was emotionally close and to create a sense of fear. A minority of patients need to hurt themselves (poke their eyes, pull their hair, dig holes in their skin or oral mucosa, stick pins or pencils into their arms, crack their joints until they hurt, and on and on). While the ejection of a tic may lead to short-term gratification, the child soon feels the mounting of renewed tension to which he will inevitably and perhaps shamefully capitulate. This cycle of tension, motor or phonic tic action, amelioration of anxiety and mounting crescendo of tension in varying loci of the body may be repeated many times an hour and lead to paroxysms of physically exhausting tics.

It is of interest that extraneous sensory stimuli may, at times, exacerbate tics. Parents of children with GTS, and adult patients with the syndrome, report that bright flashing lights, loud background noise, or a combination of intense sensory loading and excitement (as in an amusement park) will increase tics, as will watching rapidly changing, exciting events on television or in the movies. This sensory provocation of ticking may be related to the premonitory experiences of GTS; increased sensory input seems to overcome the stimulus barrier and to trigger more tics. Speculatively, we may wonder if the neurobiological correlates of this phenomenon may be related to the recruitment of sensory–motor, cortico–thalamocortical brain circuits[5].

THE ROLE OF FANTASY

To try to understand what has been taking place inside themselves and between them and their families, children elaborate fantasies about their inner world and the workings of their mind-brains. They picture their bodies and minds. As a mode of self-understanding, these fantasies help them cope with the intrusion into consciousness, and then into action, of ideas and acts which are and are not their own. Often, in their first layering, these constructions are built upon the theories about the biochemistry of the brain which are offered to them by well-meaning physicians and their parents. In such medical fairy-tales, the child is taught that 'dopamine' and 'neurotransmitters' are mysterious and uncontrollable forces. As retold by one boy: 'My problem, the tics, are 'cause of too much dopamine sensitivity . . . the chemicals in my brain are too over wild'. Occasionally, the child is taught that his brain has been 'damaged' and that there are 'abnormal pathways' in his head.

Psychoanalytically informed clinicians are fully aware of the pitfalls of explaining: we can never be quite sure of what children and adults take in and take away from 'explanations' and how they will make use of what is offered. How surprised we sometimes are when we hear patients re-present what they have learned from us about the genetics and neurochemistry of GTS; even thoughtful clarifications may bring new dimensions of confusion. From another perspective, these 'confusions' are another source of information about the dynamic functioning of the mind to which the clinician has a privileged access.

For children in the midst of the bewildering experience of medicalization of their tic symptoms, our current concepts—genes, neuromodulators, brain circuits—and our scientific methods—brain imaging, blood sampling, urine tests—are amalgamated with what they have learned from *Where the Wild Things Are* and their own dreams. The source of the child's crazy thoughts and bizarre actions becomes conceptualized as another part of the self or as a dominating, secondary will: an illness or disease surrounded by an array of fantasies about who or what was the cause, where it is located and what is its precise pathological process. Beneath scientific rhetoric children may experience life as if an evil witch had cast her spell. They, and their parents, may wait for the prince's magic to free them from possession and they are quite ready for professional help in the many forms it may be offered, both conventional and otherwise. When there is clinical improvement, we and our medications may be granted more credit than deserved.

Often, the child becomes a vigilant observer of the internal forces which compel his tics and impulsions. To master these forces, the source of the distressing symptoms, he directs attention to the urges and uses conscious will-power to control the split-off, internal agency, the alien introject of the secondary will. This defensive splitting may be useful for the child. Through splitting his normal self from his urge to spit, bark, pull faces and the like, the child manages to maintain a degree of coherence. He stands over and against his disowned impulses and acts. But to maintain this splitting requires constant vigilance and exertion of control. In the process, the child's energies are drained and his difficulties in concentration are compounded. In spite of this, it has seemed that children do best when they are allowed to maintain this type of splitting, where the child is not constantly encouraged to take responsibility and to inhibit his tics. It is helpful for the child to know that others understand he cannot stop. Yet, among the most tragic patients are those where such a disavowal goes too far. When disavowal overcarries, the patient may feel he has lost control over himself and has merged with his illness. These individuals may be blocked, at the core of their beings, in achieving the sense of ownership of the self which comes with owning up to and taking responsibility for what they do[6].

The breaking down between the voluntary and the involuntary in our mental lives, the emergence of primitive rage, the loss of control leave a wake of anxiety and sometimes panic, if but for one instant frozen in time and memory. Fortunately and more often, the processes which allow for symbolization and sublimation, the processes of inhibition and creative camouflage, usually prevail over the raw expression of forbidden urges.

Understanding these processes of the psychopathology of everyday life provides a context for conceptualizing the everyday experiences of patients with GTS. In GTS, just those processes of modulation which normally are called upon to maintain equanimity fail repeatedly. For GTS patients, crazy ideas and action tendencies invade the normal matrix of experience hundreds of times a day. The normal filtering mechanisms are overly permeable to contents of unconscious fantasy, rage and sexual drive; the barrier between preconsciousness and consciousness, just as the barrier between perception and action, is attenuated, and the internal structures, the mental dikes, which demarcate boundaries are constantly in need of repair. What can a 7-year-old boy make of his tics and odd thoughts? Just at the phase of life when third graders are mastering the latency age tasks of giving structure to experience—internalizing rules; fashioning their superegos through internalized values and their ego-ideals around super-heroes; feeling competent in sports, reading and writing; understanding the sequence of seasons, the regularity of schedules and the rules of school and friendship—the child with GTS is plagued by disorder. He counts and recounts, does and undoes, holds back and gives in to terrifying desires. He feels weird, crazy and on the verge of losing control.

PHILOSOPHICAL PERSPECTIVES

But when a child with GTS feels weird, what is he feeling, how does he know it, how can he find the words to tell us what is on his mind, and how do we understand what he is experiencing? The study of questions such as these lies on the border between empirical research on GTS and the philosophy of mind. By exploring this terrain, we can perhaps clarify our understanding of the predicament of the child with GTS in forming a picture of his own mind and body and those of others[7].

The philosopher's model of mind assumes an orderliness of experience, a shared regularity in the relations between events and what humans normally feel and say about their feelings. From many different angles, Wittgenstein and those who have worked in his path have tried to illuminate how the language of emotions (sensations, beliefs, intentions)—in short the language of psychology—is learned and practised within the *forms of life* which are distinctly human and which we share. Within these communally shared forms of living, the 'rules' of usage and of self- and other-understanding are the grammar of average expectable experience. In this context, utterances ('I hurt') replace our primitive cries ('ouch') and pain-behaviour (jumping up, holding our mouth)[8]. We learn how to speak of being angry and to ascribe feelings to others within our forms of social relations. Speech about feelings, our own and others', is congruous with conventions which guide feelings towards others as people. In this natural psychology, we do not infer a person is in pain from his writhing and moaning. To the contrary, we feel compassion for someone and reach out to help him and we move from this experience of concern to a description of his (underlying) pain and suffering. We relate to people as having feelings, not on the basis of their behaviour but because of who we are and who they are. That is, we naturally relate to others as people.

For children with GTS, these forms of life break down. They yell out curses when they are not angry and touch their mothers sexually when they are not aroused; they stick out their tongues to friends and smooch a stranger. Their assertions do not, in the normal way, replace their behaviour (as 'I am in pain' replaces shrieking with pain) and the disconnections between display and feelings confuse others who cannot understand the child's actions in the normal way. The surface of the child's behaviour is not mapped by the grammar of intentions nor does the ordinary discourse of emotions and feelings convey what he is experiencing.

Clinically, we might hypothesize, the child with GTS is handicapped not only in making sense of himself but in the complementary process as well: learning and understanding the third-person language of emotions and sensations, seeing things from the inside of the other. Children learn to describe another's suffering along with learning how to express their own feelings; their personal experience with pain and sorrow, as with varied forms of pleasure and satisfaction, is relevant to their subtle and sensitive understanding of what another individual is going through. But if the internal world of a child or adolescent is incongruous with that of others—in just the ways it is for children with GTS—the task of empathic understanding may be far more difficult and sometimes insurmountable.

At times, individuals who are severely afflicted with GTS seem not fully to grasp their impact on others or their needs. Narcissism and self-centredness are issues, of course, for many children with chronic illness, physical or mental, and arise from a variety of sources. It is hard to be altruistic when one is suffering or to feel good about one's self or concerned about others when one's own body has not been a source of pleasure. Yet, in addition to these general and expected causes of self-centredness, the narcissistic preoccupation of some patients with GTS seems to reflect deeper and more pervasive difficulties in areas which are the central concern of the philosophy of mind: the cognitive and affective task of understanding one's mind (intentions, aversions, desires, beliefs, etc.) and the mind of others. They are not secure in decoding the rules which govern the inner lives of others. If this is so, we might be able to understand, from a new and more sympathetic angle, why it is so urgent for some individuals who are afflicted with severe GTS to maintain themselves as a dominating topic in their lives.

In important ways, children with GTS are all too aware of how their minds and bodies work. But, for those most severely afflicted, they cannot make sense of their experiences, of their intentions, desires, and sensory phenomena; or they try to make sense of these inner processes by regarding a portion of their minds and bodies as foreign or wholly 'other'. They know they play a role even in relation to the 'other' inside themselves, but defining this role eludes language. We have hypothesized that persistent interferences of these types—with normal unfolding of a sense of body and with the normal experiences of consciousness—skew the ways in which children conceptualize how others tick and thus their 'theory of mind'.

What does a child experience when he recognizes that his wish to poke at his mother's breast and his rage at her comes from inside himself but are not under his control? That he wishes for what he dreads having fulfilled? That instead of protecting his body from harm he is compelled to gouge out his own eye and burn his own hand? The phenomenology of GTS illuminates processes which usually are only inferred. Over the course of clinical engagement, one can see how obsessions and compulsions take shape around aggressive, destructive and sexual urges, and how fantasies can be created to counteract even more frightening fantasy and the terror involved in the experience of intrusive mental processes. Patients with GTS can describe their self-representations: hated aspects of the self are placated and there is repeated capitulation to urges. The self is split and during periods of catastrophic ticking it is fragmented.

Tics, obsessive thoughts and compulsions present themselves to consciousness as unwilled interferences in the normal unfolding of experience and desire. Through the mobilization of defences and fantasies, such as intellectualization and denial, adolescents and adults will attempt to ward off the anxiety associated with loss of control, frightening impulses, and discontinuities in thinking and action. Generally, these defensive manoeuvres succeed in maintaining the 'symptoms' as disturbing but not self-permeating or dominating burdens.

IMPACT ON ISSUES OF IDENTITY AND CHARACTER

The adolescents and young adults who do worst, as whole people, are those whose tics, obsessive thoughts and rituals have led to traumatic disruptions of fundamental developmental processes concerned with the self and its representations. Their 'irrepressible symptoms' profoundly shape and deform their characters. Their disorder distorts relations with families and peers, forges internalized object relations, and moulds intra-psychic representations of drives and other strong effects in general. In this way, GTS takes hold of character formation and the individual develops an identity of being a 'victim' which may also make him entitled to feeling he should be treated as an exception[9,10]. This self-system serves as an organization that aggregates much of life's experience into a tortured whole and explains any personal limitations in motivation or responsibility. The 'victim of GTS' may hand over major decisions to physicians and other caregivers or to fate, and all of life's misfortunes become read as subtexts of having an illness which deprives one of self-control. The goal of treatment of patients with GTS is to prevent this from happening.

FAMILY PERSPECTIVES

For a child with GTS, life within the family will deviate in very important ways from what normally can be anticipated[11]. The individual with GTS generally will provide ambivalent pleasure for his or her parents, pose special challenges for his or her siblings, and experience different, indeed unique, problems in his or her role as offspring, brother or sister, husband or wife, father or mother. That an individual with GTS will pose such challenges to families, and experience difficulties in trying to be a rewarding and beloved member and creator of a family, is almost self-evident. As a serious, chronic illness, GTS presents realistic strains on family functioning. Yet, over and above such nonspecific factors, GTS disrupts family life in ways that often are more difficult to overcome. These stresses relate to the natural history of the disorder, its symptoms, the familial nature of the condition, the possibility of suppressibility, inadequate public information, and the types of treatment offered[1,12]. After many years of perfectly normal development, children who will eventually have GTS slowly develop symptoms that grow upon parental awareness as worthy of note. Their simple childhood tics fail to disappear. At dinner time, a father will reprimand a child for making a noise, a mother will scold the boy for making funny faces. Tension mounts: soon, there is hardly a time when the family assembles that the child is not scolded for his noises, gestures, or facial expressions. Parents generally are more sensitive to their children's shortcomings as well as assets than are others; thus parents may experience the child's tics as more disruptive, odd appearing, or louder than do others. Each tic may be felt as painful by the parents, who may try to look away or ignore its occurrence for some period of time but then lose their temper and reprimand the child. In spite of parental response, tics worsen, with one type of tic leaving and others taking its place. Some of these may be very odd, such as bending down to touch the floor, making faces, sticking out their tongue, hawking, spitting, coughing and the like. Their peculiarity makes the family increasingly uncomfortable, edgy and worried. As they progress from the appearance of the first 'childhood' tic to the reassuring pronouncement by family doctor or a paediatrician that this is just a 'nervous habit' to the ultimate realization that the child is suffering from GTS, the child and family may feel very much alone and confused. Children may experience the onset of GTS as so bewildering that they may feel they are going crazy; parents may have the same worries. Occasionally, parents will resort to physical aggression, such as spanking or striking their children, or to bribes and threats. The years that pass between onset and diagnosis may shape patterns of interaction that are long-lived, as well as bitter memories of abuse and guilt. In front of their very eyes, parents see their lovely children dissolve into anxious, preoccupied tickers and they feel impotent, angry and hurt.

For those children whose tics are preceded by attentional and behavioural problems—whose problems may later be the most severe—the onset of the tics may follow upon several years of tension between parents and children. The hyperactive, disruptive, inattentive and naughty 4-year-old child can wreak havoc on a family. Parents may feel the child is wilfully or intentionally mean, and the child may be excluded from nursery school, day care, and play groups, and ostracized by other children and families. Exhausted mothers naturally will feel furious and are likely to have scolded and disciplined the child. Thus the onset of tics is within a matrix, in such cases, of already existing negative interactions. Such children are likely to feel that they are 'bad' and 'mean' or 'unloving'; it is at a surprisingly early age that children are able to take in and make a part of themselves the reactions that they have elicited in others. The unfolding of tics may be seen by both child and parent as an expression of the child's anger.

Whether the child has had, or concurrently develops, attentional and behavioural difficulties along with the tics, or whether the tics appear in a child who was a 'perfect angel', the tics are often quickly related to issues surrounding anger and aggression. Parents will feel angry with their children; they will feel that they are doing what they are doing out of spite, and children will feel anger with themselves and with others.

ASSESSMENT AND TREATMENT

The assessment and treatment of children (and adults) with GTS require a thoughtful understanding of them in relation to the important people in their world. This type of assessment involves understanding the way in which GTS patients relate to their parents, the patients' internal pictures of their role and the parents' responses to them, and the parents' understanding of the causes of their children's basic troubles and associated problems. By 'family dynamics' we mean the ways in which each person in a family has a powerful impact on others, the balance between love and hatred, the ways in which needs are satisfied or frustrated, the recognition of the individuality of each family member, the modes for expression of irritations and sharing of fondness. Dynamics include the channels and efficacy of communication (who talks to whom, when, about what, and with what effect), and how thoughts and feelings are expressed in addition to talking (thoughtfulness, caring, forgetting, doing favours, sabotaging the other's plans, etc.). To what degree do family members feel that their basic needs are satisfied, that they are being as effective as they would like to be, that they find it fulfilling to be at home? When things become too much to bear, what escape valves exist for each member, and at what cost are they used? Is family life a haven of security or a jungle with beasts lurking here and there? Does the child feel he or she can retreat into the family to be protected or is this where the most sharply felt wounds are inflicted? Does the father come home or go to a bar to unwind? Where is the child sent when the noises become too much, or are they never felt as too much? Where does the child go to do his or her tics? Does the child feel most comfort when unleashing the pent-up symptoms alone? Are there other relatives who can buffer the nuclear family—grandparents who can step in, aunts who can be visited for meals—or others in the community who can be counted upon? Is the family isolated or part of a larger network? Can they trust or are they a combat unit against the larger world? What takes place between the siblings that is fun, and what happens when they get out of hand? How do brothers and sisters explain the GTS patient's symptoms to their friends, or do they avoid bringing them into the house? Do they worry that they will develop GTS, or even fear that the GTS symptoms are contagious?

Understanding the workings of a family does not result from a single interview, however long and sensitive. Most often, it is based upon reports of various family members, observations of how they actually relate in front of the clinician, and months of involvement. The physician becomes entrained in the family dynamics and experiences, along with the family, the ways in which they treat each other (and the physician as a transference figure) and outsiders (and how this makes the physician feel, in the countertransference).

Almost without exception, families feel a sense of relief in telling their story. This family story—the childhood and family experiences of the parents, the continuing involvement with their parents and siblings, and how the children fit into their dreams and now their agonies—is also, almost without exception, richer and more varied than one would predict from the 'social surface'. As the story is spun, the child takes on a history that precedes birth, stretching back to the childhood of the parents and their sense of what sort of a life they wished for themselves, and moving forward to their vision of the child's future. Often, this story is very poignant, with sadness, illness, loss and disappointment that may still be sharply felt even though 'objectively' in the historical past.

The child's GTS symptoms are thus not isolated medical phenomena, but meaningful: they take on their meaning in relation to the specifics of how the family is considered and the fantasies and aspirations of the parents and others.

The overriding goal of all treatments of GTS is to help patients to move forward. It is to help children feel good about themselves and succeed in the tasks of life—learning, working, making friends, falling in love, dealing with losses; it is to help adults succeed as workers, lovers and parents. The clinician working with families in which there is GTS thus must help parents keep their eyes on the basic target: to help their offspring move ahead. To achieve this, the parents must be able to balance realistic concern for their children and their special needs, with realistic assessment of what they can accomplish in spite of their problems. By and large, this means that parents must be helped to see through the tics—to see their children with tics as children, and not as patients or as burdens. Adults must be helped to recognize what they can achieve, in spite of their lifelong troubles. These are not easy clinical tasks. Sometimes parents must be helped to be not too worried or concerned, and to encourage their children into entering social and other situations where they might be embarrassed, just as adults must be willing to expose themselves. Through work with the family, the child's symptoms can become less encrusted with the feelings, fantasies, dashed hopes and angers that have grown up over many years or decades. In some deep way, this often means that the mysterious symptoms of GTS are again made into 'nervous habits' that the child is allowed to have, rather than horrible evidence of some basic defect in the child, the parents, or the entire family.

ACKNOWLEDGEMENTS

Portions of this chapter are based on, Tourette's syndrome: Developmental psychopathology of a model neuropsychiatric disorder of childhood, *Strecker Monograph Series XXVII*, 1990 by Donald J. Cohen[2]; and, Family functioning and Tourette syndrome, by Donald J. Cohen, Sharon I. Ort, James F. Leckman, Mark A. Riddle, and Maureen T. Hardin, first published in 1988 by John Wiley & Sons as a chapter in *Tourette Syndrome and Tic Disorders: Clinical Understanding and Treatment*[11]. We are grateful for the permission to use them here.

REFERENCES

1. Cohen, D. J. and Leckman, J. F. (1994) Developmental psychopathology and neurobiology of Tourette's syndrome. *J. Am. Acad. Child Adolesc. Psychiatry*, **33**, 2–15.
2. Cohen, D. J. (1990) Tourette's syndrome: Developmental psychopathology of a model neuropsychiatric disorder of childhood. *Strecker Monograph Series XXVII*, Philadelphia, pp. 1–64.
3. Bliss, J. (1980) Sensory experiences of Gilles de la Tourette syndrome. *Arch. Gen. Psychiatry*, **37**, 1343–1347.
4. Leckman, J. F., Walker, D. E. and Cohen, D. J. (1993) Premonitory urges in Tourette's syndrome. *Am. J. Psychiatry*, **150**, 98–102.
5. Leckman, J. F., Pauls, D. L., Peterson, B. S., Riddle, M. A., Anderson, G. M. and Cohen, D. J. (1992) Pathogenesis of Tourette's syndrome: Clues from the clinical phenotype and natural history. *Adv. Neurol.*, **58**, 15–24.
6. Cohen, D. J. (1980) The pathology of the self in primary childhood autism and Tourette's syndrome. *Psychiatr. Clin. North Am.*, **3**, 383–402.
7. Cohen, D. J. (1990) Tourette's syndrome: a model disorder for integrating psychoanalytic and biological perspectives. *Int. Rev. Psychoanal.*, **18**, 195–209.
8. Wittgenstein, L. (1958) *Philosophical Investigations*. Blackwell, Oxford.
9. Freud, S. (1916) Some character-types met with in psycho-analytic work. In *Complete Psychological Works of Sigmund Freud*, Vol. 14 (J. Strachey, Ed.). Hogarth Press, London, pp. 310–333.
10. Wolff, E. (1988) Psychotherapeutic interventions with Tourette's syndrome. In *Tourette Syndrome and Tic Disorders: Clinical Understanding and Treatment* (D. J. Cohen, R. Bruun and J. F. Leckman, Eds). John Wiley and Sons, New York, pp. 207–222.
11. Cohen, D. J., Ort, S. I., Leckman, J. F., Riddle, M. A. and Hardin, M. (1988) Family function and Tourette syndrome. In *Tourette Syndrome and Tic Disorders: Clinical Understanding and Treatment* (D. J. Cohen, R. Bruun and J. F. Leckman, Eds). John Wiley and Sons, New York, pp. 179–196.
12. Cohen, D. J., Detlor, J., Shaywitz, B. A. and Leckman, J. F. (1982) Interaction of biological and psychological factors in the natural history of Tourette's syndrome: A model of childhood neuropsychiatric disorders. *Adv. Neurol.*, **35**, 31–40.

4 Obsessive–Compulsive Disorder in Children and Adolescents

ROBERT A. KING
and
LAWRENCE SCAHILL
Yale Child Study Center, Yale University School of Medicine, New Haven, Connecticut, USA

DEFINITION AND DIAGNOSTIC CRITERIA

Obsessions are recurrent thoughts or images that are experienced as intrusive, unwanted, distressing and difficult to suppress. *Compulsions* are repetitive behaviours or mental acts which the subject feels driven to perform to reduce anxiety or distress or to prevent feared outcomes, but which are recognized as excessive or unrealistic. To meet the DSM-IV criteria for obsessive–compulsive disorder (OCD), compulsions or obsessions must be severe enough to cause marked distress, to consume more than one hour per day, or to interfere significantly with routine functioning[1]. Although perceived intrusiveness, senselessness, distress and unresponsiveness to efforts at suppression are the hallmarks of obsessions and compulsions in adults, these features may not be fully expressed or difficult to elicit in children[2].

EPIDEMIOLOGY

Obsessions and compulsions are common in non-referred individuals, but are less frequent, less vivid or distressing and more easily dismissed than those of OCD patients[3,4]. Once believed to be rare, the point prevalence of OCD in various nonclinical adolescent populations is 0.35–3.6%, with an additional 1.2–2.0% reporting significant subclinical symptoms[5,6]. Despite persistent symptoms, many of these cases never come to clinical attention[5,7].

As many as one-half of adult cases report onset prior to the age of 15 years. Among children with OCD, about 33–50% have their onset by the age of 9 years[8,9]. In clinical series, cases with prepubertal onset are predominantly boys, while cases with onset after puberty have a roughly equal sex ratio.

Movement and Allied Disorders. Edited by M. M. Robertson and V. Eapen

CLINICAL PHENOMENOLOGY

The onset of OCD may be abrupt or gradual.

Obsessive *contamination fears* accompanied by *compulsive washing* and avoidance of 'contaminated objects' are the commonest symptoms[8,9], often entailing protracted or ritualized washing and increasing constriction of activities. The feared contaminants may be as specific as AIDS, or in contrast, as vague as something 'sticky' or 'uncomfortable'.

Compulsive *checking* is also common and involves repetitively checking, for example, to ensure that doors are locked or that family members are safe. Such checking may be part of a more general pattern of *obsessive doubting* requiring the child to make sure that he or she didn't hurt someone's feelings, run over an animal with a bicycle, etc. Children with obsessional doubting may anxiously plague their parents with compulsive confessions or requests for reassurance regarding imagined misdeeds, bad thoughts, or feared outcomes after commonplace events such as using a public water fountain.

Other common compulsions include repetitive counting, re-reading or re-writing, religious scrupulosity (repetitive praying or worries about imagined sins), and arranging or touching in patterns. Although some compulsions may be tied to a specific worry, many compulsions are actions that are repeated until it feels 'just right'. The child may repetitively sit up and down in a chair, go back and forth through a door, or up and down stairs until he or she 'gets it right'. This sought-after sense of closure or completion may require symmetry (e.g., repeating with one limb actions done with the other or 'evening up' cuffs, sleeves, shoe lace length or tension) or repeating actions an odd or an even number of times.

Unlike many adults with OCD, children may be unable to specify the potential dreaded consequences of noncompliance with a compulsive ritual beyond a vague premonition of 'something awful happening'[8]. Simple compulsions, such as repetitive touching, or counting, may lack a discernible ideational component and may be phenomenologically indistinguishable from complex tics[10,11,12].

At the opposite pole, other children may suffer from *pure obsessions* without any accompanying behavioural or mental compulsions. These intrusive, often disturbing thoughts or images may be sexual, aggressive or self-injurious in content.

Although many children portray their obsessional thoughts as appearing 'out of the blue', careful review often reveals that many such thoughts are triggered by external cues. For example, a child with contamination fears may have such fears whenever he is near a certain person or object. The child may admit, albeit reluctantly, that the person or object may not be contaminated, but, once stimulated, the thought is difficult to dislodge and leads to subjective distress and an urge to ritualize. The performance of the ritual transiently reduces the obsessional worry. Thus, a common feature of many obsessive worries is an exaggerated perception of risk on the part of the child that is decreased by the compulsive ritual.

Although in a minority of cases, OCD may appear in the context of a compulsive or anxiously perfectionistic personality style, many children with OCD are not especially neat, overly compliant, or attentive to details outside the context of their specific symptom[2,5,8,9]. Indeed some children may be irritable or even impulsive. In children prone to obstinate struggles, it may be difficult to determine the relative mix of oppositional defiance versus compulsiveness. Many children with OCD have a current or past history of another anxiety disorder[8,9], and separation anxiety appears to be common. Other common comorbid conditions include depression and attentional difficulties.

Trichotillomania, defined as persistent hair pulling to the point of alopecia, has been speculated to be a repetitive behaviour related to OCD[13]. Although the frequency of OCD appears to be increased among children and adolescents with trichotillomania and their first-degree relatives (FDRs), most youngsters with this potentially cosmetically disfiguring condition do not have other obsessive–compulsive (OC) symptoms[13,14].

AETIOLOGY

FAMILY STUDIES

Family and twin studies suggest the existence of at least three forms of OCD.

1. A familial form related to tics.
2. A familial form unrelated to tics.
3. A non-familial form[15].

The prevalence of OC symptoms and OCD appears to be increased in the relatives of children with OCD[9,16]. The specific content of the child's and relatives' symptoms often differ, however, suggesting genetic rather than experiential influences. Cases of OCD with onset prior to 18 years of age are far more likely to have FDRs with OCD and/or tics than do cases with later onset[15].

RELATIONSHIP TO GILLES DE LA TOURETTE SYNDROME (GTS)

For many children, OCD appears clinically and aetiologically related to tics. As many as 55–90% of individuals with GTS develop substantial OC symptoms by adulthood. In many cases, it may be difficult to distinguish between complex motor tics and the compulsions or 'just right' phenomena associated with GTS[10]. Conversely, a substantial number of children presenting with obsessions or compulsions are found to have tics or a family history of tics or GTS[15,17]. The phenomenology of GTS-related OCD appears to differ from that of non-GTS-related OCD[18]. Patients with GTS are more likely to be concerned with touching, symmetry, or violent images or urges, while the latter are more likely to be concerned with contamination. Further evidence that GTS-related and non-GTS-related forms of OCD comprise distinct biological subtypes is provided by family genetic, neurochemical and drug studies (see below).

In families with a history of tic disorder, OCD appears to represent an alternative phenotypic manifestation of the putative GTS gene. Regardless of whether or not probands with tics have OCD themselves, their FDRs have a higher prevalence of OCD (both with and without tics). Although transmission appears to fit an autosomal dominant pattern, sex-specific variability in expression is evident in the greater prevalence of OCD in female relatives of GTS probands, while male relatives are more likely to manifest tics[19].

NEUROBIOLOGICAL FACTORS

Interest in the biological underpinnings of OCD has been kindled by several observations. First, the association of OCD with movement disorders (such as GTS[19], Huntington's chorea and Sydenham's chorea[20]), and with other forms of basal ganglia pathology has stimulated speculation that OCD may involve dysfunction of the basal ganglia[21]. Second, the genetic influences noted above also suggest the importance of biological factors. Third, patients with OCD have an unexpectedly high frequency of mild neurological abnormalities[22]. Although neuropsychological abnormalities have been reported in OCD subjects, the variability of these findings may reflect aetiologically heterogeneous samples[23].

The effectiveness of serotonin reuptake inhibitors (SRIs) in the treatment of OCD has focused much attention on the role of serotonin[24,25]. Although the importance of serotonin in the pathophysiology of OCD gains support from pharmacological challenge studies, serotonin probably does not act alone, but rather in concert with other neurotransmitter systems, including dopamine[24,25]. The serotonergic and dopaminergic neurotransmitter systems have close anatomical and functional interactions, especially in the basal ganglia. In both humans and animals, dopaminergic stimulants, such as cocaine and amphetamine, can induce both repetitive and compulsive behaviours[25,26].

The central role of the basal ganglia in the storage and regulation of complex motor schemas is reflected in the multiple parallel circuits connecting the striatum, cortex and thalamus[21], circuitry, which has also been implicated in the pathophysiology of GTS[12]. The positive response of certain severe, refractory cases of OCD to neurosurgical interruption of these same circuits provides further evidence of their role in the pathophysiology of OCD.

These converging lines of evidence have led to speculation that OCD is due to a failure of inhibition in cortico-striatal-thalamic-cortical circuits, with a consequent inappropriate release of fixed action patterns or difficulty in appropriately terminating them[12,21,27,28]. (Hence the OCD patient's subjective difficulty in achieving the feeling that an action is complete or 'just right'.) A neuroethological perspective further proposes that many common compulsions resemble an exaggeration or dysregulation of key mammalian behavioural routines such as grooming (cleaning, trichotillomania), nesting (hoarding) and avoiding danger (checking)[27]. Trichotillomania and similar behaviours in animals (e.g., acral lick dermatitis in dogs, pathological feather-pulling in birds) have been speculated to be examples of dysregulated grooming behaviour.

Animal studies suggest that neurohormonal systems also play an important role in the regulation of these basic behavioural routines, especially those involved in pair-bonding and reproduction[28,29]. Neurosecretory peptides, such as arginine, vasopressin and oxytocin, have also been implicated in the pathobiology of OCD. The finding that cerebrospinal fluid oxytocin is elevated only in the subset of patients with OCD who had *no* personal or family history of tic disorders underlines the biological heterogeneity of the disorder[30].

Functional neuroimaging studies, including those following challenge with provocative stimuli, have also pointed to increased metabolic abnormalities in the caudate, the cingulate, and orbitofrontal cortical regions of OCD subjects[31–33]. Of particular interest is the finding that following effective drug or behavioural treatment, improvement in OCD symptoms was accompanied by normalization of this regional hypermetabolism[31].

THE ROLE OF ANTINEURONAL ANTIBODIES

A theoretically and clinically important biological subtype of OCD has been proposed by Swedo and Kiessling[34], who suggest that a spectrum of childhood behavioural and movement disorders, including OCD, may be mediated by antineuronal antibodies. These investigators found an increased prevalence of OC symptoms and OCD in children with Sydenham's chorea[20]—a disorder often accompanied by abrupt onset of behavioural changes, emotional lability and impulsivity. They also found in a clinical series of children with OCD that about one-third had choreiform movements early in their course. Several children were identified for whom acute onset or exacerbation of OCD was accompanied by positive streptococcal throat cultures and elevated antistreptococcal and antineuronal antibodies. In one case, the OCD exacerbation was accompanied by onset of dystonic tics and chorea. In other studies, the same investigators have identified a series of children with GTS whose periods of symptom exacerbation correlated with increased antistreptococcal and antineuronal antibodies. Beyond the clinical implications of these findings, the existence of such 'phenocopies' reflecting the influence of environmental factors (e.g. streptococcal or other infections) and possible genetic factors (e.g. those controlling predisposition to producing cross-reacting auto-antibodies in response to infection) may confound family genetic studies of OCD and related movement disorders.

ASSESSMENT AND DIFFERENTIAL DIAGNOSIS

The diagnostic evaluation of children with OCD includes a careful assessment of current and past symptoms and comorbid conditions, as well as the child's overall psychosocial functioning; a detailed review of the child's medical, developmental and family histories is also essential[9,35].

Repetitive or ritualistic behaviours and recurrent worries are common in children at various stages of development[2,36–38]. Thus, the first step in the assessment of OCD in children is to distinguish between normal childhood rituals and routines, anxious worries, and pathological rituals and obsessional thoughts[2,37]. Many normal children develop *bedtime rituals* and *superstitious routines*. These may serve to bind mild anxiety, especially at times of transition or uncertainty, but usually do not involve substantial distress. School-age children's *repetitive games, rituals, and activities* are pleasurable, suppressible, and non-impairing. *Anxious worries* are generally related to current experience or specific stressful contexts, such as an upcoming school examination, athletic activity, or separation. Otherwise normal children may manifest *transient obsessional or compulsive phenomena* at stressful points in normal development, such as the preschool child faced with strong parental pressures regarding cleanliness or aggression, or the adolescent who tries on, in passing, an ascetic stance[2].

In contrast, *pathological obsessions and compulsions* are recurrent and intrusive thoughts and urges that are distressing, bothersome, and experienced as senseless or appearing 'out of the blue'. Children are often secretive or embarrassed about these symptoms and may attempt to deny, minimize, or explain them away. Beyond identifying specific symptoms, it is important to assess their context, frequency and degree of associated distress and impairment, as well as the child's efforts (if any) to resist them and the success of such efforts. The child's attitude and degree of insight into the symptoms must also be assessed.

One important dimension of assessment concerns the degree to which parents have become entangled with the child's symptoms. This is a common feature of OCD in children and often seriously impairs family life[9].

Children with *pervasive developmental disorders (PDD)* often manifest stereotypic behaviours and routines, as well as unusual preoccupations (e.g. fans, machines) that parents may describe as 'obsessive–compulsive'[2]. The cognitive and language difficulties characteristic of PDD often complicate assessment of the child's attitude towards these preoccupations and repetitive behaviours. Despite being a source of functional impairment or disturbing to others, these symptoms seen in children with PDD generally do not cause distress to the child. Moreover, such children's rigid insistence on routines usually occurs in the context of a more general difficulty with transitions and demand for sameness.

Given the close association of GTS and OCD, it is important to enquire about *motor and phonic tics*. In some cases it may be difficult to disentangle compulsive habits from complex tics. Both tics and compulsions may be preceded by premonitory physical sensations, urges, and mental perceptions that persist until the action is completed[10–12]. These subtle GTS phenomena are less commonly reported by children either because they are absent or, if present, young children may not be capable of describing them. In general, complex tics can be ruled out if there is no history of simple tics.

Even when tics are present, it is worth while to enquire if the repetitive habits are accompanied by specific fears or at least a vague discomfort that 'something bad might happen' if the ritual is not performed[9].

While focusing on the child's OC symptoms, it is important not to neglect the overall context of the child's functioning and developmental adaptation to his or her family, school and social environment. A careful developmental history is necessary to identify areas of delay or difficulty. Assessing the presence of depression, irritability, impulsivity, anxiety and aggression are essential to planning effective comprehensive treatment[35].

Once the diagnosis of OCD has been established, instruments such as the Children's Yale–Brown Obsessive–Compulsive Scale (CYBOCS) can be used to establish symptom severity. This semi-structured clinician-rated instrument is a modified version of the original adult instrument and has shown reliability and validity as well as sensitivity to change[39,40].

Medical history should review the major organ systems, including perinatal history and head injury. Recent findings linking streptococcal infections to movement disorders and OCD suggest that a history of streptococcal exposure should also be obtained[34]. In cases with recent acute onset or with exacerbations following streptococcal or other infections, a throat culture for streptococcal and anti-streptococcal and anti-nuclear antibody titres may be useful. In such cases, the presence of choreiform movements or tics should also be noted.

A careful medical and psychiatric family history, especially regarding tics, OCD and other anxiety disorders, may help to clarify diagnosis and guide treatment. It is important to note relatives with sub-clinical conditions, such as the uncle who 'outgrew' childhood tics or a grandmother with 'fanatical' but ego-syntonic cleaning.

TREATMENT

PHARMACOLOGICAL TREATMENT

The pharmacological treatment of OCD has been revolutionized by the development of the SRI clomipramine (CMI) and a host of newer and more specific SRIs, including fluoxetine, paroxetine, fluvoxamine and sertraline[25]. Various double-blind and open trials of these agents suggest that about 60% of children and adolescents experience some improvement of OCD symptoms. As no one agent appears to be consistently superior, the initial choice of anti-obsessional agent is best made in terms of the presence of comorbid diagnoses and each drug's side effects and pharmacokinetics[41].

The principal side effects of SRIs in children include disinhibition, agitation, restlessness and transient insomnia[42,43]. These side effects may often be mitigated or avoided by careful dose adjustment. In addition to lowering the seizure threshold, CMI shares the anti-cholinergic and potentially cardiotoxic side effects of the other tricyclic antidepressants and requires periodic electrocardiogram (ECG) and blood level monitoring.

Up to 10–12 weeks at an adequate dose level may be required before improvement of OCD symptoms is apparent[25]. Failure to respond may be due to too low a dose or too brief a trial; on the other hand, given the potential latency of response, it is important to avoid increasing the dose too quickly or higher than necessary. Children who fail to respond to one SRI may well respond to another.

Predictors of response to the various SRIs have not been well defined. Patterns of non-response may reflect the likely biological and aetiological heterogeneity of OCD. Supporting evidence for the existence of biological subtypes of OCD comes from the finding that individuals with OCD who have a personal or family history of tics appear to have a poorer therapeutic response to SRIs than do those without such a history[44]. Furthermore, incomplete responders with a history of comorbid tics appear particularly likely to show further improvement of OCD symptoms when a neuroleptic, such as haloperidol or pimozide is given in addition to an SRI[44]. (Preliminary clinical experience suggests that risperidone may also be a useful augmentation agent (McDougle *et al.*, unpublished data).) Controlled trials have failed to find that the addition of lithium or buspirone provides consistent augmentation of the anti-obsessional response to the SRIs[25].

Clonazepam, either alone or in conjunction with an SRI, has proven useful for OCD in small open trials with adults and in a case report in an adolescent[45].

SRIs also appear to be useful in reducing repetitive behaviours and aggression and improving social functioning in children and adults with autism and related PDDs[46].

In controlled trials for the treatment of trichotillomania, CMI has proven more effective than desipramine. The utility of the more specific SRIs, either alone or with neuroleptic or buspirone augmentation, is less clear[13]. As relapse is common, even in responders maintained on medication, a combination of medication and behavioural treatment (see below) appears optimal.

Preliminary clinical experience with a small number of cases suggests that streptococcal-related cases of OCD may respond poorly to SRIs but may benefit from plasmapheresis[47]. These cases are characterized by acute onset or exacerbation of OCD following a streptococcal infection accompanied by elevated anti-streptococcal and anti-neuronal antibodies. Experimental approaches to the treatment of such cases have included plasmapheresis and penicillin prophylaxis[34].

Despite the dramatic advances provided by the SRIs, the limitations of a purely pharmacological approach are highlighted by the failure of a substantial number of children to experience sufficient relief from anti-obsessional medication and the relapse of as many as 64–89% of responders within a few weeks of discontinuing CMI.

BEHAVIOURAL TREATMENT

Behaviour therapy has demonstrated its effectiveness in the treatment of adults with OCD[48,49], but it has not been well studied in children. As adult studies have consistently shown, exposure and response prevention are the most effective behavioural techniques. *Exposure* involves gradual confrontation with events or situations that stimulate obsessional ideas and, presumably, the urge to perform rituals. *Response prevention* consists of delaying the performance of the ritual while monitoring the initial rise and eventual fall of anxiety that predictably occurs even if the ritual is not performed.

Behaviour therapy typically begins with a careful rank ordering of anxiety-producing events or situations. Once the hierarchy is established, exposure and response prevention techniques are gradually introduced for events and situations of low intensity and progressively extended to progressively more intensely provocative stimuli. Through systematic exposure with response prevention, patients learn that their anxiety will subside with continued confrontation with the provoking stimulus even if the compulsion is not performed. Recent reports have suggested that these techniques are feasible in the treatment of children and adolescents with OCD[50–52].

Although these behavioural techniques have been successfully employed in treating children and adolescents with OCD, developmental and motivational factors may complicate their use in this population. For example, the proposal that exposure to anxiety-producing stimuli could actually result in a reduction of anxiety may be difficult for younger children to comprehend or accept. In addition, successful behaviour therapy usually requires practice outside the formal therapy sessions. Problems of compliance may arise when either the child or family are insufficiently motivated or organized or when the treatment becomes embroiled in oppositional struggles. Finally, it is common for parents to be intricately involved in their child's OC symptoms. When this has occurred, specific interventions aimed at extricating the parents from their participation in the child's rituals may be necessary.

Preliminary results from a randomized clinical trial comparing CMI versus behavioural treatment in children and adolescents suggest comparable efficacy for the two modalities[52]. Which method produces more enduring benefits is not, as yet, known. As many children relapse following discontinuation of anti-obsessional medication, it may be useful to introduce behavioural treatment even with drug responders.

A specific adaptation of behavioural treatment, employing habit reversal techniques, has been developed for the treatment of trichotillomania in children and adolescents[53].

PROGNOSIS

The natural history of OCD in the general population is unclear. It is possible that more severe or persistent cases come to clinical attention, while many milder or more transient cases do not. In a two-year follow-up of a community adolescent population, most cases of OCD or subclinical OCD persisted and continued to cause distress, even though they never came to clinical attention[7].

The often chronic and debilitating prognosis of OCD has improved since the introduction of SRI treatment. A 2–7 year follow-up of children treated with SRI and/or behaviour therapy found that although 80% were improved from baseline, 70% were still on medication and 43% still met criteria for OCD. Only 11% were completely asymptomatic, and of these, one-half were still on medication. Presence of a tic disorder and parental psychopathology were predictors of poorer outcome[17]. The specific constellation of symptoms manifested by any given patient varies widely over time[54].

Given the relative frequency of OCD in the general population and its apparent chronicity in clinical samples, more needs to be learned about the disorder's range of outcomes and their determinants.

REFERENCES

1. American Psychiatric Association (1994) *Diagnostic and Statistical Manual for Mental Disorders*, 4th Ed. American Psychiatric Association, Washington, DC.
2. King, R. A. and Noshpitz, J. D. (1991) *Pathways of Growth: Essentials of Child Psychiatry, Vol. 2—Psychopathology*. John Wiley, New York.
3. Rachman, S. and deSilva, P. (1978) Abnormal and normal obsessions. *Behav. Res. Ther.*, **16**, 233–248.
4. Apter, A., Fallon, T., King, R. A. *et al.* (1995) Obsessive compulsive characteristics: From symptoms to syndrome. Submitted for publication.
5. Flament, M. F., Whitaker, A., Rapoport, J. L. *et al.* (1988) Obsessive–compulsive disorder in adolescence: An epidemiological study. *J. Am. Acad. Child Adolesc. Psychiatry*, **27**(6), 764–771.
6. Zohar, A., Ratzoni, G., Pauls, D., Apter, A., Bleich, A., Kron, S., Rappaport, M., Weizman, A. and Cohen, D. (1992) An epidemiological study of obsessive–compulsive disorder and related disorders in Israeli adolescents. *J. Am. Acad. Child Adolesc. Psychiatry*, **31**, 1057–1061.
7. Flament, F. M., Koby, E., Rapoport, J. L., Berg, C. J., Zahn, T., Cox, C., Denckla, M. and Lenane, M. (1990) Childhood obsessive–compulsive disorder: A prospective follow-up study. *J. Child Psychol. Psychiatry*, **31**, 363–380.
8. Swedo, S. E., Rapoport, J. L., Leonard, H., Lenane, M. and Cheslow, D. (1989) Obsessive–compulsive disorder in children and adolescents. *Arch. Gen. Psychiatry*, **46**, 335–341.
9. Riddle, M. A., Scahill, L., King, R. A., Hardin, M. T., Towbin, K. T., Ort, S. I., Leckman, J. F. and Cohen, D. J. (1990) Obsessive–compulsive disorder in children and adolescents. *J. Am. Acad. Child Adolesc. Psychiatry*, **29**, 766–772.
10. Leckman, J. F., Walker, W. K., Goodman, W. K., Pauls, D. L. and Cohen, D. J. (1994) 'Just right' perceptions associated with compulsive behaviors in Tourette's syndrome. *Am. J. Psychiatry*, **151**, 675–680.
11. Leckman, J. F., Walker, D. E. and Cohen, D. J. (1993) Premonitory urges in Tourette's syndrome. *Am. J. Psychiatry*, **150**, 98–103.
12. Cohen, D. J. and Leckman, J. F. (1994) Developmental psychopathology and neurobiology of Tourette's syndrome. *J. Am. Acad. Child Adolesc. Psychiatry*, **33**, 2–15.
13. Swedo, S. E. (1993) Trichotillomania. *Child Adolesc. Psychiatr. Clin. North Am.*, **2**(4), 685–694.
14. King, R. A., Zohar, A. H., Ratzoni, G., Binder, M., Kron, S., Dycian, A., Cohen, D. J., Pauls, D. L. and Apter, A. (1995) An epidemiological study of trichotillomania in Israeli adolescents. *J. Am. Acad. Child Adolesc. Psychiatry*, in press.
15. Pauls, D. L., Alsobrook, J. P. II, Goodman, W., Rasmussen, S. and Leckman, J. F. (1995) A family study of obsessive compulsive disorder. *Am. J. Psychiatry* (In press).
16. Lenane, M. C., Swedo, S. E., Leonard, H., Pauls, D. L., Sceery, W. and Rapoport, J. L. (1990) Psychiatric disorders in first degree relatives of children and adolescents with obsessive–compulsive disorder. *J. Am. Acad. Child Adolesc. Psychiatry*, **29**, 407–412.
17. Leonard, H. L., Lenane, M. C., Swedo, S. E., Rettew, D. C., Gershon, E. S. and Rapoport, J. L. (1992) Tics and Tourette's disorder: A 2- to 7-year follow-up of 54 obsessive–compulsive children. *Am. J. Psychiatry*, **149**, 1244–1251.
18. Holzer, J. C., Goodman, W. K., McDougle, C. J., Boyarsky, B. K., Leckman, J. F. and Price, L. H. (1994) Differential symptoms in obsessive–compulsive disorder

with and without a chronic tic disorder. *Br. J. Psychiatry*, **164**, 469–473.
19. Pauls, D. L., Raymond, C. L., Leckman, J. F. and Stevenson, J. M. (1991) A family study of Tourette's syndrome. *Am. J. Hum. Genet.*, **48**, 154–163.
20. Swedo, S. E., Rapoport, J. L., Cheslow, D. L. *et al.* (1989) High prevalence of obsessive–compulsive symptoms in patients with Sydenham's chorea. *Am. J. Psychiatry*, **146**, 246–249.
21. Wise, S. P. and Rapoport, J. L. (1989) Obsessive–compulsive disorder: Is it basal ganglia dysfunction? In *Obsessive–Compulsive Disorder in Children and Adolescents* (J. L. Rapoport, Ed). American Psychiatric Press, Washington, DC, pp. 327–344.
22. Hymas, N., Lees, A., Bolton, D., Epps, K. and Head, D. (1991) The neurology of obsessional slowness. *Brain*, **114**, 2203–2233.
23. Otto, M. W. (1990) Neuropsychological approaches to obsessive–compulsive disorder. In *Obsessive–Compulsive Disorders: Theory and Management* (M. A. Jenike, L. Baer and W. E. Minichiello, Eds). Yearbook Medical Publishers, Chicago, pp. 132–148.
24. Goodman, W. K., McDougle, C. J., Price, L. H. *et al.* (1990) Beyond the serotonin hypothesis: A role for dopamine in some forms of obsessive–compulsive disorder? *J. Clin. Psychiatry*, **51** (Suppl), 36–42.
25. McDougle, C. J., Goodman, W. K., Leckman, J. F. and Price, L. H. (1993) The psychopharmacology of obsessive–compulsive disorder: Implications for treatment and pathogenesis. In *Psychiatric Clinics of North America*, Vol. 16(4). (D. L. Dunner, Ed). W. B. Saunders, Philadelphia, pp. 749–766.
26. Borcherding, B. G., Keysor, C., Rapoport, J. L. *et al.* (1990) Motor/vocal tics and compulsive behaviours on stimulant drugs: Is there a common vulnerability? *Psychiatry Res.*, **33**, 83–94.
27. Swedo, S. E. (1989) Rituals and releasers: An ethological model of OCD. In *Obsessive–Compulsive Disorder in Children and Adolescents* (J. L. Rapoport, Ed). American Psychiatric Association, Washington, DC, pp. 269–288.
28. Insel, T. R. (1992) Toward a neuroanatomy of obsessive–compulsive disorder. *Arch. Gen. Psychiatry*, **49**, 739–744.
29. Leckman, J. F., Goodman, W. K., North, W. G., Chappell, P. B., Price, L. H., Pauls, D. L., Anderson, G. M., Riddle, M. A., McSwiggan-Hardin, M. T., McDougle, C. J., Barr, L. C. and Cohen, D. J. (1994) The role of central oxytocin in obsessive–compulsive disorder and related normal behavior. *Psychoneuroendocrinology*, **19**(8), 1–27.
30. Leckman, J. F., Goodman, W. K., North, W. G., Chappell, P. B., Price, L. H., Pauls, D. L., Anderson, G. M., Riddle, M. A., McSwiggan-Hardin, M. T., McDougle, C. J., Barr, L. C. and Cohen, D. J. (1994) Elevated cerebrospinal fluid levels of oxytocin in obsessive–compulsive disorder. Comparison with Tourette's syndrome and healthy controls. *Arch. Gen. Psychiatry*, **51**, 782–792.
31. Baxter, L., Schwartz, J., Bergman, K., Szuba, M., Guze, B., Mazziotta, J., Alazraki, A., Selin, C., Ferng, H. K., Munford, P. and Phelps, M. (1992) Caudate glucose metabolic rate changes with both drug and behavior therapy for obsessive–compulsive disorder. *Arch. Gen. Psychiatry*, **49**, 211–218.
32. Rauch, S., Jenike, M., Alpert, N., Baer, L., Breiter, H., Savage, C. and Fischman, A. (1994) Regional cerebral blood flow measured during symptom provocation in OCD using oxygen 15-labelled carbon dioxide and positron emission tomography. *Arch. Gen. Psychiatry*, **51**, 62–70.
33. Baxter, L. R. Jr. (1992) Neuroimaging studies of obsessive–compulsive disorder. *Psychiatr. Clin. North Am.*, **15**(4), 871–884.
34. Swedo, S. E. and Kiessling, L. S. (1994) Speculations on antineuronal antibody-mediated neuropsychiatric disorders of childhood. *Pediatrics*, **93**(2), 323–326.
35. King, R. A. and Cohen, D. J. (1994) Psychotherapy with children and adolescents

with neuropsychiatric disorders: ADHD, OCD, and Tourette's syndrome. In *Review of Psychiatry*, Vol. 13 (J. M. Oldham and M. B. Riba, Eds). American Psychiatric Press, Washington, DC, pp. 519–539.

36. Leonard, H. (1989) Childhood rituals and superstitions: Developmental and cultural perspectives. In *Obsessive–Compulsive Disorder in Children and Adolescents* (J. L. Rapoport, Ed). American Psychiatric Press, Washington, DC, pp. 289–309.
37. Leonard, H. L., Goldberger, E. L., Rapoport, J. L., Cheslow, D. L. and Swedo, S. E. (1990) Childhood rituals: Normal development or obsessive–compulsive symptoms? *J. Am. Acad. Child Adolesc. Psychiatry*, **29**(1), 17–23.
38. Carter, A. S., Pauls, D. L. and Leckman, J. F. (1995) The development of obsessionality: Continuities and discontinuities. In *Developmental Psychopathology*, Vol. 2 (D. V. Cicchetti and D. J. Cohen, Eds). John Wiley & Sons, New York, pp. 609–632.
39. Riddle, M. A., Scahill, L., McSwiggan-Hardin, M. T., Ort, S. I., King, R. A., Cicchetti, D., Epperson, C. N. and Goodman, W. K. (1995) *The Children's Yale–Brown Obsessive–Compulsive Scale: Preliminary Report of Reliability and Validity*. Manuscript submitted for publication.
40. Riddle, M. A., Scahill, L., King, R. A., Hardin, M. T., Anderson, G. M., Ort, S. I., Smith, J. C., Leckman, J. F. and Cohen, D. J. (1992) Double-blind, crossover trial of fluoxetine and placebo in children and adolescents with obsessive–compulsive disorder. *J. Am. Acad. Child Adolesc. Psychiatry*, **31**, 1062–1069.
41. King, R. A., Riddle, M. A. and Goodman, W. K. (1992) Psychopharmacology of obsessive–compulsive disorder in Tourette's syndrome. In *Advances in Neurology—Tourette Syndrome: Genetics, Neurobiology, and Treatment*, Vol. 58 (T. N. Chase, A. J. Friedhoff and D. J. Cohen, Eds). Raven Press, New York, pp. 283–291.
42. Riddle, M. A., King, R. A., Hardin, M. T., Scahill, L., Ort, S. I. and Leckman, J. F. (1991) Behavioural side effects of fluoxetine in children and adolescents. *J. Child Adolesc. Psychopharmacology*, **1**, 193–198.
43. King, R. A., Riddle, M. A., Chappell, P. B., Hardin, M. T., Anderson, G. M., Lombroso, P. and Scahill, L. (1991) Emergence of self-destructive phenomena in children and adolescents during fluoxetine treatment. *J. Am. Acad. Child Adolesc. Psychiatry*, **30**, 179–186.
44. McDougle, C. J., Goodman, W. K., Leckman, J. F., *et al.* (1994) Haloperidol addition in fluvoxamine-refractory obsessive compulsive disorder: a double-blind, placebo-controlled study in patients with and without tics. *Arch. Gen. Psychiatry*, **51**, 302–309.
45. Leonard, H. L., Topol, D., Bukstein, O., Hindmarsh, D., Allen, A. J. and Swedo, S. E. (1994) Clonazepam as an augmenting agent in the treatment of childhood-onset obsessive–compulsive disorder. *J. Am. Acad. Child Adolesc. Psychiatry*, **33**(6), 792–794.
46. McDougle, C. J., Price, L. H. and Volkmar, F. R. (1994) Recent advances in the pharmacotherapy of autism and related conditions. *Child Adolesc. Psychiatr. Clin. North Am.*, **3**(1), 71–89.
47. Allen, A. J., Leonard, H. L. and Swedo, S. E. (1995) Case study: A new infection-triggered, autoimmune subtype of paediatric OCD and Tourette's syndrome. *J. Am. Acad. Child Adolesc. Psychiatry*, **34**(3), 307–311.
48. Marks, I. M. (1987) *Fears, Phobias, and Rituals: Panic, Anxiety and their Disorders*. Oxford University Press, Oxford.
49. Steketee, G. S. (1993) *Treatment of Obsessive–Compulsive Disorder*. Guilford Press, New York.
50. March, J. S., Mulle, K. and Herbel, B. (1994) Behavioral psychotherapy for

children and adolescents with obsessive–compulsive disorder: An open trial of a new protocol-driven treatment package. *J. Am. Acad. Child Adolesc. Psychiatry*, **33**(3), 333–341.

51. Scahill, L., Vitulano, L. A., Brenner, E., Lynch, K. A. and King, R. A. (1994) *Behavior Therapy in Children with Obsessive Compulsive Disorder: Preliminary Experience*. Poster presented at the American Academy of Child and Adolescent Psychiatry Annual Meeting, New York, October, 1994.
52. van Engeland, H., de Haan, E. and Buitelaar, J. K. (1994) *Behavioral Treatment of Children and Adolescents with Obsessive–Compulsive Disorder*. Paper presented at the International Association of Child and Adolescent Psychiatry and Allied Professions, San Francisco, CA, July, 1994.
53. Vitulano, L., King, R. A. and Scahill, L. (1992) Behavioral treatment of children with trichotillomania. *J. Am. Acad. Child Adolesc. Psychiatry*, **31**, 139–146.
54. Rettew, D. C., Swedo, S. E., Leonard, H. L., *et al.* (1992) Obsessions and compulsions across time in 79 children and adolescents with obsessive–compulsive disorder. *J. Am. Acad. Child Adolesc. Psychiatry*, **31**, 1050–1056.

5 Attention Deficit Disorder

GERALD S. GOLDEN
University of Pennsylvania School of Medicine, Philadelphia, USA

Attention deficit disorder (ADD), or attention deficit hyperactivity disorder, is a commonly encountered clinical problem, affecting as many as 6–10% of school-age boys[1]. It is diagnosed significantly much less commonly in girls, the male-to-female ratio being 5:1. A large gender difference is consistent from study to study, even though it is recognized that girls may have inattention without motor hyperactivity, and so the diagnosis may not be made as readily. Management of ADD is difficult and relies principally on the use of psychostimulant drugs, supplemented with behavioural strategies and environmental manipulation[2]. Complexities of diagnosis and treatment are compounded by the frequent comorbidity between ADD and some movement disorders, particularly tic disorders, and the overlap in symptoms between these two conditions[3]. In addition, the medications used to treat ADD may adversely affect the movement disorder[4].

ATTENTION DEFICIT DISORDER (ADD)

The nosology of this condition has changed over the years. The terms hyperactivity, hyperkinesis, or the hyperkinetic syndrome, focused on the increased motor activity that often brings the child to clinical attention. The condition was formalized in the *Diagnostic and Statistical Manual of Mental Disorders* (Third edition), *DSM-III*, as attention deficit disorder, with the proviso that the condition could occur with or without hyperactivity. A revision of this diagnostic manual, *DSM-III-R*, combined these two variants under the single term, attention deficit hyperactivity disorder[5a]. The term attention deficit disorder, or ADD, will be used in this discussion for convenience.

As there are no readily available and consistently useful biological markers for ADD, an operational definition is used and is based on three clinical features[5a]. A short attention span and impulsivity are the two invariant components of the diagnosis; hyperactivity may or may not be present. These symptoms must be viewed in a developmental context, as young children have a short attention span and are impulsive when compared to older children. It is both the absolute degree of the symptoms, and their developmentally inappropriate nature, that are important in diagnosis.

Symptoms should be present before the age of 7 years and must be present

Movement and Allied Disorders. Edited by M. M. Robertson and V. Eapen

in most social, school and work situations. The child who does not have symptoms until he is older may not, in fact, have ADD. Similar behaviours are seen in children with high degrees of anxiety, those from chaotic social settings, and those with chronic illnesses or side effects of certain medications. If symptoms are only present in one social setting, it raises the strong possibility of a specific response to interactions raised by that situation.

The introduction of DSM-IV has changed the name to attention-deficit/hyperactivity disorder and modified slightly the diagnostic criteria[5b]. Symptoms are now grouped as either inattention or hyperactivity–impulsivity. At least six symptoms must be present from either group to mke a diagnosis. In addition, there must be clear evidence of a clinically significant impairment in social, academic or occupational functioning. Other diagnostic criteria are essentially unchanged.

The diagnosis is based primarily on the history given by the child's parents, and this should be supplemented by narrative statements from the teacher or others who have worked with the child. A number of rating scales for parents and teachers are available[6]. Although these allow the rater to focus on the most common behavioural symptoms, they are subject to observer bias and the different perceptions among observers as to what constitutes developmentally inappropriate levels of attention span, impulsivity and hyperactivity. This can present problems with interrater reliability. A family history of similar behavioural characteristics is often present, especially among male relatives[7].

The common belief has been that the symptoms of ADD ameliorate, and often disappear, at the time of adolescence. There is now increasing awareness that the cardinal symptoms of ADD, especially the short attention span and impulsivity, may continue into adulthood[8]. As chronic tic disorders also continue into adult life in many patients, the diagnostic and treatment issues that arise as a result of the comorbidity of the two conditions are not restricted to childhood.

Routine physical and neurological examinations are generally normal in patients with ADD. Although there is an increase in non-localizing ('soft') neurological signs such as poor co-ordination and synkinetic movements, these have no specific diagnostic value[9]. Signs of the movement disorder obviously may be present.

Neuropsychological testing is a useful approach for documenting the short attention span and impulsivity. The most common technique is through analysis of standard psychological tests, such as the Wechsler scales, that show specific patterns of distractibility if it is present[10]. In addition, tests of attention and impulsivity, particularly continuous performance tests of various types, may be helpful; errors of omission are an index of distractibility, and errors of commission result from impulsivity. Computer administered versions of continuous performance tests are available, although the principles are the same.

Electroencephalography, neuroimaging studies and blood studies add nothing to the clinical diagnosis. Evoked potential and electrophysiological brain mapping studies, and positron emission tomography are providing interesting research results, but are not appropriate for routine clinical use.

Children with ADD often perform poorly in school. This may be a direct outcome of the attention deficit with inability to pay attention in class, secondary to a suboptimal learning environment, because of negative responses by teachers and peers to the child's behaviour, or the result of an associated learning disability[11]. The interactions between these disorders are complex, but need to be clarified in order to develop an appropriate curriculum for the child.

TREATMENT OF ADD

A decision to treat ADD hinges on a critical assessment of the impact of the symptoms on the school-age child's adjustment at home, at school and with peers, or the older individual's interpersonal relationships and job performance[12]. If the symptoms and associated problems are mild, behavioural approaches to therapy may be useful. If symptoms produce significant interference with the person's life, however, psychostimulant drugs are the mainstay of treatment. However, it is important to evaluate critically treatment indications and treatment response, as normal children may show an increase in attention span and a decrease in motor activity when given psychostimulants. A response to these drugs does not, therefore prove the diagnosis of ADD. In addition, there is also a high rate of placebo response as with treatment of any behavioural symptoms.

Methylphenidate and dextroamphetamine are the most commonly used drugs. Medication is effective in 80% of the children treated, and improvement in attention span and decrease in impulsivity show dose-related responses[13]. There is some evidence, however, that high doses may have a negative effect on cognitive skills[14]. These drugs rarely cause severe systemic toxicity, although appetite suppression may be associated with weight loss and decreased linear growth[15]. Catch-up growth is satisfactory during drug holidays. The most frequent side effects are behavioural, with increased hyperactivity or lethargy and depression.

The long-term prognosis for children with ADD is less clear. Those children who have no signs of comorbid conditions, such as conduct disorder or oppositional disorder, generally have a good outcome[16]. The presence of other psychiatric or behavioural problems, however, is associated with a high frequency of adjustment problems and psychiatric disorders in adulthood[17]. As noted, ADD may continue into adult life.

ADD AND MOVEMENT DISORDERS

Clinical features of ADD and other behavioural and neuropsychological problems have been reported in some children with Gilles de la Tourette syndrome (GTS) for more than a decade[18]. The majority of studies in the US find 40–50% of children with GTS manifesting symptoms of ADD[3,19,20]. A study of an entire cohort in Israel, all recruits screened for induction in the Israel Defence Force during a single year, found the rate of ADD in individuals with GTS to be 8.3%, compared with a population point prevalence of 3.9% in individuals without GTS[21]. Whether this represents the application of different diagnostic criteria, or a true population difference, is not clear.

Issues related to making a diagnosis of ADD in an individual with GTS are complex[22]. Several possible relationships can be defined:

1. The co-occurrence of GTS and ADD occurs at random, and the two disorders are not related biologically.
2. GTS and ADD are manifestations of the same gene, or closely linked genes, with variable expressivity of one or the other set of symptoms.
3. GTS with ADD and GTS without ADD are different conditions.
4. The features of GTS produce difficulty in sustaining attention, causing problems which cannot easily be distinguished from ADD.

Random co-occurrence of the two conditions is not supported by the data available. ADD occurs in 5–10% of the general population, but in 40–50% of individuals with GTS. Even the study from Israel, which showed a lower than expected prevalence of ADD in the overall study population and in those subjects with GTS, demonstrated an increased prevalence of ADD in the group with GTS[21].

The hypothesis that the features of GTS cause problems which appear like those of ADD also cannot be supported. ADD first becomes manifest in the preschool years, while the mean age of onset of GTS is 7 years. A history of treatment with psychostimulant drugs prior to the onset of the tic disorder has been reported[23–25]. In addition, it is unusual for symptoms of ADD to first become apparent after the diagnosis of GTS is made[20].

The hypothesis of a genetic relationship between GTS and ADD has been put forward[26–27]. Studies using a structured questionnaire as the data acquisition tool, demonstrated a significant increase in ADD in relatives of probands with GTS. There was also an increase in ADD in those relatives who had chronic tics.

This genetic hypothesis has been questioned by other investigators who demonstrated nearly identical rates of GTS among relatives of probands with GTS, with or without ADD[28]. The rate of ADD was greatly increased among relatives of probands with GTS and ADD, as compared to patients with GTS alone. However, analysis showed that in families in which the proband had both conditions, the two traits segregated independently.

More recent work, using a larger subject population, concluded that ADD, learning problems, stuttering and speech problems were not by themselves variants of GTS[22]. These data also indicated that GTS might be aetiologically related to ADD in some individuals. Relatives of patients with GTS are at increased risk for ADD. There appeared to be a group in which GTS and ADD were independent traits and another group in which ADD is secondary to GTS.

There does not appear to be a specific relationship between ADD and other movement disorders. Children with mental retardation or pervasive developmental disorder may manifest stereotyped movements and show characteristics of ADD, but these are most likely independent results of underlying neuropathological or neurochemical abnormalities.

PSYCHOSTIMULANTS AND TIC DISORDERS

Psychostimulant drugs are the primary therapeutic agents for the treatment of ADD, but the use of these drugs in patients with chronic tic disorders, particularly GTS, may be fraught with difficulties. An exacerbation of both motor and vocal tics in patients with pre-existing tic disorders has been described following institution of therapy with psychostimulant drugs, and there have been reports of the first manifestations of the tic disorder beginning when therapy was initiated. Early reports consisted of cases and retrospective series which demonstrated that many children with tic disorders had at some time received treatment with psychostimulant drugs[23–25]. As these case series were published before the full extent of the co-occurrence of GTS and ADD was known, in retrospect, a history of treatment with these agents should not have been unexpected.

The risk of tics appearing, or worsening if already present, in a large series of children with ADD who were treated with psychostimulant drugs is low. In fact, only approximately 1% of a group of children showed such effects. In the majority of cases the tic frequency decreased, or tics disappeared, when medication was discontinued[29]. In a smaller study, approximately 7% of children treated with psychostimulants for ADD developed GTS[30]. The risk of developing a tic disorder was not changed by a family history of GTS or a prior personal history of this tic disorder. There was no difference in the type of medication (methylphenidate, Dexedrine, or pemoline) or dosage, between those who developed a tic disorder and those who did not. Pemoline has been reported to induce choreoathetosis, as well as cause an exacerbation of tics in patients with chronic tic disorders, and induce the onset of symptoms of GTS[31–33].

Methylphenidate is effective in treating the symptoms of ADD in children with GTS[34,35]. Improvement of hyperactive and disruptive behaviours is dose related, and there is no evidence of a dose effect on the severity of motor tics. In fact, these investigators found that the lowest frequency of vocal tics occurred when the patient was on the highest dose of methylphenidate. Only one boy developed an exacerbation of motor tics on an operationally defined 'minimal effective dose'[35]. The authors point out that the variability of symptoms of GTS make it difficult to correlate the severity of the tic disorder with drug dose at any point in time.

Attempts have been made to find drugs that are effective in treating ADD without the risk of exacerbation of tics that is sometimes seen with psychostimulants. Clonidine, a centrally acting α_2-adrenergic receptor agonist, was reported to be effective in the treatment of behavioural disturbances in patients with GTS[36]. Additional studies showed the drug to be useful in improving attention span and reducing impulsivity and hyperactivity in patients without tics[37], and to improve symptoms without exacerbating tics in patients with GTS[38]. Not all investigators could replicate these results in double-blind studies, however[39]. A potential problem with clonidine is that high doses, up to 0.6 mg/day, are required and may cause sedation and postural hypotension.

A retrospective chart review of 54 children treated with clonidine over a 4-year period has supported the efficacy of this drug[40]. The drug was effective in treating ADD in 72% of patients, and tics in 75% of patients. Positive results were greatest in patients with both tics and ADD; 96% of this group had a good treatment response.

A clonidine patch, which provides continuous transdermal administration of the drug, is available. Administration by this means can assure a steady blood level of the agent, although the blood level may not be sustained for many days. An open study used the clonidine patch with 270 patients[41]. In this group, 210 patients had GTS, 41 had ADD and 19 had conduct disorder. Improvement of half or more of the symptoms occurred in 40% of patients and there was some improvement in 61.5%. Worsening of symptoms was found in 12%. The major side effect was skin irritation which was seen in 30%, and required therapy to be discontinued in 16%. Some patients developed headache, nausea or depression.

Tricyclic antidepressants have been found to be useful in the treatment of ADD in controlled studies[42]. A child who developed GTS after 4 years of treatment with methylphenidate, and who had an exacerbation of symptoms when methylphenidate was reintroduced after it had been discontinued, showed improvement of ADD, without an increase in tics, when treated with imipramine 50 mg/day[43]. A retrospective review of 33 patients, 30 with chronic tic disorder and ADD and three with tics only, demonstrated significant improvement in tics in 82% of patients and improvement in ADD in 80% when treated with desipramine[44]. There were no serious side effects. The average dose level was 127 mg/day (3.5 mg/kg/day). A previous report using a lower mean dose of 68 mg/day reported improvement of symptoms of ADD in 71% of patients, but no change in the tic disorder[45]. It is possible that higher doses of desipramine are required to achieve improvement in both sets of symptoms.

A chart review of patients treated with nortriptyline showed results similar to those reported with desipramine[46]. There were 12 patients; 92%

had significant improvement in ADD and 67% had improvement of their tic disorder. The mean dose was 105 mg/day with a weight corrected mean dose of 2.8 mg/kg/day.

Clomipramine was found ineffective in the control of tics[47]. A child with GTS and ADD who developed self-abusive behaviour following institution of treatment with clomipramine has been reported.[48]

An open trial of deprenyl, a monoamine oxidase inhibitor, was carried out with 29 patients who had GTS and ADD and who were unresponsive to the usual treatments for ADD[49]. Improvement in the symptoms of ADD occurred in 90% of patients at an average daily dose of 8.1 mg/day. No serious side effects occurred and only two patients had an exacerbation of their tics.

Bupropion, an aminoketone antidepressant, was found to exacerbate tics in four patients with GTS and ADD[50]. The authors suggest that this drug is not a useful alternative for the treatment of patients with both conditions.

TREATMENT STRATEGIES

There is no single approach to the treatment of the patient with both a tic disorder and ADD, or the child who first manifests tics when a psychostimulant drug is introduced for the treatment of ADD. Any treatment strategy may require a compromise that is then accepted or rejected based on an assessment of the impact of each of the two disorders on the patient's ability to function in important life areas including home, school, work and social interpersonal interactions.

If tics appear during treatment of ADD with psychostimulant drugs, the next step is to discontinue the psychostimulant and reassess the patient's ability to adjust to life circumstances. It is important to remember that a temporary rebound in the symptoms of ADD following cessation of therapy may occur, especially if large daily doses of medication had been required. Judgements about the need for the medication should be delayed for several days. Behavioural strategies and environmental manipulation should be next attempted. If the results are unsatisfactory, however, the patient must be managed as any other with both disorders.

One strategy is to focus on the ADD if the tics are not a major social adjustment problem for the patient. There does not appear to be any difference in the potential for exacerbating tics when comparing methylphenidate, dextroamphetamine or pemoline, so the choice is largely based on the preference of the physician. Advantages of psychostimulants are their effectiveness in a high percentage of cases, an extensive literature on the use of these drugs that has accumulated over many years, and a low incidence of serious systemic side effects. One disadvantage of pemoline is the delay of several weeks before a therapeutic response is seen, and the inability to assess rapidly small changes in drug dose. The minimal dose of psychostimulant that provides satisfactory improvement in the symptoms of ADD should be used. It is also important to continue to employ behavioural approaches to treatment, as a multimodal approach seems to be most effective.

Some clinicians change to clonidine if psychostimulants significantly increase tic frequency. Others would use clonidine as the first drug, as it does not exacerbate the tic disorder. Issues in the use of clonidine relate to the smaller likelihood of adequate improvement of symptoms of either the tic disorder or behaviour, as well as the side effects of clonidine. High doses of the drug, in the range 0.4–0.6 mg/day are required, and these often produce sedation. Postural hypotension is less common. The clonidine transdermal patch may provide a more steady rate of drug administration, but is associated with a high incidence of skin reddening.

A third approach relies on tricyclic antidepressants. These drugs, if used at an adequate dose level, appear to be as effective as psychostimulants in the treatment of ADD and may improve tics in some patients. There have been concerns raised about cardiotoxicity of these drugs, with reports of sudden death in children taking tricyclic compounds. The risk is low, but this possibility has inhibited the use of these drugs by some practitioners.

The experience with other drug classes, such as monoamine oxidase inhibitors, is too limited to allow recommendations to be made at this time. If psychostimulants are necessary for adequate treatment but cause an unacceptable exacerbation of tics, and if other drugs have not been effective, primary treatment with the psychostimulant and the addition of a dopamine receptor blocker to decrease the tics may be required.

REFERENCES

1. Safer, D. J. and Krager, J. M. (1988) A survey of medication treatment for hyperactive/inattentive students. *JAMA*, **260**, 2256–2258.
2. Satterfield, J. M., Satterfield, B. T. and Cantwell, D. P. (1981) Three-year multimodal treatment study of 100 hyperactive boys. *J. Pediatr.*, **98**, 650–655.
3. Erenberg, G., Cruse, R. P. and Rothner, A. D. (1986) Tourette syndrome: an analysis of 200 pediatric and adolescent cases. *Cleve. Clin. Q.*, **53**, 127–131.
4. Gadow, K. D. and Sverd, J. (1990) Stimulants for ADHD in child patients with Tourette's syndrome: the issue of relative risk. *J. Dev. Behav. Pediatr.*, **11**, 269–271.
5. (a) American Psychiatric Association (1987) *Diagnostic and Statistical Manual of Mental Disorders*, 3rd ed, revised. American Psychiatric Association, Washington, DC, pp. 49–53. (b) American Psychiatric Association (1994) *Diagnostic and Statistical Manual of Mental Disorders*, 4th ed. American Psychiatric Association, Washington, DC, pp. 78–85.
6. Conners, C. K. (1985) Rating scales and checklists for child psychopharmacology. *Psychopharmacol. Bull.*, **21**, 809–812.
7. Biederman, J., Faraone, S. V., Keenan, K., Knee, D. and Tsuang, M. T. (1990) Family-genetic and psychosocial risk factors in DSM-III attention deficit

disorder. *J. Am. Acad. Child Adolesc. Psychiatry*, **29**, 526–533.

8. Biederman, J., Faraone, S. V., Spencer, T., Wilens, T., Norman, D., Lapey, K. A. A., Mick, E., Lehman, B. K. and Doyle, A. (1993) Patterns of psychiatric comorbidity, cognition, and psychosocial functioning in adults with attention deficit hyperactivity disorder. *Am. J. Psychiatry*, **150**, 1792–1798.
9. Schonfeld, I. S., Shaffer, D. and Barmack, J. E. (1989) Neurological soft signs and school achievement: the mediating effects of sustained attention. *J. Abnorm. Child Psychol.*, **17**, 575–596.
10. Kaufman, A. (1981) The Wechsler intelligence scales for children—revised and learning disabilities assessment: state of the art. *J. Learn. Disabil.*, **14**, 520–526.
11. Shaywitz, S. E., Schnell, C., Shaywitz, B. A. and Towle, V. R. (1986) Yale children's inventory (YCI): an instrument to assess children with attention deficits and learning disabilities. I. Scale development and psychometric properties. *J. Abnorm. Child Psychol.*, **14**, 347–364.
12. Shaywitz, B. A. and Shaywitz, S. E. (1994) Learning disabilities and attention disorders. In *Pediatric Neurology: Principles and Practice* (K. F. Swaiman, Ed). Mosby, St Louis, pp. 1138–1143.
13. Sebrechts, M. M., Shaywitz, S. E., Shaywitz, B. A., Jatlow, P., Anderson, G. M. and Cohen, D. J. (1968) Components of attention, methylphenidate dosage, and blood levels in children with attention deficit disorder. *Pediatrics*, **77**, 222–228.
14. Brown, R. T. and Sleator, E. K. (1979) Methylphenidate in hyperactive children: differences in dose effects on impulsive behavior. *Pediatrics*, **64**, 408–411.
15. Mattes, J. A. and Gittleman, R. (1983) Growth of hyperactive children on maintenance regimen of methylphenidate. *Arch. Gen. Psychiatry*, **40**, 317–321.
16. Epstein, M. A., Shaywitz, S. E., Shaywitz, B. A. and Woolston, J. L. (1991) The boundaries of attention deficit disorder. *J. Learn. Disabil.*, **24**, 78–86.
17. Gittleman-Klein, R., Manuzze, S. D., Shenker, R. and Bonaqura, N. (1985) Hyperactive boys almost grown up. *Arch. Gen. Psychiatry*, **42**, 937–947.
18. Cohen, D. J., Detlor, J., Shaywitz, B. A. and Leckman, J. F. (1982) Interaction of biological and psychological factors in the natural history of Tourette syndrome. A paradigm for childhood neuropsychiatric disorders. In *Advances in Neurology*, Vol. 35, *Gilles de la Tourette Syndrome* (A. T. Friedhoff and T. N. Chase, Eds). Raven Press, New York, pp. 31 40.
19. Bornstein, R. A., Stefl, M. E. and Hammond, L. (1990) A survey of Tourette syndrome patients and their families: the 1987 Ohio survey. *J. Neuropsychiatr. Clin. Neurosci.*, **2**, 275–281.
20. Park, S., Como, P. G., Cui, L. and Kurlan, R. (1993) The early course of the Tourette's syndrome clinical spectrum. *Neurology*, **43**, 1712–1715.
21. Apter, A., Pauls, D. L., Bleich, A., Zohar, A. H., Kron, S., Ratzoni, G., Dycian, A., Kotler, M., Weizman, A., Gadot, N. and Cohen, D. J. (1993) An epidemiologic study of Gilles de la Tourette's syndrome in Israel. *Arch. Gen. Psychiatry*, **50**, 734–738.
22. Pauls, D. L., Leckman, J. F. and Cohen, D. J. (1993) Familial relationship between Gilles de la Tourette's syndrome, attention deficit disorder, learning disabilities, speech disorders, and stuttering. *J. Am. Acad. Child Adolesc. Psychiatry*, **32**, 1044–1050.
23. Golden, G. S. (1977) The effect of central nervous system stimulants on Tourette syndrome. *Ann. Neurol.*, **2**, 69–70.
24. Lowe, T. L., Cohen, D. J., Detlor, J., Kremenitzer, M. W. and Shaywitz, B. A. (1982) Stimulant medications precipitate Tourette's syndrome. *JAMA*, **247**, 1729–1731.
25. Erenberg, G., Cruse, R. P. and Rothner, A. D. (1985) Gilles de la Tourette's syndrome: effects of stimulant drugs. *Neurology*, **35**, 1346–1348.

26. Comings, D. E. and Comings, B. G. (1984) Tourette's syndrome and attention deficit disorder with hyperactivity: are they genetically related? *J. Am. Acad. Child Psychiatry*, **23**, 138–146.
27. Knell, E. R. and Comings, D. E. (1993) Tourette's syndrome and attention-deficit hyperactivity disorder: evidence for a genetic relationship. *J. Clin Psychiatry*, **54**, 331–337.
28. Pauls, D. L., Hurst, C. R., Kruger, S. D., Leckman, J. F., Kidd, K. K. and Cohen, D. J. (1986) Gilles de la Tourette's syndrome and attention deficit disorder with hyperactivity. *Arch. Gen. Psychiatry*, **43**, 1177–1179.
29. Denckla, M. B., Bemporad, J. R. and MacKay, C. M. (1976) Tics following methylphenidate administration. *JAMA*, **235**, 1349–1351.
30. Goldstein, I. J., Adesman, A. R. and Lipkin, P. H. (1991) Tics and dyskinesias in stimulant use for attention-deficit hyperactivity disorder. *Pediatr. Res.*, **29**, 9A.
31. Mitchell, E. and Matthews, K. L. (1980) Gilles de la Tourette disorder associated with pemoline. *Am. J. Psychiatry*, **137**, 1618–1619.
32. Briscoe, J. G., Curry, S. C., Gerkin, R. D. and Ruiz, R. R. (1988) Pemoline-induced choreoathetosis and rhabdomyolyis. *Med. Toxicol.*, **3**, 72–76.
33. Sallee, F. R., Stiller, R. L., Perel, J. M. and Everett, G. (1989) Pemoline-induced abnormal involuntary movements. *J. Clin. Psychopharmacol.*, **9**, 125–129.
34. Sverd, J., Gadow, K. D. and Paolicelli, L. M. (1989) Methylphenidate treatment of attention-deficit hyperactivity disorder in boys with Tourette's syndrome. *J. Am. Acad. Child Adolesc. Psychiatry*, **28**, 574–579.
35. Gadow, K. D., Nolan, E. E. and Sverd, J. (1992) Methylphenidate in hyperactive boys with comorbid tic disorder: II. Short-term behavioral effects in school settings. *J. Am. Acad. Child Adolesc. Psychiatry*, **31**, 462–471.
36. Cohen, D. J., Detlor, J., Young, J. G. and Shaywitz, B. A. (1980) Clonidine ameliorates Gilles de la Tourette syndrome. *Arch. Gen. Psychiatry*, **37**, 1350–1357.
37. Hunt, R. D., Minderaa, R. B. and Cohen, D. J. (1986) The therapeutic effect of clonidine in attention deficit disorder with hyperactivity: a comparison with placebo and methylphenidate. *Psychopharmacol. Bull.*, **23**, 111–114.
38. Leckman, J. F., Hardin, M. T., Riddle, M. A., Stevenson, J., Ort, S. and Cohen, D. J. (1991) Clonidine treatment of Gilles de la Tourette's syndrome. *Arch. Gen. Psychiatry*, **48**, 324–328.
39. Goetz, C., Tanner, C., Wilson, R., Carroll, V., Como, P. and Shannon, K. (1987) Clonidine and Gilles de la Tourette syndrome: double-blind study using objective rating measures. *Ann. Neurol.*, **21**, 307–310.
40. Steingard, R., Biederman, J., Spencer, T., Wilens, T. and Gonzalez, A. (1993) Comparison of clonidine response in the treatment of attention-deficit hyperactivity disorder with and without comorbid tic disorders. *J. Am. Acad. Child Adolesc. Psychiatry*, **32**, 350–353.
41. Comings, D. E., Comings, B. G., Tacket, T. and Li, S. (1990) The clonidine patch and behavior problems. *J. Am. Acad. Child Adolesc. Psychiatry*, **29**, 668.
42. Biederman, J., Baldessarini, R., Wright, V., Knee, D. and Harmatz, J. (1989) A double-blind placebo controlled study of desipramine in the treatment of attention deficit disorder. I. Efficacy. *J. Am. Acad. Child Adolesc. Psychiatry*, **28**, 777–784.
43. Dillon, D. C., Salzman, I. J. and Schulsinger, D. A. (1985) The use of imipramine in Tourette's syndrome and attention deficit disorder: case report. *J. Clin. Psychiatry*, **46**, 348–349.
44. Spencer, T., Biederman, J., Keman, K., Steingard, R. and Wilens, T. (1993) Desipramine treatment of children with attention-deficit hyperactivity disorder and tic disorder or Tourette's syndrome. *J. Am. Acad. Child Adolesc. Psychiatry*, **32**, 354–360.

45. Riddle, M., Hardin, M., Cho, S. C., Woolston, J. L. and Leckman, J. (1988) Desipramine treatment of boys with attention-deficit hyperactivity disorder and tics: preliminary clinical experience. *J. Am. Acad. Child Adolesc. Psychiatry*, **27**, 811–814.
46. Spencer, T., Biederman, J., Wilens, T., Steingard, R. and Geist, D. (1993) Nortriptyline treatment of children with attention-deficit hyperactivity disorder and tic disorder or Tourette's syndrome. *J. Am. Acad. Child Adolesc. Psychiatry*, **32**, 205–210.
47. Caine, E. D., Polinsky, R. J., Ebert, M. H. *et al.* (1979) Trial of clomipramine and desipramine for Gilles de la Tourette syndrome. *Ann. Neurol.*, **5**, 305–306.
48. Cruz, R. (1992) Clomipramine side effects. *J. Am. Acad. Child Adolesc. Psychiatry*, **31**, 1168–1169.
49. Jankovic, J. (1993) Deprenyl in attention deficit associate with Tourette's syndrome. *Arch. Neurol.*, **50**, 286–288.
50. Spencer, T., Biederman, J., Steingard, R. and Wilens, T. (1993) Bupropion exacerbates tics in children with attention-deficit hyperactivity disorder and Tourette's syndrome. *J. Am. Acad. Child Adolesc. Psychiatry*, **32**, 211–214.

6 Juvenile Wilson's Disease: the Neurological Syndrome

JOHN M. WALSHE
University College London School of Medicine, UK

> Nature is nowhere accustomed more openly to display her secret mysteries than in cases where she shows traces of her workings apart from the beaten path; nor is there any better way to advance the proper practice of medicine than to give our minds to the discovery of the usual laws of nature by careful investigation of cases of rarer forms of diseases. For it has been found in almost all things that what they contain of useful or applicable nature is hardly perceived unless we are deprived of them, or they become deranged in some way.
>
> William Harvey, 1657

HISTORICAL BACKGROUND

How true this statement is becomes at once clear when we stop to consider the immense increase in knowledge of both the normal and the pathological physiology of those diseases which Garrod called 'inborn errors of metabolism' but which are now classified as inherited metabolic disorders. Hepatolenticular degeneration, Wilson's disease, the subject of this chapter, is but one example of many such conditions.

Wilson's immensely long original account of this disease[1], probably more often quoted than read, is remarkable in the accurate description of the neurological signs and symptoms considering that he, personally, saw only four such patients. He summarized the symptom complex as follows '... generalized tremor, dysarthria and dysphagia, muscular rigidity and hypertonicity, emaciation, spasmodic contractions, contractures, emotionalism ... Although cirrhosis of the liver is constantly found in this affection, and is an essential feature of it, there are no signs of liver disease during life'. This last statement is surprising when it is realised that one of his patients died of bleeding oesophageal varices whilst another had an attack of jaundice shortly before the onset of neurological symptoms. Of the two additional case reports he found in the hospital records, one developed oedema, ascites and purpura during the course of her illness. In view of the accuracy of most of Wilson's other clinical observations, it is also surprising that he failed to observe the corneal pigment, the Kayser–Fleischer rings,

Movement and Allied Disorders. Edited by M. M. Robertson and V. Eapen

that are so characteristic of the disease which bears his name. He also failed to comment on the generalized cortical atrophy apparent in the brain section from a patient when compared with a normal brain (Figures 66 and 67 of his article). Wilson's search through the literature revealed an additional seven cases all showing the same or a very similar symptom complex. Their ages at presentation ranged from 9 to 26 years running a course, to death, from 4 months to 7 years.

A few years later the importance of the liver pathology was discussed by Bramwell[2] who described a sibship in which four of seven children died of liver cirrhosis between the ages of 9 to 14 years and he suggested that this might well be '. . . a preliminary stage of Wilson's disease and such cases may from time to time occur without the development of lenticular degeneration'. Pollock[3], in 1917, described the finding of Kayser–Fleischer rings in a patient with Wilson's disease although Wilson himself denied the association as late at 1922[4].

Having covered both the neurological and hepatic aspects of this disease, brief mention must be made of the biochemical lesion, the role of copper in pathogenesis. Wilson considered the disease to be 'familial' but not hereditary; he suggested that a toxin was elaborated in the liver which had a specific action on the lenticular nucleus '. . . Possibly it is chemical and of the nature of a lipoid'[1]. It was in fact Rumpel[5], very shortly after Wilson's original publication, who reported finding excess copper in the liver of a patient dying of this disease. The next clue, the significance of which was not appreciated, came when Siemerling and Oloff[6] described the association of Kayser–Fleischer rings and sun flower cataracts, and commented on the similarity of these cataracts to those caused by the deposition of a copper-containing foreign body in the eye. In the late 1920s and in the 1930s a number of authors reported single cases in which excess copper was found in either liver or brain. It was not, however, until Cumings[7] in 1948 produced convincing evidence that copper, in excess, was to be found in both brain and liver, was it fully realised that the metal must be associated with the pathogenesis of the disease. The copper theory, if such it may be called, was not at once generally accepted; in fact it became the centre of controversy. Uzman and his associates published a series of articles in which they proposed that the primary metabolic defect was one of protein or amino acid metabolism, and copper was deposited as a secondary phenomenon in damaged tissues[8–12]. However, in view of the response to treatment with copper chelating agents and the failure, using more modern techniques, to find any evidence of unusual amino acids or peptides in the urine of patients with Wilson's disease[13,14], the Uzman hypothesis of an abnormal protein metabolism has been abandoned. Very recent gene cloning[15,16] must eventually lead to a fuller understanding of the pathogenesis of this disease. The controversies over therapy, which have at times reached a similar intensity, will be mentioned in a later section.

THE MOVEMENT DISORDERS OF WILSON'S DISEASE

Wilson's disease is protean in its manifestations and no two patients are ever quite the same. The hepatic presentation has been described in some detail elsewhere[17,18] and is not germane to the present chapter.

Wilson believed the signs to be due to basal ganglia involvement and he considered this to be a pure lenticular nucleus syndrome. However, other nuclei of the basal ganglia and brainstem are also involved as is also the cerebellum, well illustrated by the nature of the movement tremor seen in some patients. In view of the fact that spasticity and extensor plantar responses may also be seen, it seems probable that the pyramidal system must also be damaged. As excess copper is general throughout the grey matter, this is hardly surprising[19].

Having stressed the pleomorphic nature of the neurological signs and symptoms in this disease, it is still possible to separate out certain broad categories of syndrome into which most patients can be grouped. It must, however, be remembered that, in untreated patients, the disease evolves so that, eventually, most patients will become rigid with contractures. There is also a subtle overlapping of the various subtypes so that it may be difficult to decide into which group any given patient must be assigned. Denny-Brown[20] suggested that patients could be classified as either 'pseudo-sclerotic' or dystonic. The former all presented after the age of 19 and their symptoms were characterized by dysarthria and 'wing-beating tremor'; they ran a relatively chronic course. The patients with dystonia were younger, the first symptoms of the illness starting between the ages of 7 and 15 years. These patients might also show Parkinsonian features; they ran a rapid course and responded very badly to treatment. However this series comprised only 18 patients, too few to draw any firm conclusions. A recent detailed analysis[21] of the presenting symptoms of 136 patients with predominantly neurological Wilson's disease noted an age range of 9–40 years and pointed out the rarity of neurological symptoms before puberty. Some 31 of these patients gave a history of an earlier, often self-limiting, attack of liver disease. The age range for these episodes was 3–25 years. Approximately one-half of all patients (65) were classified as 'juvenile' as they were aged 16 years or younger, and these form the basis of the present analysis.

As early diagnosis, before irreversible brain damage can occur, is essential for the best management of patients with Wilson's disease, let us first consider the earliest symptoms of which juvenile patients will complain, and the signs likely to be found on physical examination. Approximately one-third will either have or give a history of liver damage or haemolysis. The commonest neurological complaint is dysarthria, often associated with drooling and an open mouth. Problems with the upper limbs, tremor or dystonia, almost invariably precede difficulty in walking;

the signs are often asymmetrical. The patient, or sometimes the parent, complains of difficulty in speaking and clumsiness with the hands. Often there is also a story of a change in personality and of a deteriorating performance at school, attributed by the teachers to laziness. In practice, this may be due either to the intellectual or the physical effects of the disease or a combination of the two. It is a sad fact that many in the teaching profession seem unable to distinguish between a pupil who *can not* and a pupil who *will not* perform to expected capacity. Such children are not infrequently referred to an educational psychologist. A detailed analysis of these varying symptoms and signs, together with the initial diagnosis are given in Tables 6.1 and 6.2. In only 80% of cases was this initial diagnosis correct. The combination of a change in personality and physical signs, which are frequently bizarre, led to the diagnosis of a psychiatric or functional illness, whilst in the remainder, either no diagnosis was made or they were incorrectly labelled with a wide variety of organic diagnoses varying from myasthenia gravis, juvenile parkinsonism, familial or essential tremor to other less likely conditions. By the time all patients were correctly diagnosed, the signs and symptoms had obviously progressed and, by and large, the clinical picture fell into one of the four main types, with an inevitable degree of overlap. The most common picture was parkinsonian (43%), closely followed by dystonia (21.5%) and chorea (20%). The classical pseudosclerotic picture with wing-beating tremor was relatively uncommon in this age group (10.7%). A small number remained unclassified. The juvenile patients showed an interesting difference from the older age group in whom the pseudosclerotic picture was more common than both the dystonic and choreic. When treatment was delayed most patients eventually became severely dystonic with contractures of all

Table 6.1. Referral diagnosis and initial symptoms in 65 juvenile patients with neurological Wilson's disease as a percentage. (Total numbers in brackets.)

	Organic	Psychiatric	No diagnosis	Wilson's disease	Total
Number of patients	23 (15)	20 (13)	18.5 (12)	38.5 (25)	100 (65)
Personality change	46.7 (7)	46.1 (6)	25.0 (3)	20 (5)	32.3 (21)
Speech defect	80.0 (12)	61.5 (8)	66.7 (8)	52 (13)	63.1 (41)
Drooling	26.7 (4)	30.8 (4)	41.7 (5)	28 (7)	30.8 (20)
Dysphagia	6.7 (1)	15.4 (2)	16.7 (2)	16 (4)	13.8 (9)
Hand tremor	53.3 (8)	53.8 (7)	41.7 (5)	44 (11)	47.7 (31)
Hand clumsy	40.0 (6)	53.8 (7)	25.0 (3)	20 (5)	32.3 (21)
Abnormal gait	26.7 (4)	53.8 (7)	25.0 (3)	32 (8)	33.8 (22)
Fall in work at school	46.7 (7)	38.5 (5)	41.7 (5)	36 (9)	40.0 (26)

Table 6.2. Referral diagnosis and recorded initial signs in 65 juvenile patients with neurological Wilson's disease as a percentage. (Total numbers in brackets.)

	Organic	Psychiatric	No diagnosis	Wilson's disease	Total
Number of patients	23 (15)	20 (13)	18.5 (12)	38.5 (25)	100 (65)
Personality change	20.0 (3)	46.1 (6)	16.7 (2)	12 (3)	21.5 (14)
Dysarthria	60.0 (9)	15.4 (2)	42.7 (5)	72 (18)	52.3 (34)
Gait abnormal	6.7 (1)	7.7 (1)	16.7 (2)	16 (4)	12.3 (8)
Eye movement abnormal	6.7 (1)	7.7 (1)	0.0 (0)	8 (2)	6.1 (4)
Drooling	20.0 (3)	7.7 (1)	42.7 (5)	36 (9)	27.7 (18)
Parkinsonian facies	13.3 (2)	23.0 (3)	16.7 (2)	32 (8)	23.0 (15)
Open mouth	6.7 (1)	23.0 (3)	0.0 (0)	12 (3)	15.4 (10)
Bradykinesia	6.7 (1)	7.7 (1)	0.0 (0)	16 (4)	9.2 (6)
Tongue abnormal	13.3 (2)	7.7 (1)	16.7 (2)	24 (6)	17.9 (11)
*UL tremor	40.0 (6)	15.4 (2)	8.3 (1)	32 (8)	26.2 (17)
*UL dystonia	0.0 (0)	15.4 (2)	42.7 (5)	28 (7)	21.5 (14)
*UL spontaneous movements	13.3 (2)	7.7 (1)	8.3 (1)	16 (4)	12.3 (8)
+LL tremor	6.7 (1)	0.0 (0)	0.0 (0)	4 (1)	3.1 (2)
+LL dystonia	0.0 (0)	15.4 (2)	42.7 (5)	20 (5)	18.5 (12)
+LL spontaneous movements	0.0 (0)	0.0 (0)	8.3 (1)	0.0 (0)	1.5 (1)
Liver disease	13.3 (2)	15.4 (2)	33.3 (4)	44 (11)	29.2 (19)

*UL = upper limit
+LL = lower limit

four limbs. The personality changes include emotional lability, inappropriate behaviour, depression with suicidal tendencies, sexual disinhibition and antisocial behaviour which may lead to a clash with the law; occasionally the picture closely mimics schizophrenia.

In seeking to make the correct diagnosis in a child with a neurological disability, the clinician should always bear Wilson's disease in mind, particularly if there is no sensory loss, the symptoms are bizarre, there is a falling performance at school or a change in personality. If there is an earlier history of liver damage or haemolysis the diagnosis becomes highly probable. In seeking to confirm this, the first step is to make a careful examination of the eyes for Kayser–Fleischer pigment[22]. If the patient has blue eyes, this is relatively simple and can be carried out with a hand lens and a good light source. The pigment always appears first in the top crescent of the limbus, then the lower crescent and these spread until they become a complete ring of brown or occasionally greenish brown colour. Over a brown iris the ring may appear grey and is more difficult to see and requires some experience; if any doubt exists the eyes must be examined, under slit lamp microscopy, by an experienced ophthalmologist. Finally, the diagnosis must be confirmed by chemical analysis which requires the service of a laboratory familiar with the necessary techniques. The determinations to be made are serum caeruloplasmin and copper, and urine copper excretion. The latter estimation is apt to be unreliable as contamination of the specimen all too often occurs during the collection period. Serum copper and caeruloplasmin concentrations are low in patients with Wilson's disease but the 'free copper', that is copper not bound to caeruloplasmin, is raised as is the urine copper excretion. As the range of normal values for these parameters quoted by different laboratories varies considerably it is difficult to give absolute figures but in my laboratory the normal serum copper concentration varies between 80 and 120 μg/dl (15–20 μmol/l) and the caeruloplasmin between 25 and 40 mg/dl in males and slightly higher in females. It must be remembered that the caeruloplasmin concentration is raised in chronic inflammatory conditions and is reduced in the face of heavy proteinuria and liver failure. The normal urine copper excretion should not exceed 30 μg/24 hours (0.5 μmol) in carefully collected specimens although most laboratories quote higher figures[23].

MANAGEMENT OF THE PATIENT WITH WILSON'S DISEASE

> As doctors say of a wasting disease, to start with it is easy to cure but difficult to diagnose; after a time, unless it has been diagnosed and treated at the outset, it becomes easy to diagnose but difficult to cure.
>
> Machiavelli, *The Prince*, 1514

Machiavelli's statement is remarkably apposite to the management of Wilson's disease, for once the disease has progressed to the state in which contractures of the limbs have occurred, it is very difficult to achieve complete functional recovery. However, before starting treatment it is wise to obtain basic data about the blood count and renal function, as these may well show abnormalities for which therapy may be blamed if the determinations are only made later. Particular attention should be paid to the white cell and platelet counts as some degree of hypersplenism may well depress these; proteinuria may also be found in untreated Wilson's disease. Penicillamine, still the drug of choice for the treatment of this disease, can depress all elements of the bone marrow and can also give rise to nephrotic syndrome, and is not infrequently blamed for causing abnormalities which were, in fact, present before the drug was administered. Other investigations can be made at leisure once treatment has been established. As Wilson's disease can affect the skeleton it is helpful to X-ray the more vulnerable joints—the knees, wrists and lumbar spine.

Some 10% of patients have pigment gallstones so that an ultrasound scan of the gallbladder is also helpful; at the same time the liver size and consistency can be assessed for evidence of cirrhosis and also for the possible presence of oesophageal varices. Nowadays, it is also customary to perform a magnetic resonance imaging (MRI) scan of the brain[24], the literature on this now being extensive. While it is helpful to know the extent of the cerebral lesions which usually involve the basal ganglia and other brain stem nuclei, the findings will not influence management so that this investigation is not essential.

There are now a number of 'anticopper' regimes which must be considered as possible therapies. The first drug to be introduced was dimercaprol, dimercaptopropanol, (BAL)[25], and both Cumings[26] and Denny-Brown and Porter[27] reported limited success with its use. This was followed by penicillamine[28] which, after 40 years' experience, remains the best tried medication and probably still the treatment of choice, although its use is somewhat limited by a relatively high incidence of unwanted side reactions, approaching 10%[29]. In the following decade Schouwink suggested that zinc salts might be useful as a result of their ability to block the absorption of copper from the gut, although they have no action in mobilizing copper already present in the tissues. This suggestion was later taken up by Hoogenraad and his associates in Holland[30,31] and by Brewer and colleagues in the US[32]. About the same time trientine (triethylene tetramine dihydrochloride) was reported to be a powerful cupriuretic[33] and this has now been shown to be an effective drug for the treatment of Wilson's disease and to have remarkably few side effects[34–36]. Finally, a further advance was made by the demonstration that ammonium tetrathiomolybdate, long known to be an 'anticopper' agent in herbivores, could also be used in the treatment of Wilson's disease[37,38].

One of the difficulties the physician must face in initiating treatment for any patient with Wilson's disease is in predicting the immediate response and also the long-term outcome. Some 20% of patients treated with penicillamine show an early increase in their symptoms which may last as long as 3 months[39] and, in rare patients, this initial deterioration may be severe and irreversible. The reason for this is not apparent and, unfortunately, not predictable. I have also seen a similar deterioration with both trientine and zinc salts. However, penicillamine is a well-tried remedy and a high percentage of patients treated with it show a remarkable improvement and are able to return to normal activities. For an adult a starting dose of 500 mg, three times a day before meals is usually satisfactory, with suitably reduced doses being used for children (20 mg/kg). Penicillamine can induce pyridoxine deficiency under certain specific circumstances, that is, during a growth spurt, pregnancy, intercurrent illness or malnutrition[40], so that it is customary to give supplements of this vitamin; 50 mg weekly is sufficient. Attempts to control the abnormal movements of Wilson's disease with one or other of the drugs used for this purpose in other neurological conditions has proved remarkably disappointing, although very occasionally benzhexol (Artane) or L-dopa may give relief. Before starting treatment, the patient should be warned of a possible increase in symptoms and told not to expect significant improvement in under 6 months, for although this may occur, it is not common, and to encourage a patient with unrealistic expectations is neither kind nor wise. In the short term a small number of patients develop an urticarial rash which is morbilliform and itchy and may be associated with microscopic haematuria. It is best managed by interrupting treatment and giving an antihistamine; once the rash has cleared, penicillamine can be restarted in a small dose, building this up gradually over the course of about a week; occasionally steroid cover is needed during this period. In the long term penicillamine can induce a wide variety of toxic reactions, most being immunologically induced. The most serious are systemic lupus and immune complex nephritis[29,42]. Approximately 10% of patients show some degree of drug intolerance, but only one-half of these require a change of therapy.

Trientine also has an excellent track record in the management of patients with Wilson's disease and has remarkably few side effects. There are rare reports of sideroblastic anaemia and it may be that it can reactivate drug-precipitated systemic lupus. It is in no way related chemically to penicillamine and hence cross-toxicity does not occur. The initial adult dose is 600 mg three times a day and correspondingly less for children. The maintenance dose is 900–1200 mg daily in divided doses. As with penicillamine, trientine is ideally taken about half an hour before food, so that a maximum blood level is achieved before dietary copper is absorbed into the circulation. Experimental studies with radiocopper have shown that a very much greater degree of copper mobilization can be achieved if the chelating agent is present in the plasma before the absorbed metal can enter its normal metabolic pathways[42]. Although trientine is only licensed for treatment of penicillamine intolerant patients, it is a very effective drug if used as the initial and only therapy, and is probably safer than penicillamine; it is, however, significantly more expensive. It probably mobilizes copper from a different fluid compartment[44].

Zinc sulphate was first given extensive clinical trials in Holland where it is now used as the drug of first choice[30,31]. The claim is made that this treatment is non-toxic and is never associated with deterioration. This is not in fact strictly the case, as anaemia, cramps, severe epigastric pain and even deterioration and death have been reported in patients so treated[45–48]. The recommended dose is 50 mg metallic zinc as the sulphate or acetate taken before meals three times daily. The eventual place of this drug in the treatment of Wilson's disease remains to be assessed, but it is certainly one of the available therapies, particularly in long-term maintenance, if others have failed or induced unacceptable side effects.

Tetrathiomolybdate is not a chelating agent but, like zinc, acts by metal-to-metal antagonism. It is probably the most powerful 'anticopper' agent available and acts not only by an almost total block of copper absorption but also by forming a very strong copper-molybdate-albumin conjugate in the body which effectively detoxifies tissue copper already present. It does not mobilize significant amounts of copper for excretion in the urine[49]. In my own series of patients, one has been taking tetrathiomolybdate successfully for 10 years; she has shown improvement in her hepatic pathology and a marked reduction in the concentration of copper in her liver. Metabolic studies in man and animals have detailed the changes in blood and urine copper which this drug can induce[49]. A dose of 50 mg twice daily will promote a negative copper balance but the use of this compound poses problems. It is not licensed as a pharmaceutical drug and there has been no toxicity testing on it, so that the physician who wishes to use it will be wise to clear this with his/her ethical committee and to explain the facts to the patient. Its use has been associated with generalized, reversible marrow depression[50]. In the light of present knowledge, tetrathiomolybdate should probably therefore only be used when other therapies have failed. With greater experience it may be found to have a major role in the management of Wilson's disease. However, its use in children and adolescents for more than short periods should be approached with caution because, in growing animals it can induce severe skeletal deformities[51,52].

Finally, brief mention must also be made of dimercaprol. It is not now used as an initial treatment, but it can be a useful addition to penicillamine in the patient with severe, advanced, dystonic Wilson's disease. It is given by deep intramuscular injection, together with local anaesthetic, in 200 mg doses twice a day for 5 days a week over a period of 8 weeks.

With these various forms of therapy available, most patients with Wilson's disease can be returned to good health, but the ultimate degree of neurological recovery will depend on the amount of brain damage inflicted before treatment is started. A very few patients will fail to respond, or will respond so slowly that quite severe disability may remain in the form of contractures or dysarthria after the disease process has come under control. In such cases orthopaedic surgery may help. Pregnancy, is not contraindicated in well-treated patients[53–55]; chelating agents do not need to be interrupted in the early stages of gestation, but pyridoxine supplements must be given to patients taking penicillamine[40].

GENETICS

Wilson's disease is an autosomal recessive disorder with the abnormal gene on chromosome 13q14.3. The gene is a putative copper transporting P-type ATPase and is very similar to the X linked gene for Menke's disease[15,16]. For practical purposes this gene has limited diagnostic value, except in families with an established index case, as there are many haplotypes[56].

In managing a family in which the diagnosis of Wilson's disease has been established, it is essential to screen all the siblings, whether older or younger than the index case, as there is a one in four chance that each individual may carry two abnormal genes. It is wise also to screen cousins and also the children of patients with late onset Wilson's disease or those, who, thanks to successful treatment, have grown into the reproductive age. A few examples of parents with Wilson's disease giving birth to children with the disease have been reported. Figure 6.1 shows the result of a gene probe study in one family in which the diagnosis of one sibling (II,2) was in doubt; the biochemical studies pointed towards presymptomatic Wilson's disease and this was confirmed by analysis of the genes. Once the homozygous abnormal state is confirmed, prophylactic treatment with a chelating agent

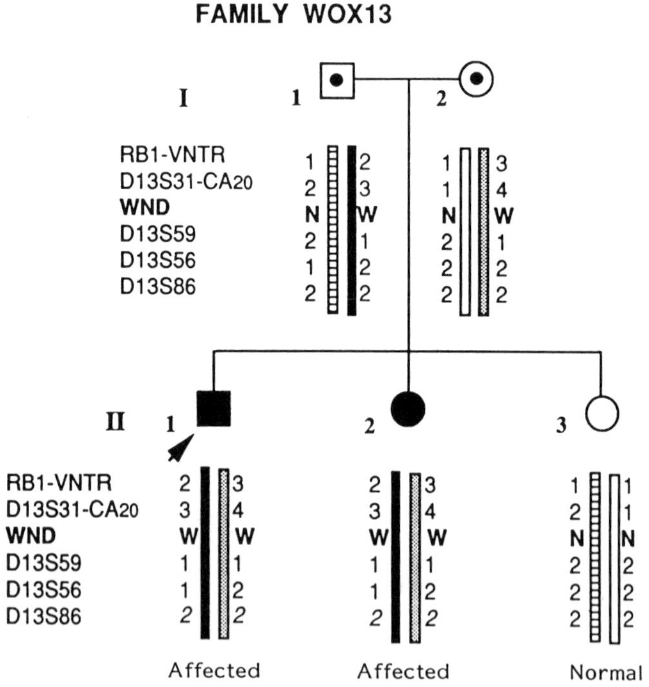

Figure 6.1. Gene study in a Wilson's disease family. The propositus was II,1. The caeruloplasmin concentrations were as follows I,1 29 mg/dl; I,2 28 mg/dl; II,1 (propositus) 9 mg/dl, II,2 14 mg/dl; II,3 34 mg/dl. Other studies on II,2, urine copper excretion and raised liver copper also pointed to Wilson's disease. This was confirmed by the gene probe. I am indebted to Professor Diane Wilson Cox for carrying out this study for me and supplying the figure

should be started without delay, as this will prevent symptoms ever developing, so long as the patient remains a good complier[57,58].

As a first screening test, the serum caeruloplasmin should be estimated. This can be compared with the normal range for the laboratory and with that of the obligate heterozygotes, the parents. Any individual who thus becomes a candidate for the diagnosis of Wilson's disease can then be given an accurate diagnosis by means of a gene probe. This very recent advance will undoubtedly simplify what has, until now, been a very difficult diagnostic problem. Where this procedure is not available, the patient under suspicion should be examined for the presence of Kayser–Fleischer rings, for evidence of hepatic or neurological disease, for urinary copper excretion and for abnormality of liver function tests. If doubt still remains, the concentration of copper in the liver must be determined. This is a situation which requires an accurate diagnosis, as a mistake can have fatal results, or subject an individual to lifelong treatment with unnecessary and potentially toxic drugs. In addition, it may well cause difficulties for both insurance and employment purposes.

REFERENCES

1. Wilson, S. A. K. (1912) Progressive lenticular degeneration: a familial nervous disease associated with cirrhosis of the liver. *Brain*, **34**, 296–509.
2. Bramwell, B. (1916) Familial cirrhosis of the liver: four cases of acute fatal cirrhosis of the liver in the same family, the patients being respectively nine, ten, fourteen, and fourteen years of age: suggested relationship to Wilson's progressive degeneration of the lenticular nucleus. *Edinb. Med. J.*, **17**, 90–99.
3. Pollock, L. J. (1917) The pathology of the nervous system in a case of progressive lenticular degeneration. *J. Nerv. Ment. Dis.*, **46**, 401–420.
4. Wilson, S. A. K. (1922) La maladie de Wilson. In *Questions Neurologiques d'Actualite* (P. Marie, Ed). Masson, Paris, pp. 1–22.
5. Rumpel, A. (1913) Ueber das wesen und die bedeutung der leberveranderungen und der pigmentierunen bei den damit verbundenen fallen von pseudosklerose, zugleich ein beitrag zur lehre von der pseudosklerose (westphal-strumpell). *Dtsch. Z. Nervenheilk*, **49**, 54–73.
6. Siemerling, E. and Oloff, H. (1922) Pseudosklerose (Westphal-Strumpell) mit Cornealring (Kayser–Fleischer) und doppelseitiger Scheinkatarakt, die nur bei seitlicher Beleuchtung sichtbar ist und die dem nach Verletzung durch Kupfersplitter enstehenden Katarakt ahnlich ist. *Klin. Wochenschr.*, **1**, 1087–1089.
7. Cumings, J. N. (1948) The copper and iron content of brain and liver in the normal and in hepatolenticular degeneration. *Brain*, **71**, 410–415.
8. Uzman, L. and Denny-Brown, D. (1948) Aminoaciduria in Wilson's disease (hepatolenticular degeneration). *Am. J. Med. Sci.*, **215**, 599–611.
9. Uzman, L. and Hood, B. (1952) The familial nature of the aminoaciduria of Wilson's disease (hepatolenticular degeneration). *Am. J. Med. Sci.*, **223**, 392–400.
10. Uzman, L., Iber, F. L., Chalmers, T. C. and Knowlton, M. (1956) The mechanism of copper deposition in the liver in hepatolenticular degeneration (Wilson's disease). *Am. J. Med. Sci.*, **231**, 511–518.

11. Uzman, L. (1957) The intrahepatic distribution of copper in relation to the pathogenesis of hepatolenticular degeneration. *Arch. Pathol.*, **64**, 464–479.
12. Uzman, L. and Jakus, M. A. (1957) The Kayser–Fleischer ring. A histochemical and electronmicroscope study. *Neurology*, **7**, 341–355.
13. Asatoor, A. M., Milne, M. D. and Walshe, J. M. (1976) Urinary excretion of peptides and hydroxyproline in Wilson's disease. *Clin. Sci. Mol. Med.*, **51**, 369–378.
14. Asatoor, A. M., Milne, M. D. and Walshe, J. M. (1983) The effect of chelation therapy on the aminoaciduria and peptiduria of Wilson's disease. *J. R. Coll. Physicians Lond.*, **17**, 122–125.
15. Bull, P. C., Thomas, G. R., Rommens, J. N., Forbes, J. R. and Cox, D. W. (1993) The Wilson's disease gene is a putative copper transporting P-type ATPase similar to the Menkes gene. *Nat. Gen.*, **5**, 327–337.
16. Petruhkin, K., Fischer, S. G., Pirastu, M., Tanzi, R. E. *et al.* (1993) Mapping, cloning and genetic characterisation of the region containing the Wilson's disease gene. *Nat. Gen.*, **5**, 338–343.
17. Scheinberg, I. H. and Sternlieb, I. (1984) *Wilson's Disease*. WB Saunders, Philadelphia and London, pp. 70–77.
18. Walshe, J. M. (1989) Wilson's disease presenting with features of hepatic dysfunction. A clinical analysis of eighty-seven patients. *Q. J. Med.*, **70**, 253–263.
19. Warren, P. J., Earl, C. J. and Thompson, R. H. S. (1960) The distribution of copper in human brain. *Brain*, **83**, 709–717.
20. Denny-Brown, D. (1964) Hepatolenticular degeneration (Wilson's disease). Two different components. *N. Engl. J. Med.*, **270**, 149–156.
21. Walshe, J. M. and Yealland, M. (1992) Wilson's disease; the problem of delayed diagnosis. *J. Neurol. Neurosurg. Psychiatry*, **55**, 692–696.
22. Cairns, J. E. and Walshe, J. M. (1970) The Kayser–Fleischer ring. *Trans. Ophthalmol. Soc. UK*, **90**, 187–190.
23. Gibbs, K. R. and Walshe, J. M. (1979) A study of the caeruloplasmin concentrations found in 75 patients with Wilson's disease, their kinships and various control groups. *Q. J. Med.*, **48**, 447–463.
24. Thuomas, K. A., Aquilonius, S. M., Bergstrom, K. and Westermark, K. (1993) Magnetic resonance imaging of the brain in Wilson's disease. *Neuroradiol.*, **35**, 134–141.
25. Peters, R. A., Stocken, L. A. and Thompson, R. H. S. (1945) British antilewisite (BAL). *Nature (Lond.)*, **15**, 656.
26. Cumings, J. N. (1951) The effect of BAL in hepatolenticular degeneration. *Brain*, **74**, 10–22.
27. Denny-Brown, D. and Porter, H. (1951) The effect of BAL (2,3dimercaptopropanol) on hepatolenticular degeneration (Wilson's disease). *N. Engl. J. Med.*, **245**, 917–925.
28. Walshe, J. M. (1956) Penicillamine. A new oral therapy for Wilson's disease. *Am. J. Med.*, **21**, 487–495.
29. Walshe, J. M. (1981) Penicillamine and the SLE syndrome. *J. Rheumatol.*, **8**, (Suppl 7), 155–160.
30. Hoogenraad, T. U., van den Hamer, C. J. A., Koevoet, R. and de Royter Korver, E. G. W. M. (1978) Oral zinc in Wilson's disease. *Lancet*, **ii**, 1262.
31. Hoogenraad, T. U., van den Hamer, C. J. A. and van Hattum, J. (1984) Effective treatment of Wilson's disease with oral zinc sulphate: two case reports. *BMJ*, **289**, 273–276.
32. Brewer, G. J., Hill, G. M., Prasad, A. S., Cossak, Z. T. and Rabbani, P. (1983) Oral zinc therapy for Wilson's disease. *Ann. Intern. Med.*, **99**, 314–320.
33. Walshe, J. M. (1969) Management of penicillamine nephropathy in Wilson's disease: a new chelating agent. *Lancet*, **ii**, 401–402.

34. Walshe, J. M. (1982) Treatment of Wilson's disease with Trientine (triethylene tetramine) dihydrochloride. *Lancet*, **i**, 643–647.
35. Scheinberg, I. H., Jaffe, M. E. and Sternlieb, I. (1987) The use of trientine in preventing the effects of interrupting penicillamine therapy in Wilson's disease. *N. Engl. J. Med.*, **317**, 209–213.
36. Dubois, R. S., Rodgerson, D. O. and Hambidge, K. M. (1990) Treatment of Wilson's disease with triethylene tetramine hydrochloride (trientine). *J. Pediatr. Gastroenterol. Nutr.*, **10**, 77–81.
37. Walshe, J. M. (1984) Copper: its role in the pathogenesis of liver disease. *Semin. Liver Dis.*, **4**, 252–263.
38. Danks, D. M. (1991) Copper and liver disease. *Eur. J. Pediatr.*, **150**, 142–148.
39. Walshe, J. M. and Yealland, M. (1993) Chelation treatment of neurological Wilson's disease. *Q. J. Med.*, **86**, 197–204.
40. Gibbs, K. R. and Walshe, J. M. (1969) Interruption of the tryptophan–nicotinic acid pathway by penicillamine induced pyridoxine deficiency in patients with Wilson's disease and in experimental animals. *Ann. N.Y. Acad. Sci.*, **166**, 158–169.
41. Frankel, J. P., Hughes, A., Lees, A. J., Stern, G. M. and Walshe, J. M. (1989) The use of apomorphine to test for dopamine responsiveness in Wilson's disease. *Lancet*, **ii**, 801.
42. Huskisson, E. C. (1981) The side effects of penicillamine therapy in rheumatoid arthritis. *J. Rheumatol.*, **8** (Suppl 7), 146–148.
43. Walshe, J. M. (1967) The physiology of copper in man and its relation to Wilson's disease. *Brain*, **90**, 149–176.
44. Walshe, J. M. (1973) Copper chelation in patients with Wilson's disease. A comparison of penicillamine and triethylene tetramine dihydrochloride, *Q. J. Med.*, **42**, 441–452.
45. Simon, S. R., Branda, R. F., Tindle, B. H. and Burns, S. L. (1988) Copper deficiency and sideroblastic anaemia associated with zinc ingestion. *Am. J. Hematol.*, **28**, 181–183.
46. Stremmel, W. (1991) Discussion. In *Wilson's Disease*. Proceedings of the fifth symposium (A. Czlonkowska and C. J. A. van den Hammer, Eds). Technical University, Delft, The Netherlands, pp. 184–186.
47. Lang, C. J., Rabas-Kolominsky, P., Englehardt, A., Korbas, G. and Konig, H. (1993) Fatal deterioration of Wilson's disease after institution of oral zinc therapy. *Arch. Neurol.*, **50**, 1007–1008.
48. Walshe, J. M. and Munro, N. A. R. (1995) Zinc induced deterioration in Wilson's disease aborted by treatment with penicillamine, dimercaprol and a novel zero copper diet. *Arch. Neurol.* **52**, 10–11.
49. Walshe, J. M. (1986) Tetrethio molybdate (MoS_4) as an anti-copper agent in man. In *Orphan Diseases and Orphan Drugs* (I. H. Scheinberg and J. M. Walshe, Eds). Manchester University Press, Manchester, pp. 76–85.
50. Harper, P. L. and Walshe, J. M. (1986) Reversible pancytopoenia secondary to treatment with tetrathio molybdate. *Br. J. Haematol.*, **64**, 851–853.
51. Spence, J. A., Suttle, N. F., Wenham, G., El-Gallad, T. and Bremner, I. (1980) A sequential study of the skeletal abnormalities which develop in rats given a small dietary supplement of ammonium tetrathio molybdate. *J. Comp. Pathol.*, **90**, 139–153.
52. Fell, B. F., Dinsdale, D. and El-Gallad, T. T. (1979) Gut pathology of rats dosed with tetrathiomolybdate. *J. Comp. Pathol.*, **89**, 495–514.
53. Scheinberg, I. H. and Sternlieb, I. (1975) Pregnancy in penicillamine treated patients with Wilson's disease. *N. Engl. J. Med.*, **293**, 1300–1302.
54. Walshe, J. M. (1977) Pregnancy in Wilson's disease. *Q. J. Med.*, **46**, 73–83.

55. Walshe, J. M. (1986) The management of pregnancy in Wilson's disease treated with trientine. *Q. J. Med.*, **58**, 81–87.
56. Thomas, G. R., Bull, P. C., Roberts, E. A., Walshe, J. M. and Cox, D. W. (1994) Haplotype studies in Wilson's disease. *Am. J. Hum. Genet.*, **54**, 71–78.
57. Sternlieb, I. and Scheinberg, I. H. (1968) Prevention of Wilson's disease in asymptomatic patients. *N. Engl. J. Med.*, **278**, 352–359.
58. Walshe, J. M. (1988) Diagnosis and treatment of presymptomatic Wilson's disease. *Lancet*, **ii**, 435–437.

7 Phenylketonuria: An Unfolding Story

ALAN J. THOMPSON
Institute of Neurology, London, UK

INTRODUCTION

Phenylketonuria (PKU) is an autosomal recessive disorder resulting from a deficiency in the enzyme phenylalanine hydroxylase and occurs in approximately 1:10 000 births in the UK[1]. Over the last 60 years there has been an increase in the understanding of the condition in terms of its biochemistry, clinical manifestations and, most importantly, its management. While the introduction of neonatal screening and dietary management have resulted in a striking reduction in the neurological complications, it has only been possible in the last decade to evaluate the true impact of these measures[2,3]. This has coincided with the availability of imaging techniques such as magnetic resonance imaging (MRI) which give a much greater insight into disorders of the white matter in the central nervous system (CNS)[4]. Recent findings have prompted a further evaluation of the approach to management.

HISTORY

The initial discovery of this disease was made by Folling in 1934[5,6], as a result of the astute observations and persistence of a mother of two children who were severely cognitively impaired. She was aware of an unusual musty smell which clung to her children, and when Folling tested their urine, it turned green, transiently but consistently, when adding ferric chloride. Efforts were then concentrated on isolating and identifying this substance in the urine which was shown to have a benzene structure with a three carbon side chain consistent with phenylpyruvic acid. Folling found eight similar cases among 430 children in institutions for educationally subnormal children, and noted that they shared a number of clinical features including fair hair, rigidity of muscles and a tendency to have a forward leaning posture. He postulated that the most likely metabolic source was phenylalanine and his next step was to develop a process which would allow the measurement of phenylalanine in the blood. This was

Movement and Allied Disorders. Edited by M. M. Robertson and V. Eapen

impossible to do directly at that time, but his fellow scientists hit upon the idea of using the bacillus *Proteus vulgaris* to change phenylalanine to phenylpyruvic acid which could be measured using a colour reaction. They found that all the patients with this clinical syndrome had higher than normal levels of phenylalanine in their blood.

The study of the disease in a larger number of patients and their families suggested an autosomal recessive mode of inheritance, and also showed that the level of phenylalanine in heterozygotes was higher than normal.

In the meantime, work was being undertaken in the areas of biochemistry, pathology and clinical description. The biochemical pathway was being slowly unravelled and an important discovery was the fact that the main catabolic pathway of phenylalanine was through hydroxylation to tyrosine. Early in the 1950s the enzyme responsible for this step, phenylalanine hydroxylase, was identified[7]. Subsequent work showed that a lack of this enzyme may result from a number of different mechanisms including, in a small proportion of patients (less than 1–3%), a lack of the co-factor tetrahydrobioptrin[8] (see Fig. 7.1).

CLINICAL MANIFESTATIONS

The initial description by Folling underlined the severe cognitive impairment which occurred in patients with PKU. He also noted that the patients had pale complexion and tended to have stiff muscles. Larger studies[9,10] demonstrated the frequency of epilepsy in patients with PKU and the frequency of upper motor neuron signs, particularly brisk reflexes with paraparesis occurring in about 5% of patients. Cowie, in 1951, also highlighted the occurrence of tremor and extrapyramidal signs including cogwheel rigidity and choreoathetosis[11]. She also made the important contribution in the same year of describing so-called 'atypical' PKU in a patient with mild cognitive impairment and low levels of phenylalanine[12].

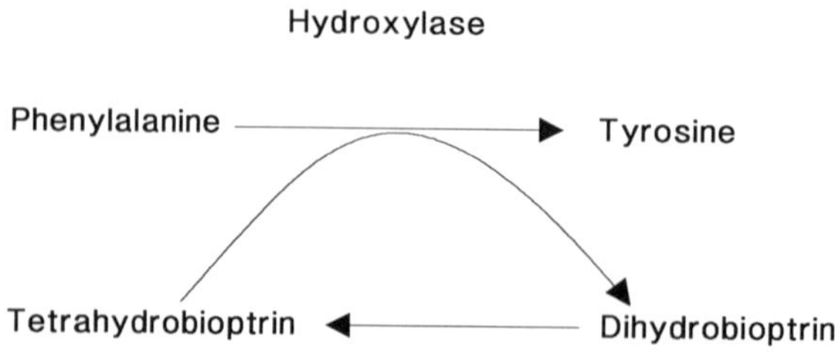

Figure 7.1. Conversion of phenylalanine to tyrosine

More recently, PKU resulting from deficiency of tetrahydrobioptrin has been shown to cause a progressive neurological disorder in which movement disorder is a prominent feature[8].

PATHOLOGY

In 1950 Alvord described pathological abnormalities in the myelin in children who had died of PKU[13], the nature of which was unclear and remains so to this day. Corsellis, three years later, underlined the frequent finding of microcephaly[14]. Others have described abnormalities of myelin, some suggesting that it is similar to that seen in the leukodystrophies[15,16]. The most recent pathological study was carried out 30 years ago by Malamud[17] who described four patients with PKU who showed a striking neurological deterioration in early adult life, all of whom had extensive myelin loss with probable relative preservation of axons. By contrast, in a further four patients who died in childhood, the most marked change was hypomyelination with numerous vacuoles interspersed among nerve fibres. Malamud suggested that while there was a failure of myelination in early childhood, some survivors developed active demyelination in late adolescence. These observations may have some relevance to findings in more recent MRI studies. However, there is some concern over the certainty with which it is possible to differentiate between primary demyelination or demyelination secondary to Walerian axonal degeneration; both may have similar appearances on light microscopy[18].

MECHANISM OF DAMAGE

The precise biochemical event which results in damage to the central nervous system remains uncertain. In animals, phenylalanine excess has been shown to increase central myelin turnover in a dose-dependent manner, leading to increased myelin destruction, and deficits in re-synthesis as phenylalanine exposure increases[19,20]. It has been suggested that in patients with pathological change, it does not relate directly to high levels of phenylalanine and its ketoacidotic derivatives, as they are not thought likely to reach sufficiently high levels to cause neurological damage. However, there may be an indirect effect as a result of competition with other amino acids, notably tyrosine and tryptophan, across the blood–brain barrier. Thus patients may have high levels of phenylalanine and low levels of tyrosine with reduction in dopamine and serotonin as a result. Damage may result from neurotransmitter deficiency[21], or, more probably, from an inhibition of brain protein and/or inhibition of myelin sulphatides.

MANAGEMENT

It became clear that whatever the precise mechanism, pathological damage and consequent neurological impairment were likely to result, either directly or indirectly, from high levels of phenylalanine and, in 1953, it was suggested that restricting phenylalanine intake would be an appropriate method of management[22]. The next major step was the appreciation that for dietary restriction to be useful it was essential that it be started as early following birth as possible and the concept of neonatal identification of patients was introduced using the now familiar Guthrie, or heel prick test[23]. It was hoped that the combination of early detection and dietary restriction would effectively prevent the occurrence of the severe neurological impairments previously described. Perceived wisdom was that this management was particularly important in the early years of development when myelin was particularly vulnerable, and that it might be appropriate to stop, or at least relax, dietary restriction at the age of 8 years or in the mid-teens. This philosophy was also taking account of practical issues in relation to diet, imposing as it did severe restrictions on the patients and involving supplements which were unpleasant to take.

While it is clear that this management has prevented the severe neurological sequelae, it is only now, 30 years following the introduction of dietary restriction, that its real effects can be seen. Reports in the literature in the late 1970s, suggesting that patients who stopped diet early may suffer some degree of cognitive impairment, albeit mild, raised the possibility that the duration of management may need to be reconsidered[24]. More recently there is evidence to suggest that cognitive and behavioural impairment may also be seen in patients who have been treated early[25].

PSYCHOLOGICAL IMPAIRMENT

For over 10 years there has been accumulating evidence of neuropsychological impairment in children with PKU, including those who have been treated early[26–28] (Table 7.1). Children and adults have mean intelligence quotients (IQs) roughly half a standard deviation lower than those of unaffected siblings[29]. The degree of intellectual impairment in early treated pre-school children is closely associated with the degree of hyperphenylalaninaemia to which the subjects have been exposed[30,31]. Long periods of unusually low phenylalanine levels have also been independently associated with worse outcome. Other studies have shown worse progress in children who stopped diet at 6 years compared with those who continued[32].

Against this background, 5 years ago, a small number of single cases were reported of patients who developed severe neurological impairment

Table 7.1. Neuropsychological impairments in early treated phenylketonuria*

Children on strict diet
Reduction in average intellectual ability (IQ > 2SD below population mean in 8–10% of subjects compared with expected 2%)
Delayed acquisition of speech
Increased frequency of behavioural problems including hyperactivity, anxiety, poor concentration
Reduced educational progress
Slowed response times and impaired executive function on neuropsychological testing

* Severity related to quality of control of blood phenylalanine concentrations. (From Medical Research Council Working Party on Phenylketonuria. *Brit. Med. J.* (1993) **306**, 115–119, with permission.)

in their late teens and early 20s[33], including seven patients from England who will be described in more detail in the next section[34].

NEUROLOGICAL AND MRI ABNORMALITIES IN YOUNG ADULTS WITH PHENYLKETONURIA

Seven patients were studied aged between 19 and 29, including five men and two women (Table 7.2). Four patients had been detected by routine neonatal screening and started on a low phenylalanine diet in infancy. Three of those were known to be well controlled on diet, although all had a low IQ at the age of 5 years. Three patients had been diagnosed in childhood because of developmental delay. Neurological deterioration was observed after cessation of diet in five patients, and during dietary treatment (but with poor control) in two. All had signs of upper motor neuron damage and the presenting features were spastic paraparesis or quadriparesis in five, epilepsy in one and a pronounced intention tremor in one. No patient had evidence of any biochemical features to suggest an abnormality of tetrahydrobioptrin metabolism. Two patients, one from each clinical group, are described in more detail.

PATIENT 1

A female aged 19 was diagnosed by routine neonatal screening and was started on a low phenylalanine diet at 13 days. Dietary control was good for 4 years (blood phenylalanine 60–400 μmol/l; normal range 40–80

Table 7.2. Summary of patients with phenylketonuria and late onset neurological deterioration

Subject	Age at diagnosis	Blood Phe* at diagnosis (μmol/l)	Age diet stopped (year)	IQ at school (WISC)†	Late neurological illness	
					Age at onset (year)	Clinical features
1	1 week	3630	18	94	13	Quadriparesis, ataxia, epilepsy
2	5 weeks	>1200	Teens	ND‡	20	Paraparesis
3	6 weeks	2880	**	64	16	Epilepsy
4	1 week	2745	18	61	19	Ataxia, hyperreflexia
5	2 years	1420	7	95	25	Quadriparesis, dystonia, epilepsy
6	15 months	1026	7	45	20	Quadriparesis, sensory changes
7	18 months	1360	7	45	15	Tremor, paraparesis, dystonia

* Phe = Phenylalanine
† WISC = Wechsler Intelligence Scale for Children (at age 5 years)
‡ ND = not done
** = Still on diet
(From Thompson, A. J., Smith, I., Brenton, D. *et al.*, *Lancet* (1990) **336**, 602–605, with permission.)

μmol/l). Subsequent control was less strict (400–700 μmol/l at 10 years, 500–1300 μmol/l thereafter). She attended normal school but at 12 years her intellectual ability deteriorated. At 13 she had two grand mal convulsions and was treated with sodium valproate. She was noted to have mild ataxia and horizontal nystagmus after the second fit. At the age of 14 she had a further fit at which time pyramidal weakness of the right leg was noted; over the next year the ataxia worsened and she developed a mild spastic paraparesis although gait was not impaired. Routine investigations and cerebrospinal fluid (CSF) examination were normal. An electroencephalogram (EEG) showed generalized spike and slow wave activity, and computed tomography (CT) suggested mild white matter atrophy. She remained stable without any further neurological deterioration and went from relaxed diet to total cessation at the age of 18 years, at which stage blood phenylalanine levels rose to 2000 μmol/l.

PATIENT 2

A female aged 24 was diagnosed at 15 months when she presented with developmental delay, hypersomnolence and infantile spasms. Dietary treatment was started but control was poor (blood phenylalanine 330–1400 μmol/l). She required special education and diet was stopped at 7 years. She remained stable until the age of 20 when she noted progressive difficulty walking and paraesthesia of her left hand. On examination she had a spastic quadriparesis with extensor plantar responses and dorsal column sensory loss in the lower limbs. Over the next 6 months her walking deteriorated and she became wheelchair bound at the age of 21. Routine blood and CSF investigations, myelography and CT were normal. Plasma phenylalanine concentration was 1533 μmol/l. She was restarted on a low phenylalanine diet and this was associated with a slow but steady recovery in her mobility, such that she was able to walk long distances unaided 2 years later.

All patients underwent T_2-weighted axial MRI brain scan on a 0.5 Tesla machine. All had abnormal high signal areas in the cerebral white matter which, although varying in size and distribution, tended to be periventricular and more common in the posterior temporal and occipital white matter (see Fig. 7.2). Discrete high signal areas were also seen in some subjects, and in one patient the high signal extended from the trigones

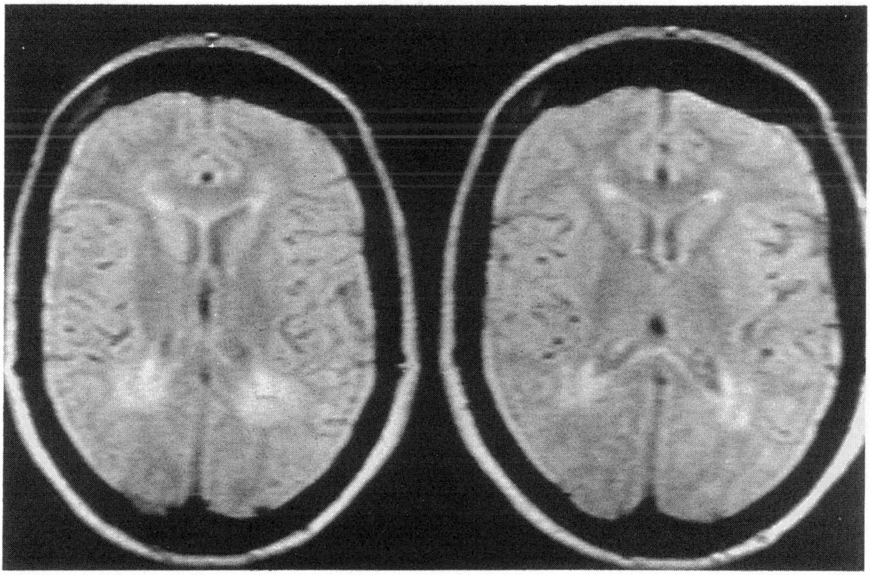

Figure 7.2. T_2-weighted axial MRI brain scan of patient 1 demonstrating areas of high signal which are predominantly periventricular and posterior

above and laterally to the subcortical white matter (see Fig. 7.3). Two patients underwent serial scanning with intervals of over 12 months between each scan. In the first there was no change noted, but in the second there was quite marked change which paralleled the clinical abnormality, and warrants more detailed description.

A 25-year-old patient was diagnosed at 18 months when he presented with developmental delay and infantile spasms. Dietary treatment was started with reasonable control although this deteriorated over the 2 years prior to cessation of diet at the age of 7 years. He attended a school for the educationally subnormal but remained neurologically stable until the age of 15 when he developed severe tremor and had generalized hyperreflexia on examination. Routine investigations were normal and an EEG showed mild diffuse abnormality. He returned to diet for a brief period. At the age of 21 he developed striking neurological deterioration. He became less communicative and was noted to have an impaired gait, right-sided dystonia and mild paraparesis. MRI showed a marked deterioration when compared with a scan done 1 year previously (Figs. 7.4a and b). He was readmitted and commenced on a strict diet which resulted in detectable clinical

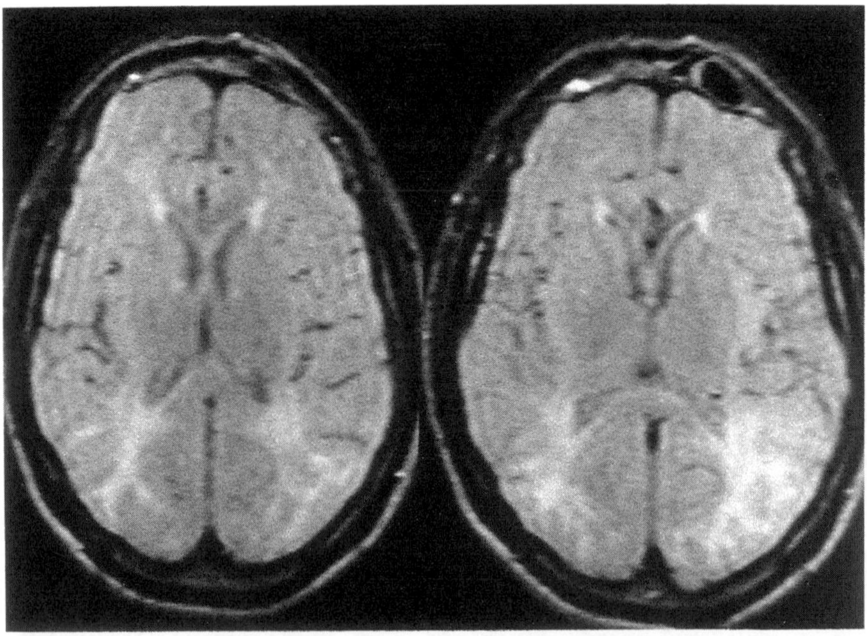

Figure 7.3. T_2-weighted axial MRI brain scan of a 24-year-old patient who was diagnosed in infancy and who had a low IQ and epilepsy from early childhood. Areas of high signal extend from the trigones above and laterally to the subcortical white matter in a distribution similar to that seen in leukodystrophy

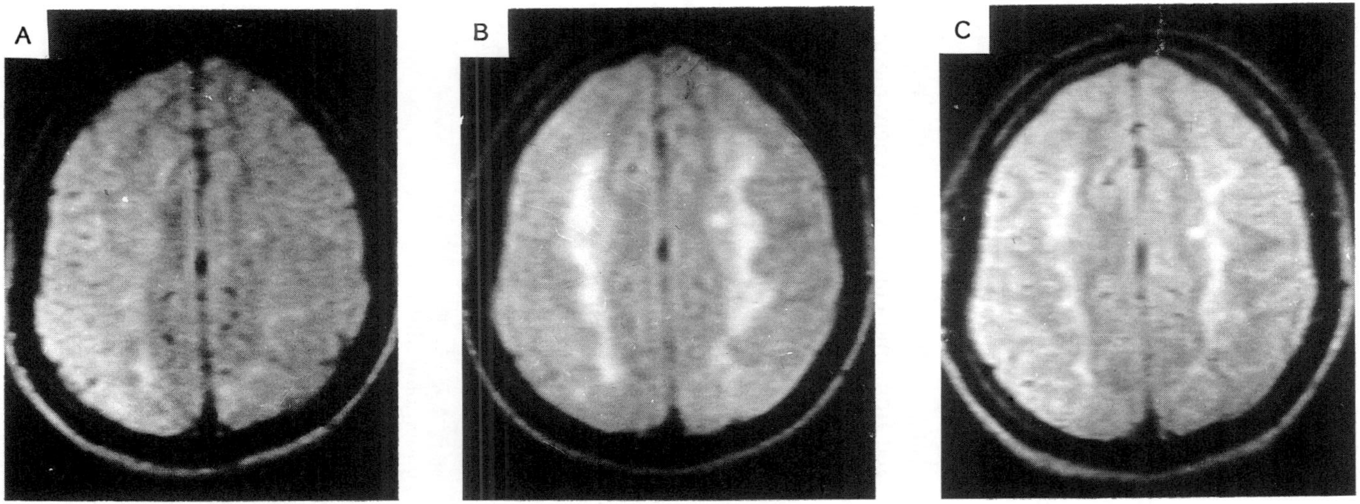

Figure 7.4. Axial T_2-weighted MRI brain scans ($SE_{2000/60}$), of a patient with reversible neurological deficit. Scans taken at one year pre-neurological deterioration (A), at time of clinical deterioration (B), and following neurological improvement on strict dietary treatment (C). Abnormal high signal areas mainly periventricular and posterior are seen in scan A, increasingly dramatically in B and resolving in C. (Reproduced from Thompson, A. J., Smith, I., Brenton, D. *et al*. (1990) *Lancet* **336**, 602–605, with permission.)

improvement within 5 days. A repeat scan done 2 months later showed considerable improvement (Fig. 7.4c).

The occurrence of neurological deterioration in patients with PKU was obviously of some considerable concern, particularly as a number of patients had been identified and treated from birth, although in all but one of these there was some evidence of cognitive impairment at an early age. The immediate questions were first, how prevalent was neurological impairment in the PKU population as a whole, and second, whether such impairment is related in any way to previous management. A third issue related to findings of abnormalities on MRI in all seven patients. As this offered a potential method of monitoring pathological change in PKU it was obviously important to determine how prevalent such abnormalities were in the PKU population, and if there was a relationship between these changes and either cognitive or neurological impairment. In an attempt to answer these questions, a pilot study was established. It included a wide cross-section of subjects aged from mid-childhood, where the majority was still receiving a reasonably well-controlled diet, to young adult life, where a high proportion was on a relaxed or normal diet (see Table 7.3)[2].

Of the 34 patients who were studied and whose data were analysed, all, with the exception of one untreated symptomless subject, had received a low phenylalanine diet until at least 7 years of age, and had been shown to have blood phenylalanine levels greater than 1200 μmol/l during a period of normal diet given after the neonatal period. Twenty-five had been detected by routine neonatal screening. Nine had been missed on the screening programme, and of these, eight had presented with developmental delay, whereas one had been identified for the first time by routine blood testing at the age of 5 years when a younger sibling was detected in the screening programme. This patient had never shown any symptoms

Table 7.3. Details of subjects undergoing MRI

	Group 1	Group 2
Number of subjects	25	9
Diagnostic phenylalanine concentration μmol/l (range)	1270–2910	1150–2960
Age at which diet started (range)	5–61 days	8 months–5 years*
Age at MRI (range)	8–30 years	14–32 years
Number of subjects on normal diet (%)	9 (36%)	7* (78%)
Age at which diet stopped (range)	7–18 years	8–20 years*
Interval between stopping diet and MRI (range)	1–17 years	3–18 years*

Group 1, early diagnosed (<4 months) by routine testing; Group 2, late diagnosed having been missed on screening
* One subject was never tested
(From Thompson, A. J., Tillotson, S., Smith, I., *et al. Brain* (1993) **116**, 811–821, by permission of Oxford University Press.)

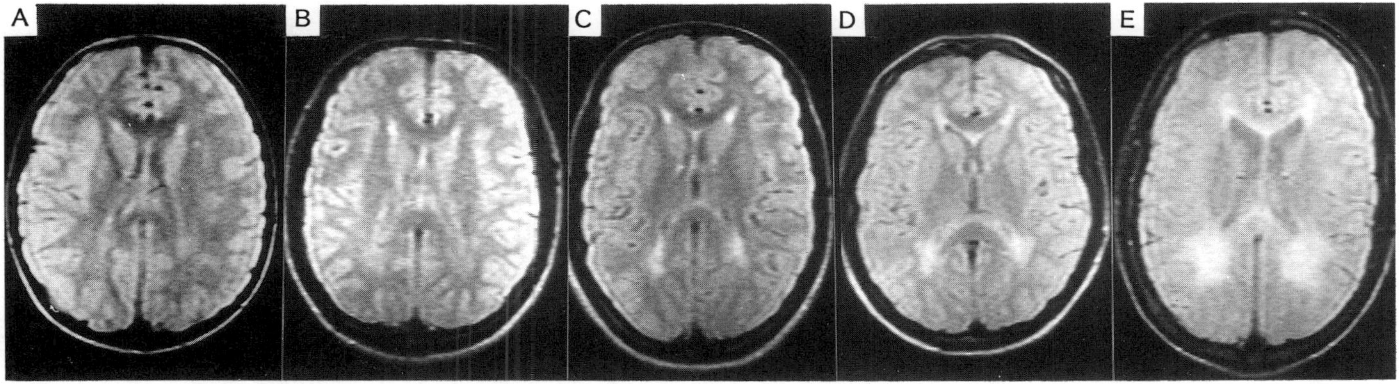

Figure 7.5. Examples of graded (1–5) abnormalities in T_2-weighted MRI scans in patients with phenylketonuria who had been diagnosed by neonatal screening. The scans considered within normal limits or equivocal were graded 0, the remainder were graded from 1 to 5 reflecting the severity of white matter abnormality, particularly posteriorly. (A) Grade 1, an 8-year-old female with a mild tremor continuing on diet; blood phenylalanine 649 μmol/l; minimal periventricular abnormalities with occasional, small discrete lesions (<5 mm). (B) Grade 2, a 23-year-old male continuing on diet; blood phenylalanine 1154 μmol/l; up to 30% parieto-occipital involvement with occasional discrete lesions (<5 mm). (C) Grade 3, a 16-year-old female who stopped diet at age 12 years; blood phenylalanine 1630 μmol/l; 30–60% parieto-occipital involvement with some small to medium sized discrete lesions (5–10 mm); septum pellucidum involved. (D) Grade 4, a 26-year-old female who stopped diet at aged 8 years; blood phenylalanine 1208 μmol/l; 50–75% parieto-occipital involvement with medium sized discrete lesions; septum pellucidum and corpus callosum involved. (E) Grade 5, a 19-year-old male with mild tremor and increased reflexes in the lower limbs, who stopped the diet at age 15 years; blood phenylalanine 1110 μmol/l; >75% parieto-occipital involvement with medium sized discrete lesions; septum pellucidum and corpus callosum involved. (Reproduced from Thompson, A. J., Tillotson, S., Smith, I. *et al*. (1993) *Brain* **116**, 811–821, by permission of Oxford University Press.)

and had received no treatment. Sixteen patients in Group 1 and two patients in Group 2 were still receiving dietary treatment at the time of the study, defined as receiving regular supplements of phenylalanine low protein substitute, not simply protein restriction alone. Details of diagnosis and follow-up, including diet and dietary control as evidenced by phenylalanine levels, were obtained from the National Phenylketonuria Register for 31 of the 34 patients[29].

All patients underwent detailed neurological examination. The most prominent neurological features were pyramidal tract signs, tremor and epilepsy, and these were graded on a predetermined scale of disability (0 = no abnormalities, 1 = physical signs only, 2 = some disability, 3 = moderate to severe disability). All patients had plasma phenylalanine and tyrosine concentrations measured, and MRI scans carried out on a 0.5 Tesla scanner with a T_2-weighted sequence (spin $echo_{2000/60}$, and 24 contiguous 5 mm slices with 128 × 256 image matrix). They were reported by a neuroradiologist who was unaware of the neurological findings and were graded from 0 to 5 according to the severity of the white matter changes (Fig. 7.5). Psychological assessments were not done during the study but data were taken from the Register using WISC/WAIS (pre-1972 births) or WISC-R and WAIS-R (1972 births onwards). Data was also available on two of the three patients not included in the register. The most recent IQ was selected for each patient and the score adjusted to a WISC-R equivalent as described previously[29].

In the analysis of data, Groups 1 and 2 were examined separately. In Group 1 ordinal logistic regression was used to assess the influence of key explanatory variables on MRI grades.

RESULTS

Group 1, 10 subjects (40%) showed some neurological abnormality consisting of brisk lower limb reflexes, tremor or epilepsy. In none did the abnormality score result in moderate to severe disability (a score of 3), the mean neurological score was 0.7. The mean IQ for this group was 98.6 (range 67–127). No patient in the group had an unequivocally normal MRI scan. Two were considered equivocal and, in one subject, movement during investigation made it difficult to grade more precisely than between 0 and 2. The mean MRI score was 0.7 (range 0–5). There was no significant relationship between neurological impairment, any factors relating to management, MRI grade or IQ. There was however a clear association between MRI grade and (1) the time that had elapsed between stopping the low phenylalanine diet, (2) phenylalanine concentration on the day of investigation, and (3) age (Table 7.4, Fig. 7.6).

Ordinal logistical regression was undertaken with MRI grade as the

Table 7.4. MRI grades of Group 1 subjects

	MRI grades		
	0–2	3	4–5
Diet status			
Strict (phenylalanine ≤700 μmol/l)	6*	0	0
Relaxed (phenylalanine >700 μmol/l)	5	4	1‡
Off <2 years	0	4	0
Off >2 years	0	0	5
Blood phenylalanine concentration (μmol/l)			
<700	6*	0	0
700–1199	5	3	0
>1200	0	5	6
Age (years)			
< 11	8*	1	0
11–16	0	3	1‡
>16	3†	4	5

* One patient moved on MRI—omitted from further analysis
† Never off diet despite age (three subjects)
‡ Worst control of subjects still on diet (one subject)
(From Thompson, A. J., Tillotson, S., Smith, I., *et al.*, *Brain* (1993) **116**, 811–821, by permission of Oxford University Press.)

ordered categorical outcome variable and with phenylalanine concentrations, age and years off diet as continuous explanatory variables. Individually, each of the three explanatory variables were significantly associated with MRI grade, however, when the other two variables were accounted for, phenylalanine remained statistically significant ($\chi^2 = 9.65$, $p = 0.0019$), as did years off diet ($\chi^2 = 4.657$, $p = 0.03$), but age was no longer significant ($\chi^2 = 0.176$, $p = 0.0675$). Using the regression model the odds of having a higher MRI score increased by a factor of 1.53 for each 100 μmol/l raise in blood phenylalanine. Likewise, for a given phenylalanine concentration, the odds of having a higher MRI group increased by a factor of 1.27 for each year off diet.

All nine late-diagnosed patients had neurological abnormalities, three of whom were moderately to severely disabled as a result, and the mean neurological score for the group was 2.3. The mean IQ was 78 with a range of 44–106. All nine subjects had abnormal MRI scans, graded between 2 and 4. Given the small number of subjects it was difficult to assess the relationship between MRI grade and other factors although the IQ level did deteriorate as the MRI abnormalities worsened. However, it was of interest that when the subjects' MRI grades were plotted against their phenylalanine concentrations, the disposition of the group did not differ substantially from that of the early treated subjects, and did not suggest therefore that their MRIs were worse in relation to their current

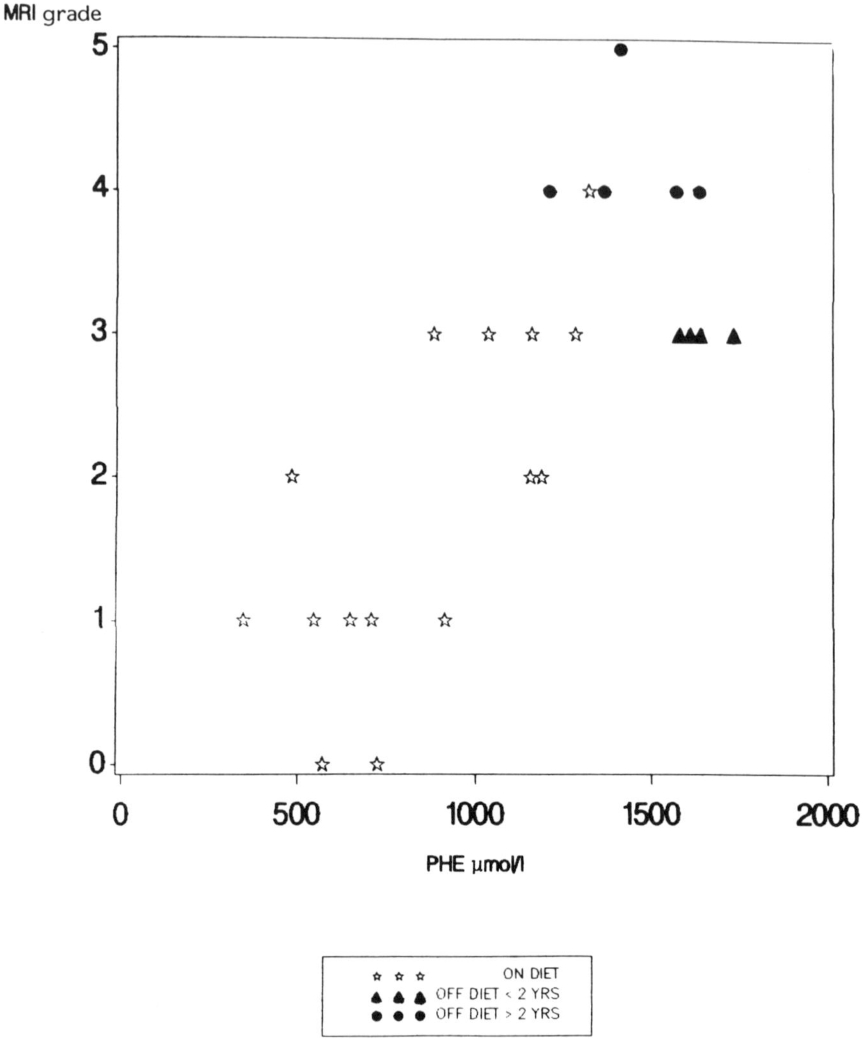

Figure 7.6. Plot of MRI grade in each subject against blood phenylalanine concentration; open stars = still on diet (receiving protein substitute); closed triangles = normal diet <2 years; closed circles = normal diet >2 years. (Reproduced from Thompson, A. J., Tillotson, S., Smith, I. *et al.* (1993) *Brain* **116,** 811–821, by permission of Oxford University Press.)

phenylalanine concentrations and diet history.

In summary, these studies indicated that while neurological impairment was common in PKU, particularly in older and less well-controlled patients, it rarely led to a significant disability, apart from a small group of whom the majority were poorly controlled. In contrast, MRI abnormalities were found in all patients over the age of 7 years as previously reported[34–36]. Although these MRI abnormalities did not relate to neurological dysfunction, they had a highly significant correlation with both the duration of exposure to high phenylalanine levels and the phenylalanine level on the day of examination. Other investigators have not found such a clear-cut relationship, but Bick and colleagues[34] did find that the worst MRI changes occurred in those patients with the highest phenylalanine levels. In this study, as in others[37], there was a high variation in the extent of abnormality among subjects, making it difficult, if not impossible, to make individual predictions. A surprising finding was that the average phenylalanine control up to the age of 8 years did not appear to be associated with the severity of MRI change, which seemed to relate more to recent biochemical events.

What then is the nature and significance of these areas of high signal on MRI? It is clear that these abnormalities were not directly related to neurological dysfunction. This should not be surprising if one considers the predominantly periventricular and parieto-occipital location of these abnormalities which would be unlikely to result in pyramidal tract signs and tremor. The former could possibly result from spinal cord involvement, although a recent study has failed to demonstrate any specific abnormality of the cord in PKU (Davies and Thompson, personal communication). The difficulty in reconciling disability with MRI abnormalities is also seen in other conditions, for example multiple sclerosis (MS)[38]. Perhaps more surprising is the lack of correlation between IQ and the extent of MRI abnormalities. However, IQ is an extremely crude estimate of cognitive function and more detailed psychometry may well show subtle changes which may correlate more closely with the extent of abnormalities on MRI. In this regard the description of an occipital syndrome by Meyding-Lamade and Lieu (1992, personal communication) is of interest. The patients in our study also underwent visual evoked potentials (VEPs) and it is of interest that the recording of all those with an MRI grade greater than 2 showed a reduced amplitude while maintaining a normal latency[39].

In considering the nature of these MRI abnormalities the most important point to make is that such change has no pathological specificity and is seen in a wide range of conditions, including those of an inflammatory, demyelinating and vascular aetiology. Areas of high signal are also seen in a significant proportion of healthy controls over the age of 50 years[40]. These MRI changes may result from a wide range of processes including inflammation and oedema, which are potentially reversible, and demyelination and axonal loss which could be associated with irreversible deficit. It is also possible that, as happens in MS, a combination of these processes occurs.

It would, however, be unwise to ignore these MRI changes in such a young group of patients, for a number of reasons. They show a strong association with dietary control, they have been shown to enlarge in association with clinical deterioration and to improve in parallel with subsequent clinical improvement, associated with strict dietary control, and they are very similar to the changes reported in patients with more severe neurological dysfunction. While it is impossible to state the precise pathological basis for these abnormalities it is likely that oedema is the underlying cause of the rapidly reversing change seen in association with clinical deterioration. This is supported by the finding by Bick and colleagues that such lesions have biexponential T_2 magnetization decay

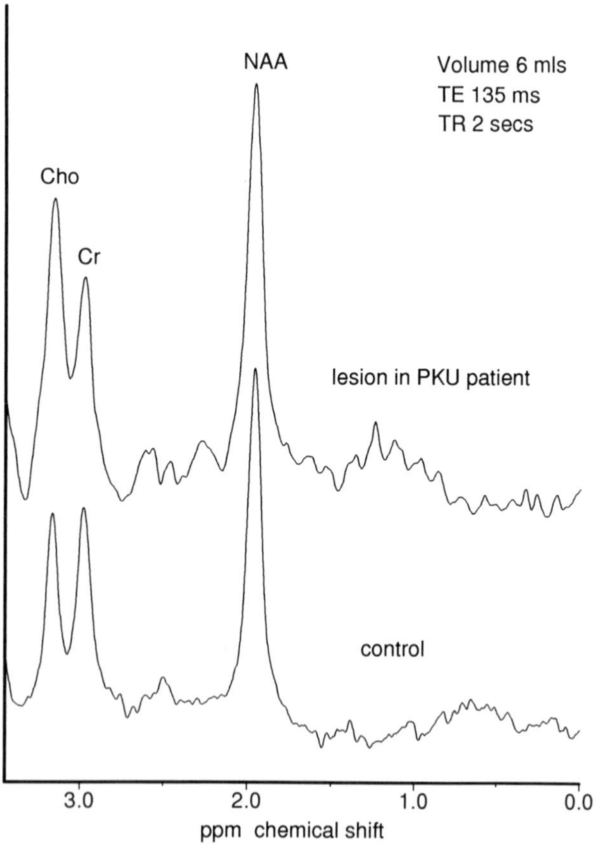

Figure 7.7. Spectra from a patient with PKU and a normal control demonstrating a normal NAA peak in the PKU patient together with a mildly elevated choline/creatine ratio. Cho = choline, Cr = creatine

curves indicating both intracellular and extracellular water compartments[41]. It is likely that the irreversible change reflects an abnormality of myelin as suggested by both animal and pathological studies[17]. Thus, a more diffuse abnormality of myelin may occur, which although sufficient to produce MRI change, may not be clinically detectable.

Clearer understanding may result from the development of imaging techniques which improve pathological specificity. Proton magnetic resonance spectroscopy (MRS) has the potential to do this. This process allows the detection of a number of biochemical constituents of the tissue, notably N-acetyl aspartate (NAA), an amino acid which in humans is contained almost exclusively within neurons and their processes[42]. It has been suggested that NAA levels may give an index of axonal loss or dysfunction. Other detectable metabolites include choline and creatine, the ratio of which is thought to give an indication of membrane turnover. A pilot study of five PKU patients with abnormal MRI has shown that there is no difference in the NAA peak in either abnormal or normal appearing white matter (NAWM) when compared with controls[43]. However an increase in the choline/creatine ratio was seen, both in lesions and NAWM, in PKU patients (Fig. 7.7). No lipid peak, which would indicate myelin breakdown, was seen in the spectra of PKU patients. These findings suggest that little axonal loss or myelin breakdown is occurring within the areas of abnormality on MRI. The increased choline/creatine ratio suggests increased membrane turnover which would be consistent with the animal studies previously discussed.

MRS may also have the potential to detect raised levels of phenylalanine in the brain[44,45], although it has been suggested that levels may not be high enough. If this is the case, MRS may have a very important role in the future looking at effect of dietary control on phenylalanine levels in the brain and the relationship to neurological dysfunction.

CURRENT MANAGEMENT STRATEGIES

How do these developments influence management? The plethora of recent findings encouraged the Medical Research Council to bring together a working party to address this issue[2,46]. It concluded that outcome in early treated subjects was not as good as anticipated and that the quality of blood phenylalanine control is relevant at every age. As a result the recommendations on dietary management emphasized early neonatal detection with immediate dietary restriction. Strict monitoring was encouraged in an attempt to keep phenylalanine levels lower than previously recommended. Finally, patients were encouraged to continue dietary control into adult life.

GENETICS

It is well known that PKU may result in a wide ranging clinical presentation with varying degrees of enzyme deficiency. This variation has recently been explained by the demonstration of over 40 mutations of the hydroxylase gene[47]. A high proportion of affected subjects are therefore compound heterozygotes rather than homozygotes. The gene for phenylalanine hydroxylase is on chromosome 12 and contains 13 exons. Association between genotype and phenotype has been observed and supported by expression studies[48]. These advances in molecular genetics mean that, by using a combination of haplotype and mutation analysis, prenatal diagnosis is now possible in the great majority of patients or parents who already have a child with PKU.

THE FUTURE

However good dietary restriction, it cannot fully substitute for the fine tuning of phenylalanine turnover normally exerted by hepatic phenylalanine hydroxylase. This is particularly the case in patients with severe enzyme deficiency in whom even a slight fever may result in raised phenylalanine levels. Aiming at 'normal' levels also runs the risk of inducing phenylalanine deficiency which may be harmful. It is clear that better therapeutic strategies will be needed if there is to be a substantial improvement in outcome in patients with PKU. Given the difficulties in implementing treatment, the human and financial costs and the concerns about neurological deterioration, PKU is a good candidate for gene therapy. This treatment strategy has had a promising start from recent successful gene transplants by Woo in an inbred strain of mouse with phenylalanine hydroxylase deficiency[49]. In the meantime more information needs to be gathered on the neurological status of early treated children from infancy onwards and more detailed assessments of progress in the realms of neurophysiology, neuropsychology and neuroimaging.

REFERENCES

1. Smith, I. (1985) The hyperphenylalaninaemias. In *Genetic and Metabolic Disease in Pediatrics* (J. K. Lloyd and C. R. Scriver, Eds). Butterworths, London, pp. 166–210.
2. Medical Research Council Working Party on Phenylketonuria (1993) Phenylketonuria due to phenylalanine hydroxylase deficiency: an unfolding story. *BMJ*, **306**, 115–119.
3. Thompson, A. J., Tillotson, S., Smith, I., Kendall, B., Moore, S. G. and Brenton,

D. P. (1993) Brain MRI changes in phenylketonuria: Associations with dietary status. *Brain*, **116**, 811–821.

4. Thompson, A. J. and Miller, D. H. (1992) Magnetic resonance imaging in clinical practice. In *Recent Advances in Clinical Neurology* Vol. 7 (C. Kennard, Ed). Churchill Livingstone, Edinburgh, pp. 199–219.
5. Folling, A. (1934) Über Ausscheidung von Phenylbrenztraubensaure in den Harn Stoffwechselanomalie in Verbindung mit Imbezillitat. *Z. Physiol. Chem.*, **277**, 169–187.
6. Folling, A. (1934) Utskillelse av fenylpyrodruesyre i urien som stoffskifteanomali i forbindelse med imbezillitat. *Nord. Med. Tidskr.*, **8**, 1054–1059.
7. Jervis, G. A. (1953) Deficiency of phenylalanine oxidizing system. *Proc. Soc. Exp. Biol. Med.*, **82**, 514–515.
8. Smith, I., Leeming, R. J., Cavanagh, N. P. C. and Hyland, K. (1986) Neurological aspects of biopterin metabolism. *Arch. Dis. Child.*, **61**, 130–137.
9. Jervis, G. A. (1937) Phenylpyruvic oligophrenia: introductory study of 50 cases of mental deficiency associated with excretion of phenylpyruvic acid. *Arch. Neurol. (Chic)*, **38**, 944–963.
10. Paine, R. S. (1957) The variability and manifestations of untreated patients with phenylketonuria (phenylpyruvic aciduria). *Paediatrics*, **20**, 290–302.
11. Cowie, V. A. (1951) Phenylpyruvic oligophrenia. *J. Ment. Sci.*, **97**, 505–531.
12. Cowie, V. A. (1951) An atypical case of phenylketonuria. *Lancet*, **1**, 272–273.
13. Alvord, E. C., Stevenson, L. D., Vogel, F. S. and Engle, R. L. (1950) Neuropathological findings in phenylpyruvic oligophrenia (phenylketonuria) *J. Neuropath. Exp. Neurol.*, **9**, 298–310.
14. Corsellis, J. A. N. (1953) The pathological report of a case of phenylpyruvic oligophrenia. *J. Neurol. Neurosurg. Psychiatry*, **16**, 139–143.
15. Poser, C. M. and van Bogaert, L. (1959) Neuropathologic observations in phenylketonuria. *Brain*, **82**, 1–9.
16. Chrome, L. (1962) The association of phenylketonuria with leukodystrophy. *J. Neurol. Neurosurg. Psychiatry*, **25**, 149–154.
17. Malamud, N. (1966) Neuropathology of phenylketonuria. *J. Neuropathol. Exp. Neurol.*, **25**, 254–268.
18. McDonald, W. I. (1966) The effects of experimental demyelination on con duction of peripheral nerve. A histological and electrophysiological study. *Brain*, **86**, 481–500.
19. Hommes, F. A. and Moss, L. (1992) Myelin turnover in hyperphenylalaninaemia. A re-evaluation of the HPH-5 mouse. *J. Inherit. Metab. Dis.*, **15**, 243–251.
20. Hommes, F. A., Eller, A. G. and Taylor, E. H. (1982) Turnover of the fast components of myelin and myelin proteins in experimental hyperphenylalaninaemia. Relevance to termination of dietary treatment of human phenylketonuria. *J. Inherit. Metab. Dis.*, **5**, 21–27.
21. Lou, H. C., Lykkelund, C., Gerdes, A. M., Udesen, H. and Bruhn, P. (1987) Increased vigilance and dopamine synthesis by large doses of tyrosine or phenylalanine restriction in phenylketonuria. *Acta Paediatr. Scand.*, **76**, 560–565.
22. Bickel, H., Gerrard, J. and Hickmans, E. M. (1953) The influence of phenylalanine intake on phenylketonuria (preliminary communication). *Lancet*, **ii**, 812–813.
23. Guthrie, R. and Susi, A. (1963) A simple phenylalanine method for detecting phenylketonuria in large populations of newborn infants. *Pediatrics*, **32**, 338–343.
24. Smith, I., Lobascher, M. E., Stevenson, J. E. *et al.* (1978) Effect of stopping low phenylalanine diet on intellectual progress of children with phenylketonuria. *BMJ*, **ii**, 723–726.

25. Smith, I., Beasley, M. G. and Ades, A. E. (1990) Intelligence and quality of dietary treatment in phenylketonuria. *Arch. Dis. Child.*, **65**, 472–478.
26. Melnick, C. R., Michals, K. K. and Matalon, R. (1981) Linguistic development in children with phenylketonuria and normal intelligence. *J. Pediatr.*, **98**, 269–272.
27. Fischler, K., Azen, C., Henderson, R., Friedman, E. and Koch, R. (1987) Psychoeducational findings among children treated for phenylketonuria. *Am. J. Ment. Defic.*, **92**, 65–73.
28. Smith, I., Beasley, M., Wolff, O. H. and Ades, E. A. (1988) Behavioural disturbance in eight year olds with early treated phenylketonuria (PKU). *J. Pediatr.*, **112**, 403–408.
29. Smith, I., Beasley, M. and Ades, E. A. (1991) Effects on intelligence of relaxing the low phenylalanine diet in phenylketonuria. *Arch. Dis. Child.*, **66**, 311–316.
30. Dobson, J. C., Williamson, M. I., Azen, C. and Koch, R. (1977) Intellectual assessment of 111 four year old children with phenylketonuria. *Pediatrics*, **60**, 822–827.
31. Koch, R., Azen, C. G., Friedman, E. G. and Williamson, M. L. (1982) Preliminary report on the effects of diet discontinuation in PKU. *J. Pediatr.*, **100**, 870–875.
32. Villasana, E., Butler, I. J., William, J. C. and Roonngta, S. M. (1989) Neurological deterioration in an adult with phenylketonuria. *J. Inherit. Metab. Dis.*, **12**, 451–459.
33. Thompson, A. J., Smith, I., Brenton, D. *et al.* (1990) Neurological deterioration in young adults with phenylketonuria. *Lancet*, **336**, 602–605.
34. Bick, U., Fahrendorf, G., Ludolph, A. C. *et al.* (1991) Disturbed myelination in patients with treated hyperphenylalaninaemia: evaluation with magnetic resonance imaging. *Eur. J. Pediatr.*, **22**, 147.
35. Tomà, P., Oddone, M., Lucigrai, G. *et al.* (1991) Phenylketonuria (PKU): brain magnetic resonance (MR) findings. *Neuropediatrics*, **22**, 174.
36. Meyding-Lamade, U. K., Pietz, J., Fahrendorf, G. and Sartor, K. J. (1992) Treated phenylketonuria: evaluation of cranial MR images and clinical data. *Neurology*, Cleveland **42**(3), 286.
37. McCombe, P. A., McLaughlin, D. B., Chalk, J. B. *et al.* (1992) Spasticity and white matter abnormalities in adult phenylketonuria. *J. Neurol. Neurosurg. Psychiatry*, **55**, 359–361.
38. Thompson, A. J., Kermode, A. G., MacManus, D. G. *et al.* (1990) Patterns of disease activity in multiple sclerosis: a clinical and magnetic resonance imaging study. *BMJ*, **300**, 631–634.
39. Jones, S. J., Turano, G., Kriss, A., Shawkat, F., Kendall, B. and Thompson, A. J. (1995) Visual evoked potentials in phenylketonuria: association with brain MRI, dietary status and intelligence quotient. *J. Neurol. Neurosurg. Psychiatry* (in press).
40. Fazekas, F., Offenbacher, H., Fuchs, S. *et al.* (1988) Criteria for an increased specificity of MRI interpretation in elderly subjects with suspected multiple sclerosis. *Neurology*, **38**, 1822–1825.
41. Bick, U., Ullrich, K., Stöber, U. *et al.* (1991) MRI white matter abnormalities in patients with treated hyperphenylalaninemia: disturbed myelination or toxic edema? *Neuropediatrics*, **22**, 174.
42. Urenjak, J., Williams, S. R., Gadian, D. G. and Noble, M. (1993) Proton nuclear magnetic resonance spectroscopy unambiguously identifies different neural cell types. *J. Neurosci.*, **13**(3), 981–989.
43. Davie, C. A., Barker, G. J., Brenton, D., Miller, D. H. and Thompson, A. J. (1994) Proton magnetic resonance spectroscopy in adult cases of phenylketonuria. *J. Neurol. Neurosurg. Psychiatry*, **57**, 1292.
44. Novotny, J., Avison, M. J., Rothman, D. L. *et al.* (1989) Detection of

phenylketonuria in the human brain. *Society of Magnetic Resonance in Medicine, Book of Abstracts*, **1**, 441.

45. Kreis, R., Pietz, J., Penzien, J., Herschkowitz, N. and Boesch, C. (1994) Unequivocal identification and quantitation of phenylalanine in the brain of patients with phenylketonuria by means of localized *in vivo* ^{1}H MRS. *Society of Magnetic Resonance in Medicine, Book of Abstracts*, **1**, 308.
46. Medical Research Council Working Party on Phenylketonuria (1993) Recommendations on the dietary management of phenylketonuria. *Arch. Dis. Child*, **68**, 426–427.
47. Konecki, D. S. and Lichter-Konecki, U. (1991) The phenylketonuria locus; current knowledge about alleles and mutations of the phenylalanine hydroxylase gene in various populations. *Hum. Genet.*, **87**, 377–388.
48. Okano, Y., Eisensmith, R. C., Guttler, F. *et al.* (1991) Molecular basis of phenotypic heterogeneity in phenylketonuria. *N. Engl. J. Med.*, **324**, 1232–1238.
49. Woo (1991) Personal communication. European Metabolic Group, Copenhagen.

8 Chorea, Athetosis, Dystonia, Tremor and Parkinsonism

KIMBERLY S. TRINIDAD
and
ROGER KURLAN
University of Rochester, NY, USA

CHOREA, ATHETOSIS

CLINICAL PHENOMENOLOGY

The term chorea, derived from the Latin word for 'dance', refers to arrhythmic (irregularly timed), random, brief, purposeless involuntary movements[1]. The disorder may be generalized or it may be confined to the extremities, trunk, face, or buccal-oral-lingual region. When facial muscles are involved, a variety of facial expressions may occur along with chewing movements, and lip and tongue protrusion[2]. Involvement of the neck and trunk leads to swaying and jerking of the head and body. Chorea of the limbs may give the appearance of restlessness as the movements flow from one body part to another. Choreic gait may have a dance-like, halting or lurching appearance. Chorea often intrudes on volitional activity so that patients are unable to maintain a sustained action for more than a few seconds. When asked to supply a constant grip to the examiner's fingers, for example, there is intermittent relaxation and tightening of the hand ('milkmaid grasp'). Similarly, patients with lingual chorea may be unable to protrude the tongue in a sustained fashion. The severity of chorea may vary from the appearance of mild fidgetiness to intense, high-amplitude movements which impair balance.

'Ballismus' describes wild flinging or throwing movements of the limbs which can be considered to represent an extreme form of chorea[3]. Ballistic movements are usually limited to one side of the body (hemiballismus), but bilateral involvement may occur. While the sudden, rapid movements of pure chorea may be seen in some childhood disorders (e.g. Sydenham's chorea), the movements are more typically combined with slower, sinuous, writhing movements of the distal parts of the extremities known as athetosis. The term 'choreoathetosis' is applied to this form of movement disorder.

Movement and Allied Disorders. Edited by M. M. Robertson and V. Eapen

PATHOPHYSIOLOGY

Continuous changes in the activation order of muscles and in the length of electromyographic (EMG) bursts are observed during choreic movements, but there is no single pattern of EMG activity that adequately characterizes chorea[4].

Like most movement disorders, chorea is thought to arise from dysfunction of the basal ganglia, most notably striatum (caudate and putamen), pallidum and subthalamic nucleus. The basal ganglia function in modifying the motor output of the cerebral cortex, act to select or focus behaviours through reinforcement of intended or ongoing activity and suppression of unwanted or interfering behaviours. As basal ganglia circuitry is currently viewed, there are two separate but interconnecting circuits which seem to be modulated by the striatum[5]. The first pathway is from cortex to striatal matrix to medial pallidum and pars reticulata, and then to thalamus and cortex. Dopaminergic input from the substantia nigra normally excites or stimulates this circuit. The second pathway is from cortex to striatal matrix to lateral pallidum to subthalamic nucleus to medial pallidum/pars reticulata, and then to thalamus and cortex. This circuit is inhibited by dopaminergic inputs. Under this conceptualization, loss of specific subgroups of neurons in the striatum would produce a loss of matrix inhibitory inputs to the lateral pallidum and result in chorea. A subthalamic nucleus lesion would produce a similar clinical effect. Using this notion of basal ganglia function, chorea may be viewed as fragments of cortically generated movements superimposed on a background of other motor behaviours[1].

A variety of neurotransmitters are used as chemical messengers within the basal ganglia. Despite growing knowledge of the chemical morphology in this brain region, a common pathophysiological mechanism for all types of chorea has not yet been identified. Excessive dopaminergic activity is thought to be important and may explain why such movements respond to agents that block dopamine receptors (i.e., neuroleptics) or deplete synaptic dopamine (e.g., reserpine, tetrabenazine). Recent attention has focused on the role of excitatory neurotransmitters.

AETIOLOGIES OF CHILDHOOD CHOREA

Chorea may be caused by a wide variety of medical disorders. The following discussion classifies choreic disorders according to their presumed aetiology or pathogenesis and emphasizes those most commonly encountered in childhood[6,7].

DEVELOPMENTAL CHOREAS (Table 8.1)

Chorea may occur as a normal physiological manifestation of infant motor

Table 8.1. Developmental choreas

Physiological chorea of infancy
Athetoid cerebral palsy
Choreiform syndrome

development, appearing most prominently during the first three months of life and gradually disappearing within the context of cortical/basal ganglionic maturation[8]. Such *'physiological chorea of infancy'* is readily distinguished from chorea resulting from perinatal brain injury or cerebral palsy which is associated with other features of cerebral dysfunction. This *'hyperkinetic'* or *'athetoid'* form of cerebral palsy is most commonly ascribed to some degree of perinatal asphyxia with or without kernicterus, but the relative roles of pre- and perinatal events remain controversial. In clinical series of patients with cerebral palsy, 25–30% of cases have been described as being hyperkinetic[9,10]. In some cases, abnormal movements may not appear for several years after birth. One possible explanation for this is that choreic movements require an anatomical substrate that is not sufficiently developed at the time of the initial injury. Progression can occur into the second decade of life, and the movement disorder may evolve into overt dystonia. There is no specific therapy for this form of choreoathetosis. If the movements are disabling, they may respond to neuroleptic therapy. Apparently representing a maturation problem, chorea may occur in preschool and early school-age children and is often accompanied by other signs of minimal brain dysfunction and postural instability (sometimes referred to as the *'choreiform syndrome'*)[11]. Presumably in these children there is defective or delayed maturation of normal basal ganglia influences on motor function.

HEREDITARY CHOREAS (Table 8.2)

The designation hereditary chorea has traditionally been used for disorders inherited in an autosomal dominant pattern, notably Huntington's disease. However, there are also a number of recessive and

Table 8.2. Hereditary choreas

Juvenile Huntington's disease
Benign familial chorea
Hereditary paroxysmal choreas
Paroxysmal dystonic choreoathetosis
Familial paroxysmal kinesiogenic choreoathetosis
Inborn errors of metabolism (e.g., gangliosidoses, lipofuscinoses, phakomatoses, Lesch–Nyhan syndrome, Hallervorden–Spatz disease)

X-linked hereditary choreas in which clinical onset usually occurs in infancy, childhood or early adolescence. These choreic disorders are generally associated with evidence of widespread cerebral dysfunction and are usually inexorably progressive. However, some of these conditions, notably Wilson's disease (see Chapter 6) are eminently treatable. Included are most of the traditional inborn errors of metabolism affecting the central nervous system, gangliosidoses, lipofuscinoses, phakomatoses, Hallervorden–Spatz disease, Lesch–Nyhan syndrome and its variants, and myoclonic epilepsy[1].

Juvenile Huntington's disease

In contrast to the early-onset hereditary choreas, those with clinical onset in late adolescence or adulthood are more commonly inherited as autosomal dominant traits and, therefore, are usually revealed in the setting of a positive family history. Huntington's disease (HD), the prototype of autosomal dominant choreas, is a neurodegenerative disorder that is manifested typically by chorea. The HD gene has recently been localized to the short arm of chromosome 4[12] and is characterized by an abnormal repeat of the trinucleotide cytosine-adenine-guanine (CAG). The illness usually emerges at an age of about 35–40 years with disorders of movement, mentation (dementia) and behaviour (depression). The clinical features reflect a progressive neuronal loss that is most prominent in the striatum.

About 10% of HD gene carriers develop signs of illness prior to the age of 20. These patients with so-called 'juvenile HD' (Westphal variant) are often distinguished from adult-onset patients by the prominence of dystonia, parkinsonism, ocular motor abnormalities, the presence of ataxia or seizures and a more rapid rate of functional decline[13]. Chorea may be minimal or absent in these patients. In 70–80% of childhood-onset cases, patients have inherited the gene from an affected father, in contrast to the expected 50% rate[12]. Molecular analysis of the HD gene indicates that the length of trinucleotide repeats closely correlates with the age at onset of the disorder; thus, the juvenile-onset cases of HD have the longest trinucleotide repeats. The inheritance of the longest repeats from male transmissions explains the observation that most juvenile-onset HD cases result from paternal inheritance. It appears that the process of spermatogenesis in males is a particular source of instability in repeat length. For full discussion of the genetics of HD, see Chapter 12.

Current treatment of HD is limited to palliation of symptoms. Disabling chorea is treated with dopamine antagonists, while bradykinesia and rigidity may respond to anti-parkinsonian drugs. Antidepressant therapy or counselling may be required for patients with depression, and neuroleptics may modify aggressive or violent behaviour. There is no treatment for the progressive dementia of HD. Severe dysphagia, which may be worsened by neuroleptic therapy, often leads to severe weight loss and may require the placement of a feeding gastrostomy tube. Genetic counselling is an important component in the management of this condition and genetic testing from blood samples is now available for the diagnosis of symptomatic and at-risk individuals, and for prenatal analysis of amniotic cells or chorionic villus samples[14].

Benign familial chorea

Benign familial chorea (or chronic juvenile chorea) has been considered a *forme fruste* of HD since it is usually dominantly inherited and shares clinical features[15]. Unlike HD, however, evidence of striatal degeneration is minimal or absent in this more benign and slowly progressive condition. Benign familial chorea typically begins in the first decade and may be evident in the first months of life. Chorea is most prevalent in the face and distal arms. The legs are less involved, although gait may be clumsy with frequent falling, particularly in the youngest children. The chorea may be associated with a postural tremor but speech and intelligence are unaffected. School performance may be impaired due to problems with arm and hand dexterity. The involuntary movements are usually persistent and non-progressive or improve with age, but in some cases there may be some worsening of chorea during adolescence. Treatment involves symptomatic therapy for the choreic movements if they interfere with daily functioning. Genetic testing can be used to distinguish this disorder from juvenile HD.

Hereditary paroxysmal choreas

In contrast to the typically continuous or progressive chorea observed in the foregoing genetic disorders, a group of hereditary paroxysmal choreic disorders has been recognized. First described by Mount and Reback in 1940, patients with *paroxysmal dystonic choreoathetosis* (PDC) experience attacks of choreic movements and dystonic posturing of the trunk and limbs which last minutes to hours[16,17]. The attacks are often preceded by a prodromal sensation of tightness or stiffness and may be provoked by a number of different factors, such as alcohol, fatigue or cold. There is no alteration of consciousness and patients are normal between episodes. The condition tends to be chronic and lifelong and is inherited in an autosomal dominant fashion in most reported families. Of the various drugs used, benzodiazepines seem to have the most predictable therapeutic effect.

In *familial paroxysmal kinesiogenic choreoathetosis* (FPKC), attacks are provoked by a sudden movement and are brief, lasting seconds to a few minutes. Episodes tend to recur many times daily[18]. Choreoathetotic movements are frequently confined to one side of the body, but they may be generalized. The condition is typically familial and autosomal dominant patterns have been reported in some families. The symptoms of FPKC usually respond readily to anticonvulsant medications, such as phenobarbital, carbamazepine, valproate or phenytoin.

INFECTIOUS/IMMUNOLOGICAL CHOREAS (Table 8.3)

Infectious and immunological choreas are thought to be mediated by antigens or antibodies (humoral or cell-mediated), immune complexes, bacterial toxins or direct invasion by a pathogen. *Sydenham's chorea* is the most widely recognized choreic sequelae of infection and is thought to develop as a late complication of streptococcal pharyngitis[19]. Less than one-third of patients, however, give the expected history of pharyngeal infection. The incidence of Sydenham's chorea has declined with the widespread use of antibiotics. Recent outbreaks in some areas have been ascribed to the emergence of new strains of group A streptococcus and aggressive treatment of streptococcal infections remains of prime importance in preventing rheumatic complications.

Patient's with Sydenham's chorea are usually between 5 and 15 years of age and there is a strong female preponderance. The streptococcal infection usually precedes the movement disorder by 1–6 months. Although chorea is usually generalized, some patients (about 20%) have unilateral involvement (hemichorea) on initial presentation. Involuntary movements may be accompanied by dysarthria and personality changes, particularly irritability and obsessive–compulsive behaviour, or a frank confusional state. The chorea typically worsens over 2–4 weeks, persists for a variable period of time, and then resolves spontaneously over 3–6 months. In about one-quarter of patients, chorea recurs, usually within two years.

Since Sydenham's chorea usually begins long after the initial infection,

Table 8.3. Infectious/immunological choreas

Sydenham's chorea
Systemic lupus erythematosis
Scarlet fever
Diphtheria
Pertussis
Typhoid fever
Viral encephalitis
Neurosyphilis
Mononucleosis
Bacterial endocarditis
Sarcoidosis
Periarteritis nodosa
Bechet's syndrome
Schönlein–Henoch purpura
Multiple sclerosis

laboratory studies such as antistreptolysin antibody titres, erythrocyte sedimentation rate and throat culture are often unrevealing and the diagnosis is made by history and clinical presentation. Once Sydenham's chorea is diagnosed, patients should be evaluated for evidence of rheumatic cardiac disease.

The pathophysiology of Sydenham's chorea remains unknown but antibodies to striatal and subthalamic neurons have been identified[20,21]. Neuroleptics can be used to treat disabling chorea, but there is no known specific therapy to shorten the duration of the choreic episode. Many clinicians recommend treatment with penicillin when the diagnosis is made, even without a positive culture for streptococcus. Long-term subsequent prophylactic treatment to prevent rheumatic complications of dental and other procedures may also be recommended.

Chorea is a rare manifestation of *systemic lupus erythematosus* (SLE)[22]. In a review of 36 published cases, the age at onset was 20 years or less in 64% of patients, and in 30% of patients, chorea was the presenting symptom[23]. The duration of chorea may vary from days to years and the chorea may be episodic. The chorea usually presents in a hemidistribution, although generalized chorea may occur. SLE-related vasculopathy or autoimmune, cytotoxic antibodies reacting with neuronal antigens have been proposed to be possible mechanisms responsible for the development of chorea. It has also been suggested that the lupus anticoagulant (antiphospholipid antibody) has a pathogenetic role in the appearance of chorea[24]. Therapy is generally directed at the primary disease.

DRUG-INDUCED/TOXIC CHOREAS (Table 8.4)

With the decline in the incidence of Sydenham's chorea, drugs are now considered the most common cause of chorea in children. The number of

Table 8.4. Drug-induced/toxic choreas

Neuroleptics
Tardive dyskinesia
Withdrawal–emergent syndrome
Psychostimulants
Anticonvulsants
Oral contraceptives
Steroids
Antihistamines
Tricyclic antidepressants
Alcohol intoxication and withdrawal
Carbon monoxide
Manganese
Toluene (glue sniffing)

drug-induced and toxic causes of chorea has expanded considerably in recent years due to improved recognition of these largely iatrogenic conditions and to the increasing use of psychoactive medications in children[1]. The importance of these disorders is underscored by the fact that eliminating exposure to the drugs will eventually result in a reduction or resolution of the movement disorder. However, the choreic sequelae of chronic neuroleptic administration (see below) may be permanent or very long-lasting, emphasizing the need for caution when using these drugs. Non-toxic dosages of medications commonly prescribed in childhood, including noradrenergic stimulants, anticonvulsants and oestrogens, may induce chorea in individuals who have seemingly normal basal ganglia function. Among the toxins that can cause chorea, alcohol is a prime offender, usually in the setting of alcohol withdrawal.

Perhaps the best-known category of drug-induced chorea is that associated with neuroleptic treatment. In addition to children requiring antipsychotic therapy, others at risk include cancer patients receiving the antiemetic medications metoclopramide or prochlorperazine and patients being treated for Gilles de la Tourette syndrome. *'Tardive dyskinesia'* refers to the development of abnormal involuntary movements in patients treated chronically with neuroleptic medications. Choreic movements involving the face, such as lip smacking, chewing or tongue protrusion, are most common. Chorea may also involve the neck, trunk and limbs. Patients are typically exposed to neuroleptics for several months prior to the onset of dyskinesias, but the duration of treatment may be much briefer. The incidence of tardive dyskinesia in children is unknown, but one study of 41 children and adolescents treated with neuroleptics found the disorder in three patients[25]. The treatment of tardive dyskinesia involves discontinuation of the offending agent if possible. Up to one-third of patients will have resolution of symptoms within 3 months of stopping the drug, but the movement disorder may persist for years[26]. Medications that deplete dopamine, such as reserpine and tetrabenazine, have been effective in improving dyskinesias for some patients. Some patients have also benefited from treatment with benzodiazepines, baclofen and valproic acid. Patients may first experience transient chorea or other involuntary movements upon discontinuation of neuroleptic therapy, a condition which has been referred to as the *'withdrawal emergent syndrome'*. The movements are indistinguishable from those of tardive dyskinesia and resolution usually occurs within a few months of the cessation of neuroleptic therapy.

METABOLIC/ENDOCRINE/NUTRITIONAL CHOREAS (Table 8.5)

Chorea is an occasional manifestation of metabolic disorders, such as electrolyte abnormalities, hypoglycaemia, hyperglycaemia, and hepatic and renal failure. Chronic, rather than acute, metabolic disturbances more

Table 8.5. Miscellaneous choreas

Metabolic disorders
Hyponatraemia, Hypernatraemia
Hypoglycaemia, Hyperglycaemia
Hypocalcaemia
Hypomagnesaemia
Hepatic encephalopathy
Renal encephalopathy
Endocrine disorders
Hyperthyroidism
Hypoparathyroidism
Pseudohypoparathyroidism
Chorea gravidarum (in pregnancy)
Addison's disease
Nutritional disorders
Vitamin B12 deficiency (infants)
Beriberi
Pellagra
Post-traumatic
Brain tumors
Post-operative (cardiovascular surgery)
Cerebrovascular (stroke, haemorrhage, arteriovenous malformation, migraine, polycythemia vera)

commonly lead to the development of chorea. Hyperthyroidism is a sufficiently common cause of chorea to warrant the screening of thyroid function in individuals with chorea of undetermined cause.

MISCELLANEOUS CHOREAS

A variety of traumatic insults and tumours of the brain may produce chorea. Choreic movements have been reported in infants and children following a variety of cardiovascular procedures, presumably due to impaired cerebral perfusion affecting the basal ganglia. In a recent review, Medlock and colleagues found that over a 10-year period during which 668 children underwent open cardiac surgery, eight (1.2%) developed post-operative chorea[27]. The onset of chorea was 3–12 days following surgery. Three patients had transient and five had persistent chorea. None of the patients was developmentally normal 22–130 months following surgery. The authors found a strong association between postoperative chorea and deep hypothermia and circulatory arrest during surgery.

DYSTONIA

CLINICAL PHENOMENOLOGY

Definition

Dystonia has been defined slightly differently by several authors over the years. Herz defined dystonia as slow, sustained postures, while Denny-Brown described it as a fixed or relatively fixed attitude[28,29]. In 1984, an *ad hoc* committee of the Dystonia Medical Research Foundation whose members included A. Barbeau, D. B. Calne, S. Fahn, C. D. Marsden, J. Menkes and G. F. Wooten, defined dystonia as 'a syndrome of sustained muscle contractions, frequently causing twisting and repetitive movements, or abnormal postures'[30].

Classification

Dystonia is commonly classified by age at onset, aetiology and distribution.

Age at onset

This classification can be helpful in guiding toward particular aetiologies, as well as in determining prognosis. The *ad hoc* committee divided age at onset into three groups.

1. Childhood (0–12 years).
2. Adolescent (13–20 years).
3. Adult (>20 years).

Further subdivision of the childhood group may be helpful (see below). For idiopathic dystonia, young age at onset is associated with increased likelihood of the dystonia becoming severe and generalized[31–33].

Aetiology

Classification by aetiology can be divided into two major categories: idiopathic (primary) and symptomatic (secondary). Idiopathic dystonias may be subdivided into familial and nonfamilial (sporadic) types. Secondary dystonias are those caused by identifiable diseases; in some of these conditions, dystonia is only one of many symptoms and signs.

Body distribution

When classified according to body distribution, dystonia can be divided as focal, segmental, generalized, multifocal, and hemidystonia. Focal dystonia involves a single body part. Examples of common focal dystonias are blepharospasm which affects the eyelids, torticollis which affects the neck, and writer's cramp which affects the arm. Segmental dystonia involves two or more contiguous body parts. With cranial dystonia, two or more parts of cranial and neck musculature are affected. Axial dystonia involves the neck and trunk. Brachial dystonia refers to one arm and axial or both arms with or without axial dystonia. Crural dystonia affects one leg and the trunk or both legs with or without the trunk. Two further segmental dystonias are cranial plus brachial and cranial plus axial dystonias. Generalized dystonia is a combination of segmental crural dystonia and dystonia of any other body part. Multifocal dystonia involves two or more noncontiguous body parts such as one leg and the neck or one arm and the contralateral leg. Hemidystonia affects parts of one-half of the body. Dystonia of one leg and the ipsilateral arm would be classified as hemidystonia, as would dystonia of one leg, the trunk and the ipsilateral arm. The occurrence of segmental dystonia and hemidystonia suggests focal, structural lesions.

PATHOPHYSIOLOGY

The pathophysiology of dystonia is not well known. Co-contraction of agonist and antagonist muscles can be demonstrated by palpation of muscle bellies and by electromyography[34–36]. Contraction of remote muscles, known as 'overflow' may be found, particularly during fine movements[35]. Reciprocal inhibition is abnormal when assessing the H reflex in people with focal or segmental dystonia[36].

Dystonia is thought to be a disorder of the basal ganglia. Some conditions which cause dystonia, such as Leigh's disease and carbon monoxide intoxication, however, involve structures and pathways outside of the basal ganglia. Dystonia has been reported with structural lesions of the caudate nucleus, lentiform nuclei (particularly the putamen) and thalamus[37].

The bioamine neurotransmitter system is thought to be responsible for dystonia, most likely the dopamine system. However, more detailed information regarding the chemical pathology of dystonia is lacking.

GENETICS

Some of the dystonias are hereditary. Primary dystonia has been transmitted within families in autosomal dominant and X-linked patterns. Twenty-five percent of 40 persons with idiopathic focal dystonia studied by Waddy *et al.*, had relatives with dystonia[38]; segregation analysis suggested autosomal dominant inheritance, possibly with reduced penetrance. Fletcher *et al.*, studied 100 British families in which there was generalized, multifocal or segmental dystonia and concluded that 85% of the cases of idiopathic torsion dystonia (ITD) were due to an autosomal dominant gene with 40% penetrance and variable expression[39].

A gene for ITD, in one non-Jewish and several Jewish kindreds, has recently been localized to chromosome 9q32-q34[40,41]. The gene for the dystonia–parkinsonism syndrome in people of descent from Panay, Philippines has been localized to Xq13[42]. Some of the secondary forms of dystonia are inherited as well. For full discussion of the genetics of dystonia, see Chapter 12.

AETIOLOGIES OF DYSTONIA

The many disorders reported to cause dystonia are listed in Table 8.6. Tables 8.7–8.12 list the disorders most likely to cause dystonia in particular paediatric age groups. Because a discussion of all of these disorders is beyond the scope of this chapter, the text below reviews the primary dystonias and the most common forms of secondary dystonia.

EVALUATION

Table 8.6 includes the diagnostic tests available for specific diseases that may cause dystonia. In order to rule out the potentially treatable condition, Wilson's disease, a slit lamp eye examination should be performed and serum copper and ceruloplasmin levels should be obtained for any child with a movement disorder in whom the diagnosis is not known. Some authorities recommend liver biopsy for a child with an undiagnosed movement disorder, even when serum copper and ceruloplasmin are normal and no Kayser–Fleischer rings are evident.

TREATMENT STRATEGIES

Many authorities recommend a trial of L-dopa in all children with dystonia, as some may have a L-dopa-responsive form (see below). Children with L-dopa-responsive dystonia–parkinsonism disorder respond dramatically to small doses of the drug and there are very few side effects. One can start with one-half of a Sinemet 25/100 tablet in the morning and increase by one-half tablet every 2 days until the child is taking 1 tablet 3 times daily. Failure to respond to this dose indicates that the child does not have L-dopa-responsive dystonia.

Some other primary dystonias have specific therapies. Paroxysmal dystonic choreoathetosis may respond to clonazepam, acetazolamide or oxazepam. Phenytoin is the drug of choice for treating paroxysmal kinesiogenic choreoathetosis, but phenobarbital, carbamazepine and diazepam may be helpful as well. For the secondary dystonias, the main therapeutic approach is directed toward the primary process when possible.

Symptomatic therapy for dystonia is indicated when the disorder is

Table 8.6. Aetiologies of dystonia

Disorder	Laboratory tests
Ataxia telangiectasia	Serum IgA, alpha-fetoprotein
Benign idiopathic dystonia of infancy	
Calcifications of basal ganglia	CT, serum calcium and parathyroid
Ceroid lipofuscinosis	Skin, conjunctival or rectal biopsy
Dentato-rubro-pallido-luysian atrophy	MRI, genetic testing
Dystonic lipidosis	Fibroblast sphingomyelinase, bone marrow biopsy
Familial striatal necrosis	MRI
Galactosaemia	Qualitative or quantitative galactose-1-phosphate uridyl transferase assay
Gaucher's disease (infantile/Type 1)	Glucocerebrosidase, bone marrow biopsy
Glutaric acidaemia (Type 1)	Fibroblast or leukocyte glutaryl CoA dehydrogenase Plasma and urine glutaric acid Metabolic acidosis and ketosis
GM1 gangliosidosis	Leukocyte or fibroblast beta-galactosidase, rectal biopsy Brain imaging
GM2 gangliosidosis (Sandhoff's disease)	Leukocyte or fibroblast hexosaminidase A, B, S
Hallervorden–Spatz disease	Bone marrow biopsy, lymphocytes (cytoplasmic inclusions) MRI
Hartnup's disease	Urine amino acids
Hereditary stiff baby	
Homocystinuria	Serum and urine amino acids Methionine and homocystine
Huntington's disease	Brain imaging CAG repeat genetic testing
Idiopathic torsion dystonia	Genetic testing
Infectious/post-infectious (viral, syphilis, tuberculous meningitis, non-specific)	CSF microbiology
Krabbe's disease (globoid leukodystrophy)	MRI
Leber's disease and dystonia	CT, MRI, eye exam
Lesch–Nyhan syndrome	Fibroblast or erythrocyte hypoxanthine-guanine phosphoribosyl transferase Urine-uric acid:creatinine ratio
L-Dopa-responsive dystonia-parkinsonism	Biopterin deficiency in some
Machado–Joseph–Azorean disease (Type 1)	

continued overleaf

Table 8.6. *(continued)*

Disorder	Laboratory tests
Metachromatic leukodystrophy (sulfatide lipidosis)	Leukocyte or fibroblast Aryl Sulfatase A Urine and plasma sulfatide Nerve conduction velocities Nerve biopsy
Methylmalonic acidaemia	Serum methylmalonic acid Quantitative urine and blood organic acids Metabolic acidosis Fibroblast methylmalonyl CoA mutase Brain imaging
Neuroacanthocytosis	Serum CPK Blood smear for acanthocytes
Neuronal intranuclear inclusion disease	Brain biopsy
Nocturnal paroxysmal dystonia (paroxysmal hypnogenic dystonia)	
Paroxysmal torticollis of infancy	Caloric testing (no nystagmus)
Paroxysmal dystonic choreoathetosis	
Paroxysmal kinesigenic choreoathetosis	
Perlizaeus–Merzbacher disease	MRI
Perinatal asphyxia/anoxia (dystonic form)	± brain imaging
Perinatal kernicterus	± brain imaging
Phenylketonuria	Newborn metabolic screening
Sandifer's syndrome	Gastro-oesophageal imaging
Spasmus nutans	
Subacute necrotizing encephalomyelopathy (Leigh's disease)	Serum lactate and pyruvate Metabolic acidosis
Sulfite oxidase deficiency	Sulfite oxidase Urine and plasma amino acids S-sulfocysteine and cysteine Serum sulfite
Trauma	Brain imaging
Triosephosphate isomerase deficiency	Leukocyte or fibroblast triosephosphate isomerase
Tumor	Brain imaging
Vascular (ischaemic, haemorrhagic malformations)	Brain imaging
Wilson's disease (Hepatolenticular degeneration)	Serum copper and ceruloplasmin Slit lamp Liver biopsy

Table 8.7. Causes of dystonia at any age

Stroke (typically putamen)
Arteriovenous malformations (may or may not be in the basal ganglia)
Trauma
Tumor
Encephalitis
Drugs
phenytoin
carbamazepine
phenobarbital
neuroleptics
Toxins (e.g. manganese)

Table 8.8. Causes of dystonia in the newborn (birth to 1 month)

Paroxysmal torticollis of infancy
Hereditary stiff baby syndrome
Perinatal kernicterus
Phenylketonuria
Sulfite oxidase deficiency
Gaucher's disease (infantile/Type 1)
Pelizaeus–Merzbacher disease

Table 8.9. Causes of dystonia in the infant (1–23 months)

Ataxia telangiectasia
Benign idiopathic dystonia of infancy
Calcifications of basal ganglia
Gaucher's disease (infantile/Type 1)
Glutaric acidaemia
GM2 gangliosidosis (Sandhoff's disease)
Hartnup's disease
Hereditary stiff baby syndrome
Krabbe's disease (globoid cell leukodystrophy)
Leber's disease and dystonia
Lesch–Nyhan syndrome
Methylmalonic acidaemia
Paroxysmal dystonic choreoathetosis
Paroxysmal kinesigenic choreoathetosis
Paroxysmal torticollis of infancy
Pelizaeus–Merzbacher disease
Perinatal asphyxia/anoxia (dystonic form)
Perinatal kernicterus
Phenylketonuria (variants)
Spasmus nutans
Subacute necrotizing encephalomyelopathy (Leigh's disease)
Triosephosphate isomerase deficiency

Table 8.10. Causes of dystonia in the preschool child (2–5 years)

Ataxia telangiectasia
Benign idiopathic dystonia of infancy
Calcifications of basal ganglia
Ceroid lipofuscinosis
Gaucher's disease (infantile/Type 1)
Glutaric acidaemia (Type 1)
GM2 gangliosidosis (Sandhoff's disease)
Hartnup's disease
Hereditary stiff baby syndrome
Huntington's disease
Leber's disease and dystonia
Lesch–Nyhan syndrome
L-Dopa-responsive dystonia–parkinsonism
Metachromatic leukodystrophy (sulfatide lipidosis)
Methylmalonic acidaemia
Neuronal intranuclear inclusion disease
Nocturnal paroxysmal dystonia (paroxysmal hypnogenic dystonia)
Paroxysmal torticollis of infancy
Paroxysmal dystonic choreoathetosis
Paroxysmal kinesigenic choreoathetosis
Pelizaeus–Merzbacher disease
Perinatal asphyxia/anoxia (dystonic form)
Perinatal kernicterus
Spasmus nutans
Subacute necrotizing encephalomyelopathy (Leigh's disease)
Triosephosphate isomerase deficiency

significantly interfering with the child's functioning and/or care. Anticholinergic medications are of benefit to some children. Children who are otherwise healthy, with little other neurological involvement, often tolerate high doses of these medications with few adverse effects. Benzodiazepines, particularly clonazepam, may be helpful, but sedation and clumsiness are common dose-limiting side effects.

SPECIFIC DISORDERS

Idiopathic torsion dystonia

Idiopathic torsion dystonia (ITD) was previously termed 'dystonia musculorum deformans', the latter designation being inappropriate because the disease is not of the muscle itself, and deformity is not certain.

Childhood onset ITD is a familial disorder, with the mode of inheritance and genetics being different in different kindreds. Autosomal dominant and recessive, as well as sex-linked recessive transmission have been described and sometimes debated[43–47]. A gene for ITD, in one non-Jewish

Table 8.11. Causes of dystonia in children (6–12 years)

Ataxia telangiectasia
Calcifications of basal ganglia
Ceroid lipofuscinosis
Dystonic lipidosis
Galactosaemia
GM1 gangliosidosis
GM2 gangliosidosis (Sandhoff's disease)
Hallervorden–Spatz disease
Hartnup's disease
Huntington's disease
Idiopathic torsion dystonia
Leber's disease and dystonia
Lesch–Nyhan syndrome
L-Dopa-responsive dystonia–parkinsonism
Metachromatic leukodystrophy (sulfatide lipidosis)
Methylmalonic acidaemia
Neuronal intranuclear inclusion disease
Nocturnal paroxysmal dystonia (paroxysmal hypnogenic dystonia)
Paroxysmal dystonic choreoathetosis (non-kinesigenic)
Paroxysmal kinesigenic choreoathetosis (PKC)
Pelizaeus–Merzbacher disease
Perinatal asphyxia/anoxia (dystonic form)
Perinatal kernicterus
Subacute necrotizing encephalomyelopathy (Leigh's disease)
Wilson's disease (hepatolenticular degeneration)

and several Jewish kindreds, has been localized to chromosome 9q32-q34[40,41]. The gene for the dystonia–parkinsonism syndrome in persons of descent from Panay, Philippines has been localized to Xq13[42]; see also Chapter 12.

The dystonia usually starts between the ages of 6 and 12 years as action dystonia in one lower extremity[48–50]. The most common initial symptom is torsion dystonia involving the foot, usually plantar flexed and inverted, while walking, but not at rest or during other activities such as running or walking backwards. Symptoms often progress, varying with age at onset, site of onset, and mode of inheritance. Almost all children in whom the dystonia begins in the leg progress to have generalized dystonia within 1–5 years[50–52]. There may be less axial involvement in families showing recessive inheritance[43]. Earlier age at onset (<11 years) correlates with the eventual development of generalized dystonia, although not necessarily with the rate of symptom progression[50,51]. Maximum disability often occurs within 5–10 years, with stabilization or improvement thereafter[50]. Spontaneous remissions are described, as are recurrences, most often in the original site.

Focal dystonias that fall into the category of ITD, including spasmodic torticollis and writer's cramp, do occur in children. Most often in

Table 8.12. Causes of dystonia in the adolescent (13–18 years)

Calcifications of basal ganglia
Ceroid lipofuscinosis
Dentato-rubro-pallido-luysian atrophy
Dystonic lipidosis
GM1 gangliosidosis
GM2 gangliosidosis (Sandhoff's disease)
Galactosaemia
Hallervorden–Spatz disease
Hartnup's disease
Homocystinuria
Huntington's disease
Idiopathic torsion dystonia
Lesch–Nyhan syndrome
L-Dopa-responsive dystonia–parkinsonism
Machado–Joseph–Azorean disease (Type 1)
Metachromatic leukodystrophy (sulfatide lipidosis)
Methylmalonic acidaemia
Neuroacanthocytosis
Neuronal intranuclear inclusion disease
Nocturnal paroxysmal dystonia (paroxysmal hypnogenic dystonia)
Paroxysmal dystonic choreoathetosis
Paroxysmal kinesigenic choreoathetosis
Pelizaeus–Merzbacher disease
Perinatal asphyxia/anoxia (dystonic form)
Wilson's disease (hepatolenticular degeneration)

childhood, however, they are the initial manifestation of generalized dystonia.

Histopathological post-mortem brain examinations in several patients with ITD have been unremarkable[53–55]. Neurofibrillary tangles and mild neuronal loss within the locus ceruleus and rare neurofibrillary tangles in the substantia nigra, midbrain tegmentum and dorsal raphe were noted in a 29-year-old Jewish man with ITD[53]. Neurochemical studies and clinical experience with the pharmacology of dystonia suggest that the underlying abnormality is in the bioamine neurotransmitter system but the biochemical pathology of dystonia remains to be clarified.

There are no treatments that are specific to ITD; pharmacological therapy is largely by trial and error. Anticholinergic medications are usually the first-line agents, in gradually increasing dosages. Trihexyphenidyl in doses of 80 mg per day or higher has been effective and tolerated in children with dystonia[56,57]; high doses of anticholinergic medication early in the course of the disease may inhibit progression of dystonia[58]. Baclofen has been beneficial in some patients[59]. Botulinum toxin has Federal Drug Administration approval for use in blepharospasm and hemifacial spasm in persons older than 12 years of age, although it is being used 'off-label' in a variety of other forms of dystonia; this symptomatic treatment may be considered when therapy of focal dystonic conditions is desired.

Benign idiopathic dystonia in infancy

Willemse[60], Angelini *et al.*[61] and Deonna *et al.*[62] described dystonia during infancy that spontaneously resolved over time. Focal dystonic postures began during the first few months of life, progressed over a short period of time, then spontaneously resolved. Most involved an upper extremity or neck, although lower extremity dystonia did occur in a few patients. Angelini's cases were paroxysmal, with episodes lasting minutes to hours; in two of the nine patients, the symptoms began immediately following poliomyelitis vaccination and in one patient, symptoms began during acute benign lymphocytic choriomeningitis. Two of Angelini's patients did not experience a resolution of symptoms. A few of the patients in the three reports had pre- or perinatal complications, although they had apparently normal development before developing dystonia.

The cases reported may not represent a homogeneous clinical entity, but are grouped together because of their clinical similarities. Further studies with greater numbers of patients and longer follow-up may be helpful in understanding this clinical syndrome.

Myoclonic dystonia

Myoclonus and dystonia occur together in sporadic and autosomal dominantly inherited conditions[63,64]. In the sporadic form, prominent myoclonic jerks occur without a demonstrable electroencephalographic cortical correlate. Dystonia and myoclonus may occur in the same or distant muscles, with the myoclonic jerks frequently being superimposed upon dystonic contractions. The myoclonic jerks are 50–200 msec in duration and are irregular. Multiple medications have been tried, with a few patients responding to clonazepam, benzhexol, propranolol or lisuride.

Autosomal dominant inheritance with variable penetrance was noted in a family with myoclonus and dystonia that did not involve the lower extremities. In some persons, myoclonic jerks were associated with cortical events on electroencephalography. Ingestion of alcohol improved both the myoclonus and dystonia. The women experienced premenstrual worsening of the involuntary movements. In three patients, clonazepam was beneficial initially, although tolerance developed.

Dopa-responsive dystonia

Dopa-responsive dystonia (DRD) is an autosomal dominantly inherited condition, with gender-specific penetrance; penetrance is 15% is males and

45% in females[65]. There is no increased prevalence in the Ashkenazi Jewish population. The gene defect has not been localized; the genes for tyrosine hydroxylase[66], dopamine beta-hydroxylase[67] and the idiopathic torsion dystonia locus on 9q32-34[68] have been excluded as being genetically linked to this condition.

The pathophysiology of DRD is currently under investigation. Homovanillic acid concentration has been reduced in the cerebrospinal fluid of most patients studied[69–76]. Cerebrospinal fluid levels of biopterin (a tyrosine hydroxylase cofactor) and neopterin (a biopterin metabolite) are also reduced[69,76–79]. FD-PET scans have been normal in some subjects, although some results have suggested reduced striatal uptake of FD[80–84]. In 1993, Nygaard described the preliminary post-mortem pathological findings in a single patient with DRD[65]. There was a normal appearance and cell number, with normal tyrosine hydroxylase immunoreactivity, in the substantia nigra and striatum, and severely reduced putaminal and caudate levels of dopamine. Taken together, cerebrospinal fluid (CSF), FD-PET and neuropathological studies suggest that striatal dopaminergic cells in DRD are intact in number, but deficient in dopamine output.

DRD may be divided into two distinct clinical syndromes, one with childhood onset and the other with late adulthood onset[65]. Only the childhood onset will be discussed in this chapter. The classic presentation of the childhood onset variant is that of dystonia, usually affecting the gait, with concurrent or later development of parkinsonism and a dramatic response to L-dopa[69]. The signs and symptoms may, but not necessarily, worsen as the day progresses ('diurnal fluctuation') or increase following exertion. Early motor development is usually normal, although cases of motor delay followed by the onset of classic DRD have been described[70,85]. There have been reports of DRD in which the dystonia began in the neck or arm[86,87]. The dystonia eventually becomes generalized in most patients, some within one year[65]. The degree of disability tends to be less severe in the patients with later onset, and in these cases, parkinsonism tends to worsen in late adult life[65].

DRD often improves with very small doses of L-dopa; when a peripheral dopa-decarboxylase inhibitor is used, the required dose may be as low as 50 mg of L-dopa on alternate days. Diffuse dystonia responds to L-dopa even when symptoms have been present for many years prior to beginning treatment, although longstanding focal dystonias may be resistant to the drug[86,87]. L-dopa may be started at 50 mg per day (with a peripheral dopa-decarboxylase inhibitor) and increased every 2–3 days, as necessary. Chorea may occur with L-dopa therapy, but responds to reduction in dosage, and has not been problematic in chronic use of this medication. The response to L-dopa is typically stable over time, without motor fluctuations such as 'wearing off' and 'on–off' that often complicate treatment of Parkinson's disease and juvenile Parkinson's disease (see below)[86]. A patient with continuous response during 23 years of therapy has been reported[87].

Hereditary progressive dystonia with marked diurnal fluctuation (HPD)

Hereditary progressive dystonia with marked diurnal fluctuation is a familial, dopa-responsive dystonia that begins in childhood and is characterized by dramatic worsening as the day progresses (diurnal fluctuation). There is some debate, even among the experts, whether DRD and HPD are distinct entities, or variants of the same disorder. Segawa first reported HPD in 1972[88]. In 1993, Segawa and Nomura published a monograph defining HPD as a distinct clinical entity with the following characteristics[89].

1. Onset is in childhood.
2. Symptoms have marked diurnal fluctuation initially, although this fluctuation decreases with time.
3. Disease progression is most prominent during the first two decades and slows over time so that progression is inapparent after the fourth decade.
4. Postural limb dystonia is the main symptom, with no axial torsion or action dystonia or oculogyric crises.
5. Postural tremor at 8–10 Hz occurs in the third and fourth decades; ambulation is preserved until the advanced stage and freezing is not observed.
6. L-dopa produces marked and sustained improvement in symptoms, without dyskinesias or 'on–off'.
7. There is a predilection to the left side.
8. There is a predominance of female patients.
9. Polysomnography reveals particular abnormalities in the phasic components of sleep.
10. Memory guided and visually guided ocular saccades are abnormal.
11. Autosomal dominant inheritance with low penetrance is the most likely mode of inheritance.

Juvenile parkinsonism

Dystonia can be the first symptom of juvenile parkinsonism, although rigidity and akinesia are typically more prominent. This disorder is discussed in more detail below.

Dentatorubral–pallidoluysian atrophy (DRPLA)

DRPLA is an uncommon condition in which the dentatorubral and pallidoluysian systems degenerate simultaneously. Occurring mostly in the Japanese population, it is manifest in a variety of neurological symptoms including ataxia, dementia, myoclonus, seizures, chorea, athetosis, dystonia and ballismus. Three phenotypes have been described[90].

1. The ataxo-choreoathetoid type.
2. The pseudo-Huntington's disease type.
3. The myoclonic epileptic type.

DRPLA is most often inherited in an autosomal dominant manner, with the symptomatology varying within families[91]. Sporadic cases have been reported[92,93]. Symptoms begin in childhood or adulthood.

Pathological lesions are not entirely uniform. In all cases there is degeneration of the dentatorubral and pallidoluysian systems, but neuronal loss and atrophy have been noted in the caudate, putamen, substantia nigra, pontine tegmentum, pontine nuclei, medial longitudinal fasciculus, inferior olives, posterior columns of the spinal cord and posterior spino-cerebellar tracts[90].

Paroxysmal familial hypnogenic dystonia

Paroxysmal familial hypnogenic dystonia is characterized by brief and sometimes painful dystonic spasms which occur during non-rapid eye movement sleep. The age at onset and frequency of spells are variable. Inheritance patterns suggest autosomal dominant transmission, but sporadic cases have been reported[94]. Anticonvulsants are usually not effective; amitriptyline has been beneficial[95].

Hallervorden–Spatz disease

Hallervorden–Spatz disease is a progressive disorder characterized by childhood onset of abnormal movement and dementia. Dystonia can be the presenting symptom. This disorder is discussed in more detail below, in the section on parkinsonism.

Calcification of the basal ganglia (CBG)

Deposition of calcium in the basal ganglia has been more readily evident in the years since the advent of computed tomography. There are many conditions that are associated with basal gangliar calcifications (see Table 8.13). Often, the calcifications have no clinical correlate and are discovered incidentally.

Dystonia is sometimes seen in persons with calcifications of the basal ganglia associated with altered calcium metabolism, such as hypo-parathyroidism and pseudohypoparathyroidism. Calcifications of the basal ganglia may occur without disturbances of calcium, often in an autosomal dominant or recessive hereditary pattern; dystonia may be a prominent symptom[96–98]. A family has been described in which dystonia occurred in

Table 8.13. Conditions associated with calcifications of the basal ganglia

- Endocrinological
  - Hypoparathyroidism
    - Idiopathic
    - Secondary
  - Pseudohypoparathyroidism
  - Pseudo-pseudohypoparathyroidism
  - Hyperparathyroidism
  - Hypothyroidism
- Genetic/familial
  - Cockayne's syndrome
  - Down's syndrome
  - Tuberous sclerosis
  - Neurofibromatosis
  - Lipoid proteinosis
  - Methemoglobinopathies
  - Familial idiopathic cerebral calcifications (including Fahr's syndrome)
  - Mitochondrial disorders (including Kearn–Sayre syndrome, Leigh's disease)
- Toxic
  - Lead intoxication
  - Carbon monoxide intoxication
  - Nephrotic syndrome
- Hypoxia/anoxia at birth
- Vascular disease
  - Post-infarct
  - Post-haemorrhage
- Iatrogenic
  - Radiation therapy
  - Methotrexate therapy
- Infectious (including intra-uterine)
  - Cytomegalovirus
  - Toxoplasmosis
  - Cysticercosis
  - Acquired immune deficiency syndrome (AIDS)
  - Encephalitis (measles, chickenpox, coxsackie B, pertussis)
  - Rubella
  - Herpes
- Immunological
  - Systemic lupus erythematosus

members with calcifications and those without calcifications; other relatives had calcifications without dystonia or other extrapyramidal symptoms[98].

Dystonia with bilateral basal gangliar lucencies

The many conditions that cause bilateral basal gangliar lucencies are listed in Table 8.14. Infantile bilateral striatal necrosis (IBSN) is a rare, familial or sporadic disorder in which gastrointestinal and eating problems begin after a febrile illness[99–101]. Mental and motor retardation and regression occur,

Table 8.14. Causes of bilateral basal gangliar lucencies

Head trauma
Haemolytic-uraemic syndrome
Hereditary/metabolic
Familial holotopistic striatal necrosis
Familial dystonia with visual failure
Leigh's disease
Methylmalonic aciduria
Mitochondrial cytopathy
Wilson's disease
Hypoxia/hypotension
(and perinatal encephalopathies)
Hypoglycaemic encephalopathy
Intoxication
Methyl alcohol
Carbon monoxide
Cyanide
Infantile bilateral striatal necrosis (IBSN)
Infectious
Influenza
Vascular (ischaemia or haemorrhage)
Wasp sting encephalopathy

often accompanied by involuntary movements, including dystonia. The symptoms progress and death occurs days to years after onset, usually from respiratory compromise.

Abnormal movements, including dystonia may occur in Leigh's disease (subacute necrotizing encephalomyelitis). Blood and CSF lactate levels are usually elevated. Some children with Leigh's disease have deficiencies in the pyruvate dehydrogenase enzyme complex, while others have a deficiency of cytochrome-C oxidase[102].

Families have been reported in which individuals develop dystonia and/or subacute visual loss or asymptomatic optic atrophy, with computed tomography revealing bilateral striatal lucencies[103–104]. The dystonia, when present, begins in childhood as a focal dystonia, but progresses to become generalized. These same patients may or may not have visual loss that occurs before, during or after the onset of dystonia. Visual loss occurs in other family members without dystonia. Inheritance in some families is consistent with maternal transmission and it has been suggested that this is a mitochondrial disorder[104].

Disorders that simulate dystonia

The conditions listed in Table 8.15 cause sustained postures that may mimic dystonia. Most of them involve the head and neck, simulating torticollis. Plain X-rays reveal bone abnormalities in some of the disorders. For

Table 8.15. Disorders that simulate dystonia

Psychiatric (not as common in children as in adults)
Orthopaedic
Anterior C1-2 cervical subluxation
Bone infection or neoplasm
Rotational atlanto-axial subluxation
Congenital postural torticollis
Klippel–Feil anomaly
Neurological
Paroxysmal torticollis of infancy
Posterior fossa tumor
Syringomyelia
Bobble-head doll syndrome with third ventricular cyst
Arnold–Chiari malformation
Trochlear nerve palsy
Gastrointestinal
Sandifer's syndrome

example, fracture-dislocation of the cervical spine or a paraspinal abscess may cause deviation of the head or neck which can resemble torticollis.

Paroxysmal torticollis in infancy is characterized by episodes in which the child's head is tilted to one side, with some rotation[105,106]. The episodes begin when the child is 2–8 months old, last minutes to days and typically resolve spontaneously by 5 years of age. The child may appear otherwise completely well, although fussing and crying occurs if the head is passively moved; concomitant pallor, nausea and emesis may occur. If old enough, the child may describe vertigo. Auditory testing may be abnormal. During attacks, caloric-induced nystagmus is absent.

In Sandifer's syndrome, dystonic postures, often including the neck, are associated with gastro-oesophageal reflux[107,108]. The children commonly present with vomiting and feeding problems in infancy. Dystonic postures occur during feedings or immediately afterwards. Medical or surgical treatment of the reflux (or hiatal hernia, when present) alleviates the movement disorder. The diagnosis and therapy of Sandifer's syndrome may be complicated, as there may be an underlying neurological disorder causing, or associated with, the gastro-oesophageal reflux[109].

TREMOR

PHENOMENOLOGY

Definition

Tremor is defined as an involuntary rhythmic oscillating sinusoidal movement associated with alternating or synchronous contractions of reciprocally innervated antagonistic muscles[110–112].

Classification

Condition/situation

Tremor can be categorized into three types based on the conditions under which the movement occurs. Although nomenclature in the literature has varied, this chapter will use the following terms.

1. Resting tremor refers to the tremor being present when the body part is fully relaxed (see Table 8.16).
2. Postural tremor refers to the tremor being present when the body part is sustained in a particular posture (e.g. when the arms are held outstretched in front of the patient). This type of tremor may occur in normal persons and is then termed 'physiological tremor' (see Tables 8.17 and 8.19).
3. Kinetic tremor refers to the tremor being present when the body part is actively used in pursuit of a goal, such as writing or reaching for an object (see Tables 8.18 and 8.19).

A tremor may fit into one or more category; when the tremor is present in

Table 8.16. Causes of resting tremor

Parkinson's disease
Parkinsonism
Midbrain ('rubral') tremor: rest $<$ postural $<$ kinetic
Wilson's disease
Chronic hepatocerebral degeneration
Essential tremor (only when very severe): rest $\ll$ postural and kinetic
Mercury poisoning

Table 8.17. Causes of postural tremor

Possibly accentuated physiological tremor
Action tremor of parkinsonism
Epinephrine-induced
Thyrotoxic tremor
Anxiety tremor
Tremor of fatigue
Probably unrelated to physiological tremor
Essential tremor
Alcoholic tremor
Lithium tremor
Miscellaneous
Unrelated to physiological tremor
Cerebellar tremor
Asterixis
Post-concussive tremor

Table 8.18. Causes of kinetic tremor

Cerebellar 'outflow' tremor (dentate nucleus, red nucleus and superior cerebellar peduncle)
Wilson's disease
Acquired hepatocerebral degeneration
Drugs
Phenytoin
Toxins
Mercury
Metabolic disorders
Biopterin synthesis defect—paroxysmal 'rubral-like' tremor
Post-concussive tremor

Table 8.19. Causes of kinetic and postural tremor

Physiological tremor
Exaggerated physiological tremor
Essential tremor
Primary writing tremor
With other CNS disorders
Parkinson's disease
Parkinsonism
Idiopathic dystonia
With peripheral neuropathy
Charcot–Marie–Tooth disease (Roussy–Levy syndrome)
Other peripheral neuropathies
Cerebellar tremor
Post-concussive tremor

more than one condition, it is helpful to note in which condition the tremor is most prominent.

Frequency

Tremor can also be classified by its frequency. Electromyography can give very accurate assessment of tremor frequency; such accuracy may be useful in research, but is seldom necessary in clinical practice. Experienced observers can usually differentiate between 2–4 (slow), 4–6 (intermediate) and 8–12 (fast) Hz (cycles/sec) tremors; most tremors fall into one of these ranges.

PATHOPHYSIOLOGY

The pathophysiology of tremor is not well understood. Electromyography has demonstrated contraction of reciprocally innervated antagonistic muscle groups; the contractions usually alternate, although synchronous activity in the antagonistic muscles has been observed[113]. The anatomy, neurochemistry and pharmacology of some specific types of tremor are described below.

SPECIFIC TREMORS

Physiological tremor

All persons have a low amplitude tremor which is not always visible. The tremor is best observed when the arms are extended and the fingers outstretched; placing a sheet of paper over the hands and fingers will sometimes make the tremor more visible. The frequency of this type of tremor increases with age, being 5–6 Hz before the age of 9 years, then increasing over time to 10 Hz[114–116].

In physiological tremor, EMG studies of antagonistic muscles are usually described as normal, with an 'interference pattern'; in some persons, discrete, synchronous bursts of EMG activity may be found[113]. The mechanisms underlying physiological tremor are not well understood. Several theories have been proposed, including inherent properties of motor neuron firing, supraspinal rhythmic input to motor neurons, and oscillations in the stretch reflex causing synchronization of motor neuron discharge[117]. Ischaemic block and deafferentiation by dorsal rhizotomy do not abolish physiological tremor, suggesting that the tremor is not entirely due to oscillations in the stretch reflex servo-loop[118]. Manipulation of peripheral β2-adrenergic receptors affects physiological tremor, with pharmacological stimulation increasing tremor, and antagonism reducing tremor[119–121].

Many factors are known to accentuate physiological tremor (Table 8.20). Exacerbation of physiological tremor can be mistaken for pathological or abnormal tremor; therefore, accentuated physiological tremor should be considered in the differential diagnosis of postural or kinetic tremor, and possible exacerbating factors should be explored.

Essential tremor

The most common abnormal tremor in children is essential tremor. This tremor is fine and typically in the 8–12 Hz range; frequencies as low as 3 Hz are cited in the literature. The tremor is often present during sustension of outstretched hands, but is usually of higher amplitude during action and maximal as the limb approaches the target. The upper limbs are typically affected, with the tremor being most prominent distally. Tremor of the head may occur in the horizontal ('no–no') or vertical ('yes–yes') direction. The voice, trunk and lower extremities may also be involved, but less often[122,123]. Ethanol ingestion tends to quiet the tremor.

Table 8.20. Factors that accentuate physiological tremor

Mental state
Anger
Anxiety
Stress
Fatigue
Excitement
Metabolic
Fever
Thyrotoxicosis
Pheochromocytoma
Hypoglycaemia
Drugs
Theophylline
Beta-adrenergic agonists
Dopamine agonists
Tricyclic antidepressants
Neuroleptics
Lithium
Valproate
Thyroxine
Hypoglycaemics
Adrenocorticosteroids
Metrizamide
Cimetidine
Toxins and toxic states
Bismuth
Mercury
Lead
Arsenic
Methylbromide
Alcohol withdrawal
Benzodiazepine withdrawal
Opiate withdrawal
Dietary
Methylxanthines (coffee, tea, cola)
Monosodium glutamate

The tremor typically is insidious in onset. In familial essential tremor, the tremor tends to occur earlier than in sporadic cases, and males are affected slightly earlier than females[123]. Familial essential tremor is inherited in an autosomal dominant pattern with variable penetrance; the gene has not yet been localized[122]. Bimodal distribution of onset has been noted, with peaks at 15 and 60 years of age[122]. 'Shuddering attacks' in infants may be the manifestation of essential tremor in an immature nervous system (see below)[124].

Essential tremor usually follows a slowly progressive course, although there may be periods of rapid progression and periods during which the severity abates or is static. There have been reports of spontaneous remission in childhood, with recurrence later in life[125]. Progression is characterized by increasing amplitude and spread to other body parts.

EMG has demonstrated bursts of synchronous activity in antagonistic muscle groups[113]. The origin of essential tremor is unknown; the literature contains evidence for both peripheral and central mechanisms causing the tremor[126–132]. The beta-adrenergic system seems to have a role in essential tremor[117–121]. On post-mortem examination, there have been no consistently identified central nervous system lesions.

Although essential tremor is considered to be a monosymptomatic condition, it has been associated with a variety of other disorders. Nonspecific neurological abnormalities were noted in 17 of 81 patients examined by Larsson and Sjogren[133] and 41% of 194 patients reported by Rautakorpi[123]. Essential tremor seems to occur more often than expected by chance with dystonia, familial essential myoclonus, parkinsonism and neuropathies[134–144].

The differential diagnosis for essential tremor includes accentuated physiological tremor (see above), neuropathic tremor and tremor associated with other central nervous system (CNS) diseases. When there is a positive family history and no signs or symptoms of other CNS or systemic involvement, the diagnosis is straightforward; more complicated presentations may require further work-up to exclude other possible causes of tremor. Essential tremor is a clinically diagnosed condition; there are no laboratory tests to confirm the diagnosis.

For many people, essential tremor is embarrassing but does not significantly interfere with activities. When the tremor is problematic, therapy may be warranted. The medications most commonly used to treat essential tremor are propranolol and primidone. Benzodiazepines can be beneficial, but the potential problems of chronic therapy with this class of drugs must be considered.

Neuropathic tremor

Tremor may occur with a variety of hereditary and acquired peripheral neuropathies[141–146]. The tremor is typically distal, is in the 6–8 Hz range, and is physiologically distinct from essential and physiological tremors[147]. The pathophysiology of neuropathic tremor is not known. Several mechanisms have been proposed, including delay in the stretch reflex arc, selective loss of sensory nerve fibres and muscle weakness; a central origin and associated essential tremor have also been postulated[146]. Anti-tremor medication is generally not beneficial in neuropathic tremor; the tremor may improve, however, with treatment of the underlying neuropathy.

Post-concussive tremor

Tremor is a well-described sequelae of head trauma, particularly in children. The tremor may be postural or kinetic and is usually of large amplitude and low frequency[148,149]. Johnson and Hall surveyed severely head injured children and found that tremor occurred within 18 months of injury in 45% of the cases[148]. After a follow-up period of 3 years, 54% of the children had spontaneous resolution and 5% of the cases had worsened. The anatomical correlations of tremor following head trauma are not homogeneous. Patients have been reported with haemorrhage in the putamen or low density lesion on computed tomography (CT) in the pallidum 19 days after the event[150]. Maki *et al.* hypothesized that infarction and/or haemorrhage of the basal ganglia is caused by trauma stretching the lateral branch of the perforator of the middle cerebral artery[150]. Others have reported haemorrhages in the midbrain[148]. Propranolol and stereotactic thalamotomy have been used in persons with tremor following head trauma[149,151]. The combination of propranolol and valproate was effective in a child with tremor and myoclonic jerks following head trauma[152].

Juvenile parkinsonism

Tremor is uncommon in juvenile parkinsonism. When present, the tremor is typically postural or kinetic rather than resting, as seen in typical idiopathic Parkinson's disease (IPD). Juvenile parkinsonism is discussed in more detail below.

Shuddering attacks

Brief, sudden episodes of shuddering may occur in infants and pre-school-aged children; the attacks are often associated with emotional situations. Episodes are benign and become less frequent or resolve late in the first decade. EEG is normal during the attacks[153]. There is often a family history of essential tremor and the children themselves may develop essential tremor over time. It has been suggested that shuddering attacks represent a clinical variant of essential tremor occurring in an immature nervous system[154].

Miscellaneous rhythmic movements

Table 8.21 lists many conditions that can cause rhythmic movements. These should be considered when the movement or clinical condition is not consistent with the above tremors.

Table 8.21. Miscellaneous rhythmic movements

Psychogenic tremor
Orthostatic tremor
Rhythmic movements in dystonia (dystonic tremor)
Rhythmic myoclonus (segmental myoclonus such as palatal or branchial myoclonus, spinal myoclonus, limb myorhythmia)
Oscillatory myoclonus
Asterixis
Clonus
Epilepsy partialis continua
Hereditary chin quivering
Spasmus nutans
Head shaking in the visually impaired
Head bobbing with third ventricular cysts
Nystagmus

PARKINSONISM (AKINETIC–RIGID SYNDROMES)

CLINICAL PHENOMENOLOGY

The term 'parkinsonism' is used to describe a clinical syndrome characterized by akinesia (poverty of movement), bradykinesia (slowness of movement) and rigidity. It is important to note that akinesia and bradykinesia are separate from rigidity and are not necessarily caused by the increased tone. Parkinsonism does not necessarily include tremor.

PATHOPHYSIOLOGY

Parkinsonism is due to basal ganglia dysfunction. The complicated anatomical interactions of the basal ganglia are reviewed by Albin, Young and Penney and are beyond the scope of this chapter[5] (also see chapter 13). Disturbances of the dopaminergic nigrostriatal system have been implicated in many of the disorders causing parkinsonism. Loss of dopamine-synthesizing nigral neurons, and reduction of dopamine activity via altered metabolism, inhibition of presynaptic release and/or receptor blockade can induce the akinetic–rigid state.

SPECIFIC DISORDERS (Table 8.22)

Huntington's disease

As reviewed above, parkinsonism (rather than chorea) is the typical clinical presentation of patients with juvenile-onset Huntington's disease.

Table 8.22. Causes of parkinsonism in children

Calcifications of basal ganglia
Ceroid lipofuscinosis (juvenile/Spielmeyer–Vogt and late-onset Kufs' types)
Drugs and toxins
Carbon monoxide
Cyanide
Neuroleptics
Antiemetics
Familial tic disorder, parkinsonism, motor neuron disease and acanthocytosis
Gaucher's disease
GM1 gangliosidosis (adult type)
Hallervorden–Spatz disease
Huntington's disease
Infectious/post-infectious
Mycoplasma
Viruses
measles
varicella
polio
Japanese B
western equine
Juvenile parkinsonism
L-dopa responsive dystonia–parkinsonism
Machado–Joseph disease
Mass
AVM
tumor
Metachromatic leukodystrophy
Neuroacanthocytosis
Neuronal intranuclear inclusion disease
Perinatal kernicterus
Post-anoxia
Wilson's disease (hepatolenticular degeneration)

Juvenile parkinsonism

Juvenile parkinsonism (JP) can be defined as parkinsonism that begins before the age of 40 and responds symptomatically to L-dopa. Half of the patients have rigidity and bradykinesia without tremor; when a tremor is present, it is typically postural or kinetic rather than resting. The initial symptom is often difficulty walking, with dystonia being common in those with childhood onset. Autonomic symptoms are uncommon. Progression is slower and familial incidence higher than in classical idiopathic Parkinson's disease (IPD); autosomal dominant transmission has been reported[155]. The symptoms respond dramatically to L-dopa, although L-dopa therapy is marred by the 'wearing-off' phenomenon early on and severe dopa-induced dyskinesias[156].

The neuropathology, neurochemistry and pathogenesis of JP may be different from IPD. The substantia nigra is abnormal in all cases, but Lewy bodies are not always present[157,158]. Cerebrospinal fluid biopterin levels have been reported to be lower in JP patients than in the control population, but the significance of this finding is unclear[159].

Machado–Joseph disease

Machado–Joseph disease is an autosomal dominantly transmitted motor system degeneration. This disorder was originally described in people with ancestors from the Portuguese Azores islands, although there have now been reports in non-Portuguese families[160–163]. Based on reports of several families, Machado–Joseph disease may be divided into three or four types based on the clinical findings.

1. Type I has early age at onset and is characterized by rigidity, spasticity and dystonic posturing.
2. Type II has intermediate age at onset and is characterized by pyramidal, extrapyramidal and cerebellar deficits.
3. Type III has later age at onset and is characterized by cerebellar deficits and a peripheral neuropathy.
4. Type IV, described by some authors, is characterized by parkinsonism and a neuropathy[164–167].

Eye movement abnormalities and lid retraction occur in all types. There are no specific treatments for this disorder, although L-dopa, anticholinergics, baclofen and benzodiazepines may be of benefit to some patients[168].

Histological analysis of neural tissue reveals neuronal loss and gliosis in the substantia nigra, subthalamic nucleus, dentate nucleus, motor cranial nuclei, vestibular nucleus, nucleus dorsalis of Clarke, spinocerebellar tract and anterior horn[168]. The inferior olivary nuclei are always spared, which distinguishes this disorder from the olivopontocerebellar atrophies. The pathogenesis of Machado–Joseph disease has not been defined, nor has the gene been identified.

Hallervorden–Spatz disease (HSD)

Hallervorden–Spatz, in 1922, described a progressive disorder in which five of the twelve children in one family developed dystonia, rigidity, choreoathetosis, dementia and dysarthria[169]. Many cases have been reported in the literature.

Rigidity, bradykinesia, dystonia, chorea and sometimes tremor typically begin in childhood, between the ages of 7 and 12 years. Cognitive and behaviour changes and reduced visual acuity may be the presenting symptoms. Mental retardation and/or dementia occur in most cases[170].

Optic atrophy and/or retinitis pigmentosa occur in approximately 25% of cases, leading to loss of visual acuity. Hyperreflexia, extensor plantar responses and ataxia often occur. Symptoms progress, with death occurring an average of 11 years after the onset of symptoms[170]. Autosomal recessive inheritance is suggested by occurrence in siblings and parental consanguinity in 15% of sporadic cases[170].

The pathophysiology of HSD is not understood. Pathological studies have revealed an iron-containing pigment, neuromelanin and lipofuscin in the globus pallidus and substantia nigra; smaller amounts are also present in the red nucleus and subthalamic nucleus[171–173]. There is gliosis and loss of neurons and medullated fibres from the affected regions, particularly the internal segment of the globus pallidus and the substantia nigra reticulata. Spheroids, swollen axon fragments composed of glycoprotein, lipid and mitochondria are seen in the most affected regions; these spheroids are similar to the axonal swellings found in infantile neuroaxonal dystrophy. Increased 59Fe uptake and slowed disappearance in the basal ganglia has been found using scintillation counting in people with HSD[174]. Ferrokinetic studies, however, have not revealed abnormalities of systemic iron metabolism[172,174]. Two siblings with clinical presentations and radioactive iron studies consistent with the diagnosis of HSD were found to have sea-blue histiocytes in bone marrow and cytoplasmic inclusions in circulating lymphocytes, similar to those found in neuronal ceroid lipofuscinosis[175]. Computed tomography (CT) reveals diffuse cerebral atrophy and ventricular enlargement or increased densities in the globus pallidus[176–178]. Hypointensities on T2 and gradient echo may be seen in the globus pallidus and substantia nigra using magnetic resonance imaging (MRI)[179]. Decreased signal with central increased signal ('eye of the tiger' sign) has also been noted in the globus pallidus on MRI[180].

Medical treatment of HSD is typically not effective. Iron chelation and administration of vitamin E have not changed the progression or outcome[170,175]. Anticholinergic medication and L-dopa have transiently improved parkinsonism[170,181].

REFERENCES

1. Shoulson, I. (1986) On chorea. *Clin Neuropharmacol.*, **9** (Suppl 2), 585–599.
2. Kurlan, R. and Shoulson, I. (1988) Differential diagnosis of facial chorea. *Adv. Neurol.*, **49**, 225–237.
3. Shannon, K. M. (1990) Hemiballismus. *Clin. Neuropharmacol.*, **13**, 413–425.
4. Marsden, C. D., Obeso, J. A. and Rothwell, J. C. (1983) Clinical neurophysiology of muscle jerks. In *Motor Control Mechanisms in Health and Disease* (J. E. Desmedt, Ed). Raven Press, New York, pp. 865–881.
5. Albin, R. L., Young, A. B. and Penney, J. B. (1989) The functional anatomy of basal ganglia disorders. *Trends in Neurosci.*, **12**, 366–375.

6. Rolando, S. and DeNegri, M. (1987) Childhood choreas. In *Extrapyramidal Disorders in Childhood* (L. Angelini, G. Lanzi, U. Balottin and N. Nardocci, Eds). Excerpta Medica, Amsterdam, pp. 113–125.
7. Klawans, H. L. and Brandabur, M. M. (1993) Chorea in childhood. *Pediatr. Ann.*, **22**, 41–50.
8. Shoulson, I., Rothfield, K., McBride, M. and Kurlan, R. (1987) Physiologic chorea and dystonia of infancy. *Neurology*, **37** (Suppl), 99.
9. Hagberg, B., Hagberg, G. and Olow, I. (1975) The changing panorama of cerebral palsy in Sweden 1954–1970. *Acta Paediatr. Scand.*, **64**, 193–200.
10. Kyllerman, M., Bager, B., Bensch, A., *et al.* (1982) Dyskinetic cerebral palsy, I: clinical categories, associated neurological abnormalities and incidence. *Acta Paediatr. Scand.*, **71**, 543–550.
11. Wolff, P. H. and Hurwitz, I. (1966) The choreiform syndrome. *Dev. Med. Child Neurol.*, **4**, 160–165.
12. Gusella, J. F., MacDonald, M. E., Ambrose, C. M. and Duyao, M. P. (1993) Molecular genetics of Huntington's disease. *Arch. Neurol.*, **50**, 1157–1163.
13. Shoulson, I. (1984) Huntington's disease: a decade of progress. *Neurol. Clin.*, **2**, 515–526.
14. Gusella, J. and Young, A. B. (1993) Huntington's disease. In *Molecular Basis of Neurology* (M. P. Conneally, Ed). Blackwell Scientific, Cambridge, MA, pp. 113–127.
15. Sleigh, G. and Linderbaum, R. J. (1981) Benign (non-paroxysmal) familial chorea: paediatric perspectives. *Arch. Dis. Child.*, **56**, 616–621.
16. Mount, L. A. and Reback, S. (1940) Familial paroxysmal choreoathetosis: preliminary report in a hitherto undescribed clinical syndrome. *Arch. Neurol. Psychiatry*, **44**, 841–847.
17. Lance, J. W. (1977) Familial paroxysmal dystonic choreoathetosis and its differentiation from related syndromes. *Ann. Neurol.*, **2**, 285–293.
18. Kertesz, A. (1967) Paroxysmal kinesigenic choreoathetosis. *Neurology*, **17**, 680–690.
19. Nausieda, P. A., Grossman, B. J., Koller, W. C., *et al.* (1980) Sydenham's chorea: an update. *Neurology*, **30**, 331–334.
20. Husby, G., Van de Rijn, I., Zabriskie, J. B., *et al.* (1976) Antibodies reacting with cytoplasm of subthalamic and caudate nuclei neurons in chorea and acute rheumatic fever. *J. Exp. Med.*, **144**, 1094–1100.
21. Kiessling, L. S., Marcotte, A. C. and Culpepper, L. (1983) Antineuronal antibodies in movement disorders. *Pediatrics*, **92**, 39–43.
22. Bruyn, G. W. and Padberg, G. (1984) Chorea and systemic lupus erythematous. *Eur. Neurol.*, **23**, 278–290.
23. Herd, J. K., Medhi, M., Uzendoski, D. M. and Saldivar, V. A. (1978) Chorea associated with systemic lupus erythematosis: report of two cases and review of the literature. *Pediatrics*, **61**, 308–315.
24. Hodges, J. R. (1987) Chorea and the lupus anticoagulant. *J. Neurol. Neurosurg. Psychiatry*, **50**, 368–369.
25. Gaultieri, C. T., Quade, D., Hicks, R. E., *et al.* (1984) Tardive dyskinesia and other clinical consequences of neuroleptic treatment in children and adolescents. *Am. J. Psychiatry*, **141**, 20–23.
26. Tanner, C. M. (1992) Tardive dyskinesia. In *Textbook of Clinical Neuropharmacology and Therapeutics*, 2nd ed. (H. L. Klawans, C. G. Goetz and C. M. Tanner, Eds). Raven Press, New York, pp. 151–161.
27. Medlock, M. D., Cruse, R. S., Winek, S. J., *et al.* (1993) A 10-year experience with postpump chorea. *Ann. Neurol.*, **34**, 820–826.
28. Herz, E. (1944) Dystonia. I. Historical Review: Analysis of dystonia symptoms

and physiologic mechanisms involved. *Arch. Neurol. Psychiatry*, **51**, 305–318.
29. Denny-Brown, D. (1962) *The Basal Ganglia and their Relation to Disorders of Movement*. Oxford University Press, London, p. 78.
30. Fahn, S. (1988) Concept and classification of dystonia. *Adv. Neurol.*, **50**, 1–8.
31. Marsden, C. D., Harrison, M. J. G. and Bundey, S. (1976) Natural history of idiopathic torsion dystonia. *Adv. Neurol.*, **14**, 177–187.
32. Cooper, I. S., Cullinan, T. and Riklan, M. (1976) The natural history of dystonia. *Adv. Neurol.*, **14**, 157–169.
33. Fahn, S. (1986) Generalized dystonia: concept and treatment. *Clin. Neuropharmacol.*, **9** (Suppl 2), S37–S48.
34. Oppenheim, H. (1911) Uber eine eigenartige Krampfrankheit des kindlichen und jugendlichen Alters (Dysbasia lordotica progressiva, Dystonia musculorum deformans). *Neurologisches Zentralblatt*, **30**, 1090–1107.
35. Foerster, O. (1921) Zur Analyse und Pathophysiologie der striaren Bewegungsstorungen. *Z. Gesamte Neurol. Psychiatrie*, **73**, 1–169.
36. Rothwell, J. C., Obeso, J. A., Day, B. L. and Marsden, C. D. (1983) Pathophysiology of dystonias. *Adv. Neurol.*, **39**, 851–863.
37. Dooling, E. C. and Adams, R. D. (1975) The pathological anatomy of posthemiplegic athetosis. *Brain*, **98**, 29–48.
38. Waddy, H. M., Fletcher, N. A., Harding, A. E. and Marsden, C. D. (1991) A genetic study of idiopathic focal dystonias. *Ann. Neurol.*, **29**, 320–324.
39. Fletcher, N. A., Harding, A. E. and Marsden, C. D. (1990) A genetic study of idiopathic torsion dystonia in the United Kingdom. *Brain*, **113**, 379–395.
40. Ozelius, L., Kramer, P. L., Moskowitz, C. B., Kwiatkowski, D. J., Brin, M. F., Bressman, S. B., Schuback, D. E., Falk, C. T., Risch, N., de Leon, D. *et al.* (1989) Human gene for torsion dystonia located on chromosome 9q32-34. *Neuron*, **2**, 1427–1434.
41. Kramer, P. L., de Leon, D., Ozelius, L., Risch, N., Bressman, S. B., Brin, M. F., Schuback, D. E., Burke, R. E., Kwiatkowski, D. J., Shale, H., *et al.* (1990) Dystonia gene in Ashkenazi Jewish population is located on chromosome 9q32-34. *Ann. Neurol.*, **27**, 114–120.
42. Graeber, M. B., Kupke, K. G. and Muller, U. (1992) Delineation of the dystonia–parkinsonism syndrome locus in Xq13. *Proc. Natl. Acad. Sci. USA*, **89**, 8245–8248.
43. Eldridge, R. (1970) The torsion dystonias: Literature review and genetic and clinical studies. *Neurology*, **20** (Part 2), 1–78.
44. Eldridge, R. and Gottlieb, R. (1976) The primary hereditary dystonias: Genetic classification of 768 families and revised estimate of gene frequency, autosomal recessive form and selected bibliography. *Adv. Neurol.*, **14**, 457–474.
45. Korczyn, A. D., Kahana, E., Zilber, N., *et al.* (1980) Torsion dystonia in Israel. *Ann. Neurol.*, **8**, 387–391.
46. Eldridge, R. (1981) Inheritance of torsion dystonia in Jews. *Ann. Neurol.*, **10**, 203–204.
47. Lee, L. V., Pascasio, F. M., Fuentes, F. D., *et al.* (1976) Torsion dystonia in Panay, Philippines. *Adv. Neurol.*, **14**, 137–151.
48. Zeman, W. and Dyken, P. (1968) Dystonia musculorum deformans. In *Handbook of Clinical Neurology* (P. J. Vinken and G. W. Bruyn, Eds). North-Holland, Amsterdam, pp. 517–543.
49. Herz, E. (1944) Dystonia II. Clinical classification. *Arch. Neurol. Psychiatry*, **51**, 319–355.
50. Marsden, C. D., Harrison, M. J. G. and Bundey, S. (1974) Idiopathic torsion dystonia (dystonia musculorum deformans). A review of forty-two patients. *Brain*, **97**, 793–810.

51. Burke, R. E., Brin, M. F., Fahn, S., *et al.* (1986) Analysis of the clinical course of non-Jewish autosomal dominant torsion dystonia. *Mov. Disord.*, **1**, 163–178.
52. Angelini, L., Nardocci, N., Rumi, V. *et al.* (1989) Idiopathic dystonia with onset in childhood. *J. Neurol.*, **236**, 319–321.
53. Zweig, R. M., Hedereen, J. C., Jankel, W. R., *et al.* (1988) Pathology in brainstem regions of individuals with primary dystonia. *Neurology*, **38**, 702–706.
54. Hornykiewicz, O., Kish, S. J., Becker, L. E. *et al.* (1986) Brain neurotransmitters in dystonia musculorum deformans. *N. Engl. J. Med.*, **315**, 347–353.
55. Jankovic, J., Svendsen, C. N. and Bird, E. D. (1987) Brain neurotransmitters in dystonia. *N. Engl. J. Med.*, **316**, 278–279.
56. Fahn, S. (1983) High dosage anticholinergic therapy in dystonia. *Neurology*, **33**, 1255–1261.
57. Marsden, C. D., Marion, M. H. and Quinn, N. (1984) The treatment of severe dystonia in children and adults. *J. Neurol. Neurosurg. Psychiatry*, **47**, 1166–1173.
58. Fahn, S. (1986) Generalized dystonia: concept and treatment. *Clin Neuro-pharmacol.*, **9** (Suppl 2), S37–S48.
59. Greene, P. E. and Fahn, S. (1992) Baclofen in the treatment of idiopathic dystonia in children. *Mov. Disord.*, **7**, 48–52.
60. Willemse, J. (1986) Benign idiopathic dystonia with onset in the first year of life. *Dev. Med. Child Neurol.*, **28**, 355–363.
61. Angelini, L., Rumi, V., Lazmperti, E. *et al.* (1988) Transient paroxysmal dystonia in infancy. *Neuropediatrics*, **19**, 171–174.
62. Deonna, T., Ziegler, A. and Nielsen, J. (1991) Transient idiopathic dystonia in infancy. *Neuropediatrics*, **22**, 220–224.
63. Obeso, J. A., Rothwell, J. C. and Lang, A. E. (1983) Myoclonic dystonia. *Neurology*, **33**, 825–830.
64. Quinn, N. P. and Marsden, C. D. (1984) Dominantly inherited myoclonic dystonia with dramatic response to alcohol (abstract). *Neurology*, **34** (Suppl 1), 236–237.
65. Nygaard, T. G. (1993) Dopa-responsive dystonia: delineation of the clinical syndrome and clues to pathogenesis. *Adv. Neurol.*, **60**, 577–585.
66. Fletcher, N. A., Holt, I. J., Harding, A. E., *et al.* (1989) Tyrosine hydroxylase and levodopa responsive dystonia. *J. Neurol. Neurosurg. Psychiatry*, **52**, 112–114.
67. Schuback, D., Kramer, P., Ozelius, L., *et al.* (1991) Dopamine beta-hydroxylase gene excluded in four subtypes of hereditary dystonia. *Hum. Genet.*, **87**, 311–316.
68. Kwiatkowski, D. J., Nygaard, T. G., Schuback, D. E., *et al.* (1991) Identification of a highly polymorphic microsatelite VNTR within the agininosuccinate synthetase locus—exclusion of the dystonia gene on 9q32-34 as the cause of dopa-responsive dystonia in a large kindred. *Am. J. Hum. Genet.*, **48**, 121–128.
69. Nygaard, T. G., Marsden, C. D. and Duvoisin, R. C. (1988) Dopa responsive dystonia. *Adv. Neurol.*, **50**, 377–384.
70. Nygaard, T. G., Waran, S. and Chutorian, A. M. (1989) Unexplained cerebral palsy: dopa-responsive dystonia? (abstract) *Ann. Neurol.*, **26**, 485–486.
71. Hakamada, S., Watanabe, K., Hara, K., *et al.* (1982) A case of 'hereditary progressive dystonia with marked diurnal fluctuation.' *Brain Dev.*, **14**, 44–48.
72. Ouvrier, R. A. (1978) Progressive dystonia with marked diurnal fluctuation. *Ann. Neurol.*, **4**, 412–417.
73. Willemse, J., van Nieuwenhuizen, O., Gooskens, R. H., *et al.* (1984) Treatment of non-fluctuating progressive dystonia: a neuropharmacological approach. *Neuropediatrics*, **15**, 208–210.
74. Deonna, T. (1986) DOPA-sensitive progressive dystonia of childhood with fluctuations of symptoms: Segawa's syndrome and possible variants. Results of

a collaborative study of the European Federation of Child Neurology Societies (EFCNS). *Neuropediatrics*, **17**, 81–85.
75. Gorke, W. and Bartholome, K. (1990) Biochemical and neurophysiological investigations in two forms of Segawa's disease. *Neuropediatrics*, **21**, 308.
76. LeWitt, P. A., Newman, R. P., Miller, L. P., *et al.* (1993) Treatment of dystonia with tetrahydrobiopterin (letter). *N. Engl. J. Med.*, **308**, 157–158.
77. LeWitt, P. A., Miller, L. P., Levine, R. A., *et al.* (1986) Tetrahydrobiopterin in dystonia: identification of abnormal metabolism and therapeutic trials. *Neurology*, **36**, 760–764.
78. Fink, J. K., Barton, N., Cohen, W., Lovenberg, W., Burns, R. S. and Hallett, M. (1988) Dystonia with marked diurnal variation associated with biopterin deficiency. *Neurology*, **38**, 707–711.
79. Fink, J. K., Ravin, P., Argoff, C. E., *et al.* (1989) Tetrahydrobiopterin administration in biopterin-deficient progressive dystonia with diurnal variation. *Neurology*, **39**, 1393–1395.
80. Lang, A. E., Garnett, E. S., Firnau, G., *et al.* (1988) Positron tomography in dystonia. *Adv. Neurol.*, **50**, 249–253.
81. Martin, W. R., Stoessl, A. J., Palmer, M., *et al.* (1988) PET scanning in dystonia. *Adv. Neurol.*, **50**, 223–229.
82. Nygaard, T. G., Takahashi, H., Heiman, G. A., *et al.* (1992) Long-term treatment response and flourodopa positron emission tomographic scanning of parkinsonism in a family with dopa-responsive dystonia. *Ann. Neurol.*, **32**, 603–608.
83. Sawle, G. V., Leenders, K. L., Brooks, D. J., *et al.* (1991) Dopa-responsive dystonia: 18 FDopa positron emission tomography. *Ann. Neurol.*, **30**, 24–30.
84. Snow, B. J., Nygaard, T. G., Takahashi, H., *et al.* (1993) Positron emission tomographic studies of dopa-responsive dystonia and early-onset idiopathic parkinsonism. *Ann. Neurol.*, **34**, 733–738.
85. Allen, N. and Knopp, W. (1976) Hereditary parkinsonism-dystonia with sustained control by L-dopa and anticholinergic medication. *Adv. Neurol.*, **14**, 201–213.
86. Nygaard, T. G., Trugman, J. M., de Yebenes, J. G., *et al.* (1990) Dopa-responsive dystonia: the spectrum of clinical manifestations in a large North American family. *Neurology*, **40**, 66–69.
87. Nygaard, T. G., Marsden, C. D. and Fahn, S. (1991) Dopa-responsive dystonia: long-term treatment response and prognosis. *Neurology*, **41**, 174–181.
88. Segawa, M., Ohmi, K., Itoh, S., *et al.* (1972) Childhood basal ganglia disease with remarkable response to L-dopa, 'hereditary basal ganglia disease with marked diurnal fluctuation'. *Chiryo* (Tokyo), **24**, 667–672 cited in Reference 89.
89. Segawa, M. and Nomura, Y. (1993) Hereditary progressive dystonia with marked diurnal fluctuation: pathophysiological importance of the age of onset. *Adv. Neurol.*, **60**, 568–576.
90. Iizuka, R., Hirayama, K. and Maehara, K. (1984) Dentato-rubro-pallido-luysian atrophy: a clinico-pathological study. *J. Neurol. Neurosurg. Psychiatry*, **47**, 1288–1298.
91. Takahashi, H., Ohama, E., Naito, H., *et al.* (1988) Hereditary dentatorubral-pallidoluysian atrophy: clinical and pathologic variants in a family. *Neurology*, **38**, 1065–1070.
92. Smith, J. K., Gonda, V. E. and Malamud, N. (1958) Unusual form of cerebellar ataxia: combined dentatorubral and pallido-luysian degeneration. *Neurology*, **8**, 205–209.
93. Neuman, M. A. (1959) Combined degeneration of globus pallidus and dentate nucleus and their projections. *Neurology*, **9**, 430–438.

94. Lugaresi, E. and Cirignotta, F. (1981) Hypnogenic paroxysmal dystonia: epileptic seizure or a new syndrome? *Sleep*, **4**, 129–138.
95. Lee, B. I., Lesser, R. P., Pippenger, C. E., *et al.* (1985) Familial paroxysmal hypnogenic dystonia. *Neurology*, **35**, 1357–1360.
96. Aicardi, J. and Goutieres, F. (1984) A progressive familial encephalopathy in infancy with calcifications of the basal ganglia and chronic cerebrospinal fluid lymphocytosis. *Ann. Neurol.*, **15**, 49–54.
97. Caraceni, T., Broggi, G. and Avanzini, G. (1974) Familial idiopathic basal ganglia calcification exhibiting 'dystonia musculorum deformans' features. *Eur. Neurol.*, **12**, 351–359.
98. Larsen, T. A., Dunn, H. G., Jan, J. E., *et al.* (1985) Dystonia and calcification of the basal ganglia. *Neurology*, **35**, 533–537.
99. Jellinger, K. (1986) (Exogenous) striatal necrosis. *Handb. Clin. Neurol.*, **5**(49), 499–518.
100. Roytta, M., Olsson, I., Sourander, P., *et al.* (1981) Infantile bilateral striatal necrosis: clinical and morphological report of a case and a review of the literature. *Acta Neuropathol.*, **55**, 97–103.
101. Mito, T., Tanaka, T., Becker, L. E., *et al.* (1986) Infantile bilateral striatal necrosis: clinicopathological classification. *Arch. Neurol.*, **443**, 677–680.
102. DiMauro, S., Servidei, S., Zeviani, M., *et al.* (1987) Cytochrome C-oxidase deficiency in Leigh syndrome. *Ann. Neurol.*, **22**, 498–506.
103. Marsden, C. D., Lang, A. E., Quinn, N. P., *et al.* (1986) Familial dystonia and visual failure with striatal CT lucencies. *J. Neurol. Neurosurg. Psychiatry*, **49**, 500–509.
104. Novotny, E. J. Jr., Singh, G., Wallace, D. C., *et al.* (1986) Leber's disease and dystonia: a mitochondrial disease. *Neurology*, **36**, 1053–1060.
105. Snyder, C. H. (1969) Paroxysmal torticollis in infancy: a possible form of labyrinthitis. *Am. J. Dis. Child.*, **117**, 458–460.
106. Gourley, I. M. (1971) Paroxysmal torticollis in infancy. *Can. Med. Ass. J.*, **105**, 504–505.
107. Kinsbourne, M. and Oxon, D. M. (1964) Hiatus hernia with contortions of the neck. *Lancet*, **i**, 1058–1061.
108. Werbin, S. L., D'Souza, B. J., Hogan, W. J., *et al.* (1980) Sandifer syndrome: an unappreciated clinical entity. *Dev. Med. Child Neurol.*, **22**, 374–378.
109. Sondheimer, J. and Morris, B. A. (1979) Gastroesophageal reflux among severely retarded children. *J. Pediatr.*, **94**, 710–714.
110. Fahn, S. (1972) Differential diagnosis of tremors. *Med. Clin. N. Am.*, **56**, 1363–1375.
111. Jankovic, J. and Fahn, S. (1980) Physiologic and pathologic tremors—diagnosis, mechanism and management. *Ann. Intern. Med.*, **93**, 460–465.
112. Koller, W. C. (1984) Diagnosis and treatment of tremors. *Neurol. Clin.*, **2**, 499–514.
113. Shahani, B. T. and Young, R. R. (1976) Physiological and pharmacological aids in the differential diagnosis of tremor. *J. Neurol. Neurosurg. Psychiatry*, **39**, 772–783.
114. Marshall, J. and Walsh, E. G. (1956) Physiological tremor. *J. Neurol. Neurosurg. Psychiatry*, **19**, 260–267.
115. Marshall, J. (1959) Physiological tremor in children. *J. Neurol. Neurosurg. Psychiatry*, **22**, 33–35.
116. Marshall, J. (1961) The effect of aging upon physiological tremor. *J. Neurol. Neurosurg. Psychiatry*, **24**, 14–17.
117. Marsden, C. D. (1978) The mechanism of physiological tremor and their significance for pathological tremors. In *Progress in Clinical Neurophysiology* Vol. 5, (J. E. Desmedt, Ed.) S. Karger, Basel, pp. 1–16.

118. Marsden, C. D., Meadows, J. C., Lange, G. W., *et al.* (1967) Effect of deafferentiation on human physiological tremor. *Lancet*, **2**, 700–702.
119. Marsden, C. D., Foley, T. H., Owen, D. A., *et al.* (1967) Peripheral beta adrenergic receptors concerned with tremor. *Clin. Sci.*, **33**, 53–65.
120. Larsson, S. and Svedmyr, N. (1977) Tremor caused by sympathomimetics is mediated by beta adrenoreceptors. *Scand. J. Respir. Dis.*, **58**, 5–10.
121. Perucca, E., Pickles, H. and Richens, A. (1981) Effect of atenolol, metoprolol and propranolol on isoproterenol-induced tremor and tachycardia in normal subjects. *Clin. Pharmacol. Ther.*, **29**, 425–433.
122. Larsen, T. A. and Calne, D. S. (1983) Essential tremor. *Clin. Neuropharmacol.*, **8**, 185–188.
123. Rautakorpi, I. (1978) Essential tremor. *An Epidemiological, Clinical and Genetic Study*. (Academic dissertation). Turku, Finland. Cited in Reference 122.
124. Vanesse, M., Bedard, P. and Andermann, F. (1976) Shuddering attacks in children: an early clinical manifestation of essential tremor. *Neurology*, **26**, 1027–1030.
125. Paulson, G. W. (1976) Benign essential tremor in childhood. Symptoms, pathogenesis, treatment. *Clin. Pediatr.*, **15**, 67–70.
126. Marsden, C. D. (1984) Origins of normal and pathological tremor. In *Movement Disorders: Tremor* (L. J. Findley and R. Calpildeo, Eds). McMillan Press, London, pp. 37–84.
127. Shahani, B. T. and Young, R. R. (1978) Action tremors: A clinical neurophysiological review. In *Physiological Tremor, Pathological Tremor and Clonus. Progress in Clinical Neurophysiology*, Vol. 5. (J. E. Desmedt, Ed.). S. Karger, Basel, pp. 129–137.
128. Young, R. R. and Shahani, B. T. (1979) Single unit behavior in human muscle afferent and efferent systems. *Adv. Neurol.*, **24**, 175–183.
129. Marsden, C. D., Obeso, J. and Rothwell, J. C. (1983) Benign essential tremor is not a single entity. In *Current Concepts in Parkinson's Disease* (M. D. Yahr, Ed). Excerpta Medica, Amsterdam, pp. 31–46.
130. Lee, R. G. and Stein, R. G. (1981) Resetting of tremor by mechanical perturbations: a comparison of essential tremor and parkinsonian tremor. *Ann. Neurol.*, **10**, 523–531.
131. Lee, R. G. (1987) The pathophysiology of essential tremor. In *Movement Disorders* (C. D. Marsden and S. Fahn, Eds). Butterworths, London, pp. 423–437.
132. Ohye, C., Hirai, T., Miyazaki, M., *et al.* (1982) Vim thalamotomy for the treatment of various kinds of tremor. *Appl. Neurophysiol.*, **45**, 275–280.
133. Larsson, T. and Sjogren, T. (1960) Essential tremor. A clinical and genetic population study. *Acta Psychiatr. Neurol. Scand.*, **36** (Suppl 144), 1–176. Cited in Ref. 122.
134. Couch, J. R. (1976) Dystonia and tremor in spasmodic torticollis. *Adv. Neurol.*, **14**, 245–258.
135. Marsden, C. D., Harrison, M. J. G. and Bundey, E. (1976) Natural history of idiopathic torsion dystonia. *Adv. Neurol.*, **14**. 177–186.
136. Sheehy, M. P. and Marsden, C. D. (1982) Writer's cramp—a focal dystonia. *Brain*, **105**, 461–480.
137. Yanagisawa, N., Goto, A. and Narabayashi, H. (1972) Familial dystonia musculorum deformans and tremor. *J. Neurol. Sci.*, **16**, 125–136.
138. Johnson, W., Schwartz, G. and Barbeau, A. (1962) Studies on dystonia musculorum deformans. *Arch. Neurol.*, **7**, 301–313.
139. Baxter, D. W. and Lal, S. (1979) Essential tremor and dystonic syndrome. *Adv. Neurol.*, **24**, 373–377.

140. Korten, J. J., Notermans, S. L. H., Frenken, C. W. G. M., Gabreels, F. J. M. and Joosten, E. M. G. (1974) Familial essential myoclonus. *Brain*, **97**, 131–138.
141. Adams, R. D., Shahani, B. T. and Young, R. R. (1972) Tremor in association with polyneuropathy. *Trans. Am. Neurol. Assoc.*, **97**, 44–48.
142. Delwaide, P. J. and Schoenen, J. (1976) Non-hypertrophic familial neuropathy associated with intention tremor. A variety of Charcot–Marie–Tooth disease? *J. Neurol. Sci.*, **27**, 59–69.
143. Salisachs, P. (1976) Charcot–Marie–Tooth disease associated with 'essential tremor'. Report of 7 cases and a review of the literature. *J. Neurol. Sci.*, **28**, 17–40.
144. Said, G., Bathien, N. and Cesaro, P. (1982) Peripheral neuropathies and tremor. *Neurology*, **32**, 480–485.
145. Adams, R. D., Shahani, B. T. and Young, R. R. (1972) Tremor in association with polyneuropathy. *Trans. Am. Neurol. Assoc.*, **97**, 44–48.
146. Smith, I. S., Furness, P. and Thomas, P. K. (1984) Tremor in peripheral neuropathy. In *Movement Disorders: Tremor* (L. J. Findley and R. Calpildeo, Eds). McMillan Press, London, pp. 399–406.
147. Shahni, B. T., Young, R. R. and Adams, R. D. (1973) Neuropathic tremor. *Electroencephalogr.Clin. Neurophysiol.*, **34**, 800.
148. Johnson, S. L. G. and Hall, D. M. B. (1992) Post-traumatic tremor in head injured children. *Arch. Dis. Child.*, **67**, 227–228.
149. Andrew, J., Fowler, C. J. and Harrison, M. J. G. (1982) Tremor after head injury and its treatment by stereotaxic surgery. *J. Neurol. Neurosurg. Psychiatry*, **45**, 815–819.
150. Maki, Y., Akimoto, H. and Enomoto, T. (1980) Injuries in basal ganglia following head trauma in children. *Child's Brain*, **7**, 113–123.
151. Ellison, P. H. (1978) Propranolol for severe post-head injury action tremor. *Neurology*, **28**, 197–199.
152. Obeso, J. A. and Narbona, J. (1983) Post-traumatic tremor and myoclonic jerking. *J. Neurol. Neurosurg. Psychiatry*, **46**, 788.
153. Holmes, G. L. and Russman, B. S. (1986) Shuddering attacks: evaluation using electroencephalographic frequency modulation radiotelemetry and videotape monitoring. *Am. J. Dis. Child.*, **140**, 72–73.
154. Vanasse, M., Bedard, P. and Andermann, F. (1976) Shuddering attacks in children: an early clinical manifestation of essential tremor. *Neurology*, **26**, 1027–1030.
155. Golbe, L. I., Lazzarini, A. M., *et al.* (1993) Autosomal dominant parkinsonism with benign course and typical Lewy-body pathology. *Neurology*, **43**, 2222–2227.
156. Yokochi, M. (1993) Nosological concept of juvenile parkinsonism with reference to the dopa-responsive syndrome. *Adv. Neurol.*, **60**, 548–552.
157. Mizutani, Y., Yokochi, M. and Oyanagi, S. (1991) Juvenile parkinsonism: a case with first clinical manifestation at the age of six years and with neuropathological findings suggesting a new pathogenesis. *Clin. Neuropathol.*, **10**, 91–97.
158. Hayashida, K., Oyanagi, S., Mizutani, Y., *et al.* (1993) An early cytoplasmic change before Lewy body maturation: an ultrastructural study of the substantia nigra from an autopsy case of juvenile parkinsonism. *Acta. Neuropathol.*, **85**, 445–448.
159. Furukawa, Y., Nishi, K., Kondo, T., *et al.* (1993) CSF biopterin levels and clinical features of patients with juvenile parkinsonism. *Adv. Neurol.*, **60**, 562–567.
160. Nakano, K. K., Dawson, D. M. and Spence, A. (1972) Machado disease: a hereditary ataxia in Portuguese immigrants to Massachusetts. *Neurology*, **22**, 49–55.
161. Healton, E. B., Brust, J. C. M., Kerr, D. L., *et al.* (1980) Presumably Azorean

disease in a presumably non-Portuguese family (abstract). *Neurology*, **30**, 1084–1089.

162. Cooper, J. A., Nakada, T., Knight, R. T., *et al.* (1983) Autosomal dominant motor system degeneration in a black family. *Ann. Neurol.*, **14**, 585–587.
163. Sakai, T., Ohta, M. and Ishino, H. (1983) Joseph disease in a non-Portuguese family. *Neurology*, **33**, 74–80.
164. Romanul, F. C. A., Fowler, H. L. and Radvany, J. (1977) Azorean disease of the nervous system. *N. Engl. J. Med.*, **296**, 1505–1508.
165. Coutinho, P. and Andrade, C. (1978) Autosomal dominant system degeneration in Portuguese families of the Azores Islands. *Neurology*, **28**, 703–709.
166. Rosenberg, R. N. (1978) Joseph's disease. *Adv. Neurol.*, **21**, 33–57.
167. Rosenberg, R. N. (1992) Machado–Joseph disease: An autosomal dominant motor system degeneration. *Mov. Disord.*, **7**, 193–203.
168. Sudarsky, L., Corwin, L. and Dawson, D. M. (1992) Machado–Joseph disease in New England: clinical description and distinction from the olivopontocerebellar atrophies. *Mov. Disord.*, **7**, 204–208.
169. Hallervorden, J. and Spatz, H. (1922) Eigenartige Erkrankung im extrapyramidalen system mit besonderer beteiligung des globus pallidus und der substantia nigra. *Z. Neurol. Psychiat.*, **79**, 254–232.
170. Dooling, E. C., Schoene, W. C. and Richardson, E. P., Jr. (1974) Hallervorden–Spatz syndrome. *Arch. Neurol.*, **30**, 70–83.
171. Wigboldus, J. M. and Bruyn, G. W. (1968) Hallervorden–Spatz disease. In *Handbook of Clinical Neurology* (P. J. Vinken and G. W. Bruyn, Eds). North Holland, Amsterdam, pp. 604–631.
172. Vakili, S., Drew, A. L., Von Schuching, S., *et al.* (1977) Hallervorden–Spatz syndrome. *Arch. Neurol.*, **34**, 729–738.
173. Park, B. E., Netsky, M. G. and Betsill, W. L. (1975) Pathogenesis of pigment and spheroid formation in Hallervorden–Spatz syndrome and related disorders. *Neurology*, **25**, 1172–1178.
174. Szanto, J. and Gallyas, F. (1966) A study of iron metabolism in neuropsychiatric patients: Hallervorden–Spatz disease. *Arch. Neurol.*, **14**, 438–442 and Reference 172.
175. Swaiman, K. S., Smith, S. A., Trock, G. L., *et al.* (1983) Sea-blue histiocytes, lymphocytic cytosomes, movement disorder and 59Fe uptake in basal ganglia: Hallervorden–Spatz disease or ceroid storage disease with abnormal isotope scan? *Neurology*, **33**, 301–305.
176. Dooling, E. C., Richardson, E. P. Jr and Davis, K. R. (1980) Computed tomography in Hallervorden–Spatz disease. *Neurology*, **30**, 1128–1130.
177. Van Kirk, M. P., Larsen, P. D. and O'Conner, P. S. (1986) New computed tomography scan findings in Hallervorden–Spatz syndrome. *Neuro. Ophthalmol.*, **6**, 86–90.
178. Tennison, M. B., Bouldin, T. W. and Whaley, M. D. (1988) Mineralization of the basal ganglia detected by CT in Hallervorden–Spatz syndrome. *Neurology*, **38**, 154–155.
179. Schaffert, D. A., Johnsen, S. D., Drayer, B. P., *et al.* (1988) Magnetic resonance imaging in a patient with Hallervorden–Spatz disease (abstract). *Ann. Neurol.*, **24**, 354–355.
180. Sethi, K. D., Adams, R. J., Loring, D. W., *et al.* (1988) Hallervorden–Spatz syndrome: Clinical and magnetic resonance imaging correlations. *Ann. Neurol.*, **24**, 692–694.
181. Jankovic, J., Kirkpatrich, J. B., Blomquist, K. A., *et al.* (1985) Late-onset Hallervorden–Spatz disease presenting as familial parkinsonism. *Neurology*, **35**, 227–234.

9 Myoclonus and Infantile Spasms

FRANK M.C. BESAG
St Piers Lingfield, Surrey, UK

INTRODUCTION

Myoclonus is a neurological symptom or sign which is present in a large number of different conditions. The most common form is not pathological, occurring in the majority of normal people on falling asleep. In contrast, myoclonus may be a sign of serious hereditary, metabolic or infective conditions. It may be a consequence of epileptic discharges or may occur in conditions quite separate from epilepsy. In some individuals with epilepsy, non-epileptic myoclonus may occur or may even be induced by treatment for epilepsy. There is considerable debate about what should and should not be included within the definition of myoclonus. In keeping with the remarks of Lance[1], the present author considers that rhythmic repetitive movements belong to a separate category. For this reason, and partly for considerations of brevity, the conditions of 'palatal myoclonus' and the interesting phenomenon of epilepsia partialis continua will not be considered in this chapter. Most authors would include them, however. Infantile spasms have also been grouped under this chapter heading. There is a clinical similarity between the movements in this condition and those seen in some types of myoclonus. However, it is now accepted that there is a clear neurophysiological difference between infantile spasms and myoclonus.

The subject of myoclonus remains challenging in terms of characterization, classification and treatment. There have been few attempts to review this subject comprehensively in recent years, with the notable exception of the extensive collection of papers edited by Fahn, Marsden and Van Woert[2]. It is interesting to note that some textbooks of paediatric neurology hardly mention myoclonus, except in the context of myoclonic epilepsy. Considerable advances have been made in the definition of the syndromes of myoclonic epilepsy in childhood. The remainder of the field of myoclonus has been the subject of much less attention. This chapter will endeavour to provide an overview of both epilepsy-related and non-epileptic myoclonus.

HISTORY

The term myoclonus is generally attributed to Nikolaus Friedreich, who is more famous for the form of hereditary ataxia bearing his name. On 17

Movement and Allied Disorders. Edited by M. M. Robertson and V. Eapen

January 1878 he was asked to consult on a 50-year-old comb maker from Baden in the Heidelberg Medical Clinic. This man had been treated for pneumonia, but muscle jerks, present for the previous five years, were noted by the doctors. He was said to have shown multifocal jerking of all muscles except those of the face. Friedreich was able to distinguish this from movements seen in epilepsy, the chorea described by Sydenham in 1686, associated with rheumatic fever, and the involuntary movements described by Huntington in 1872[3]. In 1881 he published the case as a newly-described condition: 'paramyoklonus multiplex'. Hallett[4] has explained that 'klonus' referred to a quick movement, but Friedreich used the prefix 'myo' to indicate that this was not an epileptic condition. Para indicates symmetry (cf. paraplegia) and multiplex indicated that several different parts of the body were affected. The cause of this condition was uncertain but, having studied the spinocerebellar ataxia now referred to as Friedreich's ataxia, he considered that the pathology for paramyoklonus multiplex might also lie in the spinal cord. A subsequent autopsy on his patient revealed no pathology in the spinal cord.

Hallett[4] has described a number of conditions which were inappropriately called myoclonus in the late 19th century. Lowenfeld (1883, quoted in Hallett[4]) proposed shortening the name to myoklonus. Further contributions to the subject were made by Unverricht[5] and Lundborg[6]. Hallett[4] has commented that in the 22 years from Friedreich to Lundborg, myoclonus had come of age.

DEFINITION

The definition of myoclonus remains controversial. Marsden, Hallett and Fahn[7] have quoted Kinnier Wilson[8] as stating: 'the word "myoclonus" has been abused almost as much as "spasm"... although extensive [the literature on myoclonus] does not satisfy, many reports being ambiguous or meagre'.

Van Woert and Chung Hwang[9] have listed forms of myoclonus as being symmetrical or asymmetrical, synchronous or asynchronous, generalized or focal, bilateral or unilateral. The time intervals between single paroxysms or myoclonic contractions may be very variable. Facial muscles, extra-ocular muscles, head, trunk, extremity and vocal muscles may be involved. They pointed out that the intensity of the muscle contractions may be very variable in the same patient and may also vary from patient to patient. Myoclonus may be slight, or may be so powerful as to fling the patient across the room or onto the floor (massive myoclonus). The abrupt movements of myoclonus distinguish it from chorea.

It is important to distinguish myoclonus from other movements resulting from abrupt muscle contraction including tics, chorea, dystonia and tremor. Marsden *et al.*[7] have stated that tics can be controlled by an effort of will, at least temporarily, whereas myoclonus cannot. Tics are said to be accompanied by a conscious urge to move and by a sense of relief after the tic has occurred. Chorea is characterized by movements continuing in a constant flow, apparently randomly distributed over the body, with each muscle involved jerking randomly in time. In contrast, the jerks of myoclonus tend to be more repetitive, although they may be quite random in time. Dystonia is usually more easily distinguished from myoclonus because the spasms are prolonged, distorting the limb or body into characteristic postures. Marsden *et al.*[7] pointed out that both dystonia and myoclonus may coexist in the same patient. In general the dystonia takes precedence but if the myoclonus is prominent the term 'myoclonic dystonia' may be appropriate. The movement of tremor is not only rhythmical but is also said to be sinusoidal. Many authors allow the inclusion of rhythmical myoclonus but the rhythmic movement is said to be more like a 'square-wave' with intervals between each movement. Marsden *et al.*[7] also contrasts rhythmical myoclonus with the alternating contractions of agonist and antagonist muscles seen in the tremor of Parkinson's disease and some types of essential tremor. In this case electrophysiological analysis of the movement may assist in diagnosis.

Marsden *et al.*[7] have added that of all the movement disorders, myoclonus is the most difficult to encapsulate into a simple framework. They have explained that the term myoclonus means a quick movement of muscle and is used to describe muscle jerks similar to those produced by electric shocks to a peripheral motor nerve. They distinguish the term from the fasciculations resulting from peripheral nerve injury, pointing out that myoclonus is now generally restricted to movements from a central nervous system origin. The following definition was proposed: muscle jerking, irregular or rhythmic, arising in the central nervous system. Included in this definition are the movements produced not only by positive muscle contractions but also by sudden lapses of muscle contraction, as in asterixis. It is interesting to note that Marsden and Fahn[10], together with many other authors, include rhythmical movements within the definition of myoclonus, although Lance[1] commented in the concluding remarks of a volume edited by two of the same authors (Fahn, Marsden and Van Woert[10]) that rhythmic repetitive movements such as 'palatal myoclonus' also belonged to a separate category. It had already been acknowledged that the sinusoidal movements of tremor were different from the more 'square-wave' character of myoclonus. The same author has stated that the symmetrical limb movements seen in advanced cerebral diseases such as subacute sclerosing panencephalitis were considered to be a repetitive dystonia distinct from myoclonus. Lance's comments, and the volume in which they appear, were based on an international workshop on myoclonus in New York. It is refreshing, if somewhat frustrating, to note that international leaders in the field, who came together to prepare the most outstanding review of the subject in recent years, nevertheless appear to have concluded on a controversial note regarding something as basic as the definition of the condition. The consensus certainly seems to be that myoclonus is a brief involuntary muscle contraction (or relaxation) of abrupt onset, arising from the central nervous system. The origin may be in the cerebral cortex, subcortical structures or in the spinal cord. The 'segmental myoclonus' arising from the spinal cord tends to present as rhythmical movements, although Marsden *et al.*[7] have pointed out that both rhythmic and arrhythmic forms can occur. Marsden *et al.*[7] have also presented very interesting neurophysiological data supporting the concept that at least some forms of reflex movements appearing to have a simple spinal pathway can be shown, by back-summation of cortical potentials, to have cortical involvement. Segmental myoclonus will not be considered further in this chapter.

CLASSIFICATION

Undoubtedly the best and most comprehensive classification is that provided by Fahn, Marsden and Van Woert[2]. This classification, which is shown in Table 9.1, applies to all ages. A few of the diagnoses are inappropriate for children, for example Alzheimer's disease, but the classification is more remarkable for the fact that many of the subgroups either begin in childhood or are confined to the early years of life, some being fatal in infancy or childhood, for example, metabolic disorders such as non-ketotic hyperglycinaemia. However, it should be noted that some of the subgroups included in their classification are not universally accepted as myoclonus. Two examples have already been given, namely infantile spasms, which are distinct from myoclonus in the neurophysiological sense, and the jerks of subacute sclerosing panencephalitis, which many would consider as being myoclonic but some would view as being a type of repetitive dystonia[1].

One of the difficulties in providing a systematic classification lies in deciding whether this should be according to the aetiology, the clinical presentation or the neurophysiological characteristics. In some cases at least, for example in some of the myoclonic epilepsy syndromes, the classification appears somewhat arbitrary and the syndromes certainly include disparate subgroups in terms of such factors as aetiology and prognosis.

Van Woert and Chung Hwang[9] have listed five aetiological subcategories of myoclonus; familial, primary seizure disorders, brain injury, slow virus infection and miscellaneous. This classification is shown in Table 9.2.

Table 9.1. Classification of myoclonus

I Physiological myoclonus (normal subjects)
- A Sleep jerks (hypnic jerks)
- B Anxiety-induced
- C Exercise-induced
- D Hiccough (singultus)
- E Benign infantile myoclonus with feeding

II Essential myoclonus (no known cause and no other gross neurological deficit)
- A Hereditary (autosomal dominant)
- B Sporadic

III Epileptic myoclonus (seizures dominate and no encephalopathy, at least initially)
- A Fragments of epilepsy
  - Isolated epileptic myoclonic jerk
  - Epilepsia partialis continua
  - Idiopathic stimulus-sensitive myoclonus
  - Photosensitive myoclonus
  - Myoclonic absences in petit mal
- B Childhood myoclonic epilepsies
  - Infantile spasms
  - Myoclonic astatic epilepsy (Lennox–Gastuat)
  - Cryptogenic myoclonus epilepsy (Aicardi)
  - Awakening myoclonus epilepsy of Janz
- C Benign familial myoclonic epilepsy (Rabot)
- D Progressive myoclonus epilepsy: Baltic myoclonus (Unverricht–Lundborg)

IV Symptomatic myoclonus (progressive or static encephalopathy dominates)
- A Storage disease
  - Lafora body disease
  - Lipidoses, e.g. GM2 gangliosidosis, Tay–Sachs, Krabbe's
  - Ceroid-lipofuscinosis (Batten)
  - Sialidosis ('cherry-red spot')
- B Spinocerebellar degeneration
  - Ramsay Hunt syndrome
  - Friedreich's ataxia
  - Ataxia telangiectasia
- C Basal ganglia degenerations
  - Wilson's disease
  - Torsion dystonia
  - Hallervorden–Spatz disease
  - Progressive supranuclear palsy
  - Huntington's disease
  - Parkinson's disease
- D Dementias
  - Creutzfeldt–Jakob disease
  - Alzheimer's disease
- E Viral encephalopathies
  - Subacute sclerosing panencephalitis
  - Encephalitis lethargica
  - Arbor virus encephalitis
  - Herpes simplex encephalitis
  - Postinfectious encephalitis

continued overleaf

Table 9.1. *(continued)*

F Metabolic
- Hepatic failure
- Renal failure
- Dialysis syndrome
- Hyponatraemia
- Hypoglycaemia
- Infantile myoclonic encephalopathy (polymyoclonus) (± neuroblastoma)
- Nonketotic hyperglycinaemia
- Multiple carboxylase deficiency
- Biotin deficiency

G Toxic encephalopathies
- Bismuth
- Heavy-metal poisons
- Methyl bromide, DDT
- Drugs, including levodopa

H Physical encephalopathies
- Posthypoxia (Lance–Adams)
- Post-traumatic
- Heat stroke
- Electric shock
- Decompression injury

I Focal CNS damage
- Poststroke
- Post-thalamotomy
- Tumour
- Trauma
- Olivodentate lesions (palatal myoclonus)

SPECIFIC TYPES OF MYOCLONUS

Examples of non-epileptic and epileptic myoclonus will be described in the following sections. The list is by no means comprehensive.

ESSENTIAL MYOCLONUS

Friedreich's original case of 'paramyoklonus multiplex' may well have been an example of essential myoclonus. Daube and Peters[11] described a hereditary form of myoclonus which was inherited as an autosomal dominant trait in 12 cases, within two families. Arrhythmic jerks of the limbs, neck and trunk began between the ages of 1 and 20 years. They persisted throughout life. They were absent or reduced at rest and increased on action. Because they were relatively small in amplitude, they did not produce much disability. These patients were otherwise neurologically normal and were also of normal intelligence. There was no history of epilepsy and the electroencephalogram (EEG) was said to have been normal.

Table 9.2. Aetiology of myoclonus

Arrhythmic myoclonus	
I	Familial
	Hereditary essential myoclonus (paramyoclonus multiplex)
	Essential startle disease (hyperekplexia)
	Progressive myoclonic epilepsy
	Dyssynergia cerebellum myoclonica (Ramsay Hunt syndrome)
	Lipidosis, e.g. ganglioside storage diseases, Amaurotic family idiocy
II	Primary seizure disorders
	Idiopathic epilepsy
	Infantile spasms
III	Brain injury
	Postanoxic intention myoclonus
	Toxins
	Metabolic disorders
	Drug toxicity (e.g. penicillin, tricyclic antidepressants, levodopa)
IV	Slow virus infection
	Creutzfeldt–Jakob disease
V	Miscellaneous
	Opsoclonus
	Infantile myoclonic encephalopathy (polymyoclonia)
	Unusual causes of intention myoclonus
Rhythmical (segmental) myoclonus	
	Acute viral infections
	Subacute sclerosing panencephalitis (inclusion body encephalitis)
	Epilepsia partialis continua
	Nocturnal myoclonus
	Palatal myoclonus

The onset of essential myoclonus is usually after 5 years of age. Muscles of the trunk are more commonly affected than those of the limbs[12] but any territory can be involved.

In an earlier review[7] it was stated that periodic movements in sleep (nocturnal myoclonus) could be considered as a type of essential myoclonus because it is non-progressive and is not associated with other neurological pathology. Lance[1] has pointed out that the slow semi-purposive movements of sleep are thought to be a distinct entity and should not be called nocturnal myoclonus. He contrasted these movements to the 'night starts' and the startle response, which were considered to fall under the descriptive heading of myoclonus. Nocturnal myoclonus should certainly not be confused with the normal myoclonic jerk which occur in most people as they fall asleep. These are referred to as 'sleep jerks' or 'hypnic jerks'. The so-called nocturnal myoclonus consists of periodic movements involving the lower limbs which may be synchronous or asynchronous in the two limbs. The jerks occur during non-REM sleep, approximately every 30 sec and last 1.5–2.5 sec. This subject has been reviewed by Coleman *et al*[13]. Marsden *et al*[7] have pointed out that this syndrome can overlap with the restless leg syndrome.

Korten *et al.*[14] reported a family in which 12 members had essential myoclonus, seven had essential tremor and four had both disorders. The inheritance pattern was autosomal dominant. This suggests that there may be an overlap between essential myoclonus and essential tremor, at least in some cases.

Fahn and Sjaastad[15] examined 56 members of a Norwegian family in which hereditary essential myoclonus was definitely observed in nine individuals, probably in one, and possibly in a further one. Two other members had a history compatible with myoclonus but developed a permanent remission. Three of the family members with definite myoclonus also had features of mild focal dystonia, indicating an overlap between dystonia and hereditary myoclonus.

ESSENTIAL STARTLE DISEASE (HYPEREKPLEXIA)

Suhren, Bruyn and Tuynman[16] described this condition as a dominant hereditary disorder in 25 members in five generations within a single family. There was a transient congenital hypertonia in the waking state and hyperkinesia. The outstanding characteristic of this condition is the abnormal startle reaction. Subjects also have myoclonic jerks on falling asleep and were said to have excessive brainstem reflexes. Gastaut and Villeneuve[17] described a similar condition with myoclonic jerking or jumping in response to sudden noise.

METABOLIC DISORDERS

Myoclonic jerks may occur in several metabolic disorders including uraemia, hepatic coma, hypoglycaemia, hypernatraemia, hypocalcaemia, and kernicterus. For example, in renal failure asymmetrical myoclonic jerking may be seen, most obvious in the face and upper limbs.

The myoclonic jerks seen in association with inborn errors of metabolism such as nonketotic hyperglycinaemia are probably related to epileptic discharges in the brain and will be considered in the section on epilepsy.

Myoclonus, tremor, bradykinesia and rigidity have been observed one to several weeks after protein–calorie refeeding in children with protein–calorie malnutrition[18,19]. Aicardi[20] has stated that the localized jerking may be difficult to distinguish from epileptic jerking, especially from epilepsia partialis continua, which he reports having seen in two of his patients. Magnesium deficiency has been proposed as a cause for the neurological signs seen on protein–calorie refeeding.

INFECTIONS

Viral infections can result in myoclonus, with or without opsoclonus.

Subacute sclerosing panencephalitis (SSPE) was described in 1934[21]. It seems to follow early measles infection, under 2 years of age. The measles antibody is raised in the serum and in the cerebrospinal fluid. Involuntary movements, including myoclonic jerks, usually appear within 2–3 months of the onset of the illness which may typically be in late childhood or in the early to mid-teenage years. It might be argued that the myoclonus here is epileptic and should better be classified in the later section of this chapter. Alternatively, as already mentioned, some authors have suggested that the movements in SSPE should be classified as dystonic rather than myoclonic.

Children with congenital rubella[22] and occasionally with acquired rubella[23] have rarely developed a fatal encephalitis about 10 years after the initial infection, with progressive dementia, ataxia and myoclonic seizures. Again, it might be argued that this condition would more appropriately be considered in the section on epilepsy-related myoclonus.

Although Whipple disease is said to be very uncommon in children[24], neurological involvement including myoclonus has been described[25].

OPSOCLONUS AND 'DANCING-EYES' SYNDROME

Opsoclonus consists of conjugate, irregular jerking of the eyes. It is differentiated from nystagmus because it does not have fast and slow components. There are many causes, including viral encephalitis, lipidosis and 'infantile myoclonic encephalopathy'. Kinsbourne[26] described the 'ocular dance' of opsoclonus in association with irregular shock-like myoclonic jerks of the extremities, trunk and head. These were aggravated by intention and anxiety. They disappeared during sleep. The myoclonic contractions produced truncal ataxia and incoordination of limb movements. This is a non-epileptic condition with, not surprisingly, a normal EEG. Treatment with steroids may result in a dramatic response. The chaotic, rapid, sudden, irregular eye movements can occur in any direction and may be precipitated by changing fixation. Violent jerking of the limbs may occur on attempted movement. Opsoclonus–myoclonus syndrome sometimes follows a viral infection; Ichiba *et al.*[27] have reported mumps-induced cases. It is essential to consider the association with neuroblastoma, which must be sought both clinically and by investigation with ultrasound, urinary vanillyl-mandelic and homovanillic acid levels. Opsoclonus–myoclonus has also been reported with hydrocephalus and drug intoxication.

EPILEPSY AND MYOCLONUS

Outstanding contributions to the characterization of the syndromes of the myoclonic epilepsies of childhood have been made by French workers including Gastaut, Aicardi, Dravet, Baumanoir, Roger and Dulac. An excellent review of these syndromes appears in the volume edited by Roger *et al.*[28]. Aicardi[29] has stated that the nosology of the myoclonic epilepsies

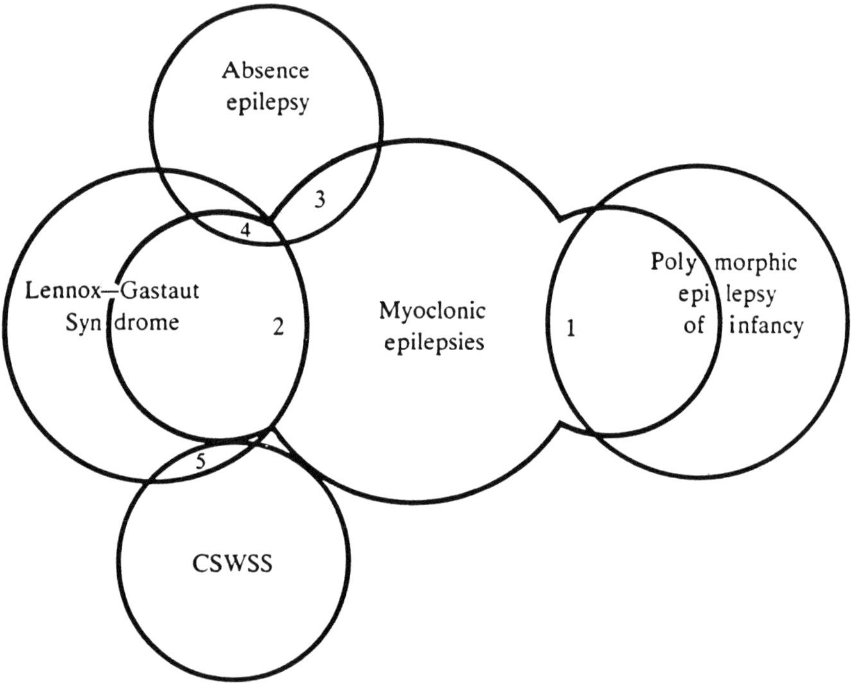

Figure 9.1. Schematic representation of the relationships between cryptogenic myoclonic epilepsy and other epileptic syndromes in infancy. (Intersections between circles and circles themselves have no quantitative significance.) (1) Myoclonic form of polymorphic epilepsy of infancy (severe myoclonic epilepsy). Myoclonic forms are probably more common than non-myoclonic ones. (2) Myoclonic variant of Lennox–Gastaut syndrome (LGS) (intermediate forms between LGS and myoclonic epilepsy). (3) Myoclonic absence epilepsy. (4) Myoclonic absence epilepsy with secondary development of LGS. (5) Transitional forms between LGS and continuous spike-waves of slow sleep (CSWSS). Doose myoclonic-astatic epilepsy is not shown because its criteria of definition differ from those used here and it probably corresponds in part to several of the syndromes shown. (After Aicardi, J. (1992) Epilepsy and other seizure disorders, In Diseases of the nervous system in childhood. *Clinics in Developmental Medicine* Nos. 115–118. MacKeith Press, London. pp. 911–1000, with permission.)

remains confused. He quotes Dravet as identifying two major groups: severe myoclonic epilepsy and benign myoclonic epilepsy, together with unclassifiable cases. He has added that other investigators, for example Lombroso[30] have cast doubts on the clear separation, instead suggesting that there is a spectrum of myoclonic syndromes with varying degrees of severity. To the myoclonic syndromes, one has to add the wide variety of precipitants leading to secondary myoclonic epilepsy, including infections, hypoxic injury, structural lesions, metabolic disorders and brain injury, including hypoxic and toxic damage. Aicardi has contributed much to demonstrating both the separation and the overlap of various epileptic syndromes. This concept is well illustrated by Fig. 9.1. The myoclonic epilepsy syndromes will be described in order of age of onset.

NEONATAL MYOCLONIC ENCEPHALOPATHY

Aicardi[31] has reviewed this subject comprehensively. The causes of the syndrome are many, and include autosomal recessive inborn errors of metabolism such as nonketotic hyperglycinaemia, methylmalonic acidaemia and propionic acidaemia. An autosomal recessive inheritance has also been suggested in cases in which no metabolic disorder was identified. The clinical manifestations include partial fragmentary erratic myoclonus, massive myoclonus, partial motor seizures and tonic infantile spasms. The EEG shows the so-called 'suppression-burst' pattern with bursts of spikes, sharp waves and slow waves separated by flattening of the EEG. The prognosis is poor, with severe neurological abnormalities and a high mortality. Half the patients died before the age of 1 year. Aicardi has made the clear distinction between this syndrome and the Ohtahara syndrome: the latter consistently includes tonic spasms and not myoclonus or partial seizures. This issue is discussed in further detail by Schlumberger et al.[32].

BENIGN MYOCLONIC EPILEPSY IN INFANTS

Dravet *et al.*[33] have made it clear that this is a rare syndrome characterized by brief bouts of generalized myoclonus occurring in the first or second year of life in normal children who often have a family history of epilepsy. The EEG shows generalized spike-and-wave or polyspike-wave discharges. The myoclonus is brief and isolated or grouped in clusters. These authors have emphasized that treatment is worthwhile and that the myoclonus is easily controlled by sodium valproate. They have suggested that the epilepsy is likely to continue and that cognitive development may be impaired if treatment is not given.

SEVERE MYOCLONIC EPILEPSY IN INFANTS

Dravet *et al.*[34] have reviewed the syndromes of severe myoclonic epilepsy in infants, originally described by them in 1982[35]. The syndrome is described as being homogeneous. There is a family history of epilepsy or febrile convulsions. The seizures begin during the first year of life as generalized or unilateral febrile clonic seizures. The average age of onset was about five months in Dravet's series. Although the onset of the myoclonus could be somewhat variable, it occurred between 1 and 4 years of age in all the children. The intensity of myoclonus varied from being barely discernible to massive myoclonus. Absences and partial seizures also occurred. EEGs showed fast generalized spike-and-wave discharges, and later exhibited variable focal and multifocal abnormalities. Photosensitivity occurred in 42% of Dravet's patients.

The seizures were very resistant to treatment. Sodium valproate, phenobarbitone and benzodiazepines have been used. Ethosuximide sometimes decreased the myoclonic attacks.

The aetiology of the condition remains unknown. The outcome tends to be poor. Neurological and mental deterioration are described in the second stage of the epilepsy. Dravet emphasized the large number of early deaths, namely 15.9%. This syndrome remains as one which is a cause for considerable concern because of its resistance to treatment and poor outcome.

MYOCLONIC ASTATIC EPILEPSY OF EARLY CHILDHOOD

The so-called Doose syndrome has been the subject of considerable discussion. Doose[36] himself has stated that this epilepsy syndrome generally has the following characteristics.

1. A genetic predisposition.
2. A mostly normal development and no neurological deficits before onset.
3. Primarily generalized myoclonic, astatic or myoclonic–astatic seizures.
4. Short absences and mostly generalized tonic–clonic seizures.
5. No tonic seizures or tonic drop attacks during daytime.
6. Generalized EEG patterns of spikes and waves with photosensitivity.
7. No multifocal EEG abnormalities.

He has agreed that there is an overlap with other syndromes such as benign and severe myoclonic epilepsy. Particular debate has centred around the overlap and difference between this syndrome and the Lennox–Gastaut syndrome. Doose has stated that Lennox–Gastaut syndrome differs from myoclonic astatic epilepsy because the following are true of the latter.

1. Genetic predisposition.
2. Mostly normal development before onset.
3. No neurometabolic or degenerative disease.
4. Usually no neurological deficit at onset.
5. Primary generalized myoclonic, astatic or myoclonic–astatic seizures.
6. Short absences and mostly generalized tonic–clonic seizures.
7. Rarely focal seizures.
8. No atypical absence seizures.
9. Tonic seizures during the night in unfavourable cases.
10. No tonic seizures or tonic drop attacks during daytime except for some rare cases with a most unfavourable course.
11. Primary generalized EEG patterns including generalized spike-and-wave discharges, photosensitivity and 4–7 cycle per second rhythms.
12. No multifocal EEG abnormalities.

The particular contrast would be with the axial tonic seizures which characteristically occur in most cases of Lennox–Gastaut syndrome.

Dulac *et al.*[37] have suggested that the series reported by Doose may comprise several subgroups, some of which correspond to syndromes described by others, for example the syndromes of severe and benign myoclonic epilepsy in infancy. Aicardi[38] has stated that the nosological situation of the various forms of myoclonic or myoclonic–astatic epilepsy remains confused. According to Aicardi[38], Doose has made is clear that he did not intend his description to be a 'rigidly defined syndrome' but wished to draw attention to a group of children with 'the wide variability of the idiopathic, generalized epilepsies of early childhood—as a result of multifactorial background responsible for electroclinical differences in presentation' (Doose[36]). Aicardi has pointed out that despite this, the Doose syndrome has tended, mistakenly, to be considered by some as a clear syndrome. Debate about the Doose syndrome continues. It is almost certainly not a single entity.

THE LENNOX–GASTAUT SYNDROME

Beaumanoir and Dravet[39] and Aicardi[38] are amongst the authors who have reviewed this important syndrome which constitutes a severe mixed epilepsy of childhood, generally resistant to antiepileptic treatment. The seizures include atypical absences, axial tonic seizures, atonic seizures and myoclonic seizures. The syndrome is also characterized by slow spike-and-wave discharges in the waking EEG (typically 2–2.5 Hz), bursts of 10 Hz discharges during sleep and poor intellectual development. Dulac *et al.*[37] have pointed out that the Lennox–Gastaut syndrome should perhaps not be classified with the myoclonic epilepsies of childhood since less than 20% exhibit myoclonus[40]. Aicardi[38] has stated that the Lennox–Gastaut syndrome is currently defined as an epilepsy syndrome characterized by multiple types of seizure including a nucleus of brief tonic, atonic and myoclonic attacks or atypical absences associated with an interictal EEG pattern of diffuse, slow spike-wave complexes. Mental retardation (learning disability) or deterioration is a very frequent but not constant feature. However, he has pointed out that some authors find this definition too inclusive and have proposed two additional criteria, namely the occurrence of generalized tonic seizures and the presence of 10 Hz EEG rhythms during sleep. Aicardi has commented that these features are not found in every case. He has emphasized that two main characteristics are generally thought to separate Lennox–Gastaut syndrome from myoclonic epilepsies proper: the presence and prominence of tonic seizures and the predominance of interictal slow spike-wave complexes. However, these features are not pathognomonic. In his review, he has also stated that the incidence is poorly known, with a frequency estimated to be between 1% and 10% of childhood epilepsies. The lower figure is probably more correct. Onset is usually between 1 and 7 years with a peak of 3–5 years. It is important to note that around 70–75% of the children with Lennox–Gastaut syndrome have a neurological abnormality, previous epilepsy or learning disability. West syndrome is estimated to precede the Lennox–Gastaut syndrome in about 17–41% of cases, according to various authors. Tonic seizures occur in 74% of cases or more.

If tonic seizures are included in the definition they must, of course, occur in 100% of cases. Aicardi[38] describes the axial tonic seizure as producing a flexor movement of the head and trunk and the axorhizomelic seizures having associated abduction and elevation of the upper limb. Atypical absence seizures are reported to occur in 13–100% of the patients. Myoclonic seizures are distinguished by spike-wave or polyspike-wave discharges in contrast to atonic seizures which tend to have the same EEG discharges as tonic seizures. Myoclonic seizures and atonic seizures are variously estimated to occur in 4–23% and 14–36% of children with Lennox–Gastaut syndrome, respectively. Episodes of nonconvulsive status epilepticus typically occur in this syndrome, the rates quoted being from 50% to 75%.

The characteristic interictal EEG pattern is of slow spike-and-wave complexes occurring singly or in groups with a frequency of 1–2.5 Hz. Although they are diffusely distributed they usually predominate over the frontocentral part of the brain. Most of the children have learning disability but 7–10% are said to remain unaffected in terms of their learning. In most of the children with Lennox–Gastaut syndrome, developmental delay is present before the onset of the syndrome, but 25–30% seemed to develop normally before the first seizure.

Beaumanoir and Dravet[39] have stated that 60% of children with this syndrome have a previous encephalopathy. Many cases, typically around 20%, are preceded by infantile spasms (West syndrome—see below).

The Lennox–Gastaut syndrome has traditionally been considered as one of the most devastating and difficult to treat syndromes of childhood epilepsy. Some more encouraging results have been obtained with the use of lamotrigine, a relatively new antiepileptic drug. In particular, Oller *et al.*[41] have reported that one-third of their patients were rendered seizure free, at least initially, when treated with lamotrigine. In the past, treatment has generally been with sodium valproate, to which some clinicians added benzodiazepines. The present author does not recommend this combination because it can, in at least some children, be very sedative.

EPILEPSY WITH MYOCLONIC ABSENCES

Myoclonic absence seizures are differentiated from other absence seizures by marked myoclonus occurring during the typical three-per-second spike-and-wave discharge. These seizures should be differentiated from the mild clonic movements which occur in typical absence seizures and which have been noticed particularly in recent years, since video/EEG recordings have been more readily available. Mild clonic movements are said to be quite common in absence seizures. In contrast, epilepsy with myoclonic absences is said to be rare; for example it has been quoted as occurring in 0.5–1% of the epilepsies observed in the selected population of the Centre Saint-Paul[42]. The mean age of onset of this type of epilepsy is said to be 7 years with a quoted range from 11 months to 12.2 years[42]. Learning disability is present before the onset of the epilepsy in a large proportion of cases: 44% in the series of 36 cases quoted by Tassinari *et al.*[42]. The myoclonic absences are prominent but other seizure types may occur, including generalized tonic–clonic seizures and additional absence seizures without severe myoclonus. In seven of the cases of the Tassinari *et al.* series, there were sudden and severe falls.

It should be noted that there was a high proportion of intellectual impairment in this group, in contrast to the situation for typical absence seizures in which intellectual development is usually normal.

ABSENCE EPILEPSY WITH EYELID MYOCLONUS

Jeavons[43] has described the association of eyelid myoclonus and absence seizures. Appleton *et al.*[44] have documented a number of cases. Panayiotopoulos[45] has expressed the strong view that this association represents a distinct epilepsy syndrome.

JUVENILE MYOCLONIC EPILEPSY

The name of Janz[46] is usually associated with this syndrome, following his publication in 1957 of 47 patients which he described as having 'impulsiv-petit mal'. Wolf[47] has recently reviewed this syndrome. The onset of juvenile myoclonic epilepsy is usually between 12 and 18 years, although the age of onset varies between 8 and 26 years, according to Janz. This syndrome is also sometimes referred to as myoclonic epilepsy of adolescence, in keeping with other reports stating an average age of onset in the mid-teenage years. The myoclonic jerks are usually, but not always, symmetrical, and may be single or repetitive. They are most prominent in the upper limbs, which go through rapid extensor jerks. The facial muscles are generally not involved. Sometimes the jerks may extend to the lower limbs. They classically occur soon after waking. Some authors have described the so-called 'flying-saucer syndrome', indicating that crockery is liable to be broken at breakfast time when it is flung from the hand in a myoclonic jerk. Most subjects seen in clinics also have generalized tonic–clonic seizures, classically also on waking. Absence seizures are also associated with juvenile myoclonic epilepsy and have been said to occur in about 10% of cases. Spikes, polyspikes and spike-and-wave discharges have been recorded in the EEGs.

The striking feature of this epilepsy syndrome is the response to sodium valproate in a large proportion of cases. In contrast to the general recommendations for epilepsy treatment, it is usually essential to treat long term. Even if the seizures have been well controlled for long periods, it is inadvisable to withdraw the sodium valproate because relapse is highly likely.

An interesting recent advance has been the suggestion that the gene for this epilepsy syndrome may be on chromosome 6[48]. However, Whitehouse *et al.*[49] have failed to confirm this.

PROGRESSIVE MYOCLONIC EPILEPSIES IN CHILDHOOD AND ADOLESCENCE

Roger *et al.*[50] have reviewed this subject and have stated that progressive myoclonus epilepsies account for about 1% of all epilepsy of childhood and adolescence. The syndrome of progressive myoclonus epilepsy covers many underlying causes. Some of these were listed by the Marseille consensus group[51] and quoted by Roger *et al.*[50] (see Table 9.3). It is interesting to note that metabolic disorders occurring in infancy and early childhood are excluded from some of the classifications. Amongst the important causes are the familial condition of Unverricht–Lundborg disease, described below, Lafora body disease, characterized by deposits of

Table 9.3. Classification and diagnosis of progressive myoclonus epilepsy cases at the Centre Saint-Paul (1960–1990) and at the Neurological Institute in Montreal

	Centre Saint-Paul (Marseille France) 1960–1990	Neurological Institute (Montreal/Canada) (Berkovic *et al.*, 1989)
Unverricht–Lundborg Baltic type	0	9
Unverricht–Lundborg Mediterranean type	47	0
MERRF	2	13
Lafora disease	33	12
Ceroid-lipofuscinosis:		
infantile type	0	0
late-infantile type	7	34
intermediate type	2	0
juvenile type	2	8
adult type	0	2
Action myoclonus—renal failure syndrome	0	4
Childhood Huntington's disease	2	0
Gaucher's disease	1	0
Unclassified	7	2
Total	103	84

polyglycans in biopsies of skin or liver, mitochondrial encephalomyopathy with ragged red fibres (MERRF) in muscle biopsies, and metabolic diseases including sialidosis, Gaucher disease and ceroid lipofuscinosis (Batten disease and its variants). It is also of particular interest to note that an infantile myoclonic form of Huntington's disease can present early in childhood, after about 3 years of age, with epilepsy including massive myoclonic jerks, rather than the choreiform movements seen in adulthood. Inheritance is by autosomal dominant transmission from the paternal side. Early death is common, between 4 and 6 years after onset.

The classic example of progressive myoclonic epilepsy is the so-called 'Baltic myoclonus' or Unverricht–Lundborg disease, recently reviewed by Koskiniemi[52]. Although it was first described in Estonia and is notably prevalent in the Baltic area, cases have been described world-wide. Several cases have been carefully documented in Finland. The previous distinction between 'Baltic' and 'Mediterranean' types has been questioned and may be resolved by molecular genetic studies[50]. This autosomal recessive condition is characterized by the onset of myoclonic jerks usually between 6 and 15 years, with subsequent tonic–clonic seizures and massive myoclonic jerks. The typical EEG is markedly abnormal with spike-and-wave or polyspike-and-wave paroxysms and photosensitivity. Past accounts have suggested an inevitably progressive course with loss of the ability to walk, and death within 15 years. More patients now survive, possibly because the previously-used high-dose phenytoin was deleterious in contrast to the apparent benefit of sodium valproate and clonazepam. Koskiniemi[52] has stated that in some cases the condition may stop after 5–10 years and that these subjects may be able to live independently. This again raises the question of whether all the reported cases of Unverricht–Lundborg disease represent the same condition.

As a working rule, any child with severe myoclonic epilepsy should be considered to have a metabolic disorder or identifiable syndrome until proved otherwise.

OTHER CLASSES OF CHILDHOOD MYOCLONIC EPILEPSY

Dulac *et al.*[37] have described children with myoclonic epilepsy which does not fit easily into the various syndrome types already described. They examined 28 children with no previous neurological abnormalities and with an epilepsy onset after 1 year of age, distinguishing two subgroups: one had a favourable outcome and the other did not. The unfavourable group were characterized by long periods of status epilepticus with erratic myoclonus of the face and limbs, lasting several weeks. Series of tonic seizures during slow-wave sleep persisted for several years and there was very significant cognitive deterioration. In the favourable group, although they exhibited several seizure types, the epilepsy resolved, lasting a mean of 14 months. The final IQ, following the last seizure, was within the normal range in all cases except one.

INFANTILE SPASMS

Undoubtedly the classic review of this subject remains that of Jeavons and Bower[53]. The original publication by West[54] in a letter to the *Lancet* in 1841 was a description by this doctor of his own child. Jeavons and Bower[53] have pointed out that although the typical infantile spasm is a sudden, brief, generalized movement like a massive myoclonic jerk, it is often longer than a myoclonic jerk. It is the duration of the spasm that has led to the distinction of this type of seizure from the myoclonic jerk. Flexion spasms are the commonest form—the arms are flung outwards and forwards and flexion occurs at the hips. This is the so-called 'salaam' movement, which has also been described as a jack-knife movement. The onset is usually between 3 and 8 months of age, peaking at around 5 or 6 months, and is nearly always before 1 year. Males are more often affected. Flexor spasms are the commonest type of seizure, reported in 68% of the cases of Jeavons and Bower[53]. Extensor, lightning and nodding spasms have also been described but these usually occur in combination with other types. The spasms may be repeated with many, e.g. 30–100, occurring in each episode. More than one episode may occur per day. The Jeavons and Bower[53] review comments that there is a tendency for a progressive lengthening between the spasms and diminution of their severity. The spasm is often associated with a cry which may be either ictal or postictal. The classical EEG pattern is that of hypsarrhythmia. This term was introduced by Gibbs and Gibbs[55] to describe a very disorganized EEG pattern, with high-voltage random slow waves and spikes in all areas. The spike discharges may be generalized but are not rhythmically repetitive, in sharp contrast to the very regular pattern seen, for example, in absence seizures. The West syndrome comprises infantile spasms, hypsarrhythmia and learning disability.

In the study of Jeavons and Bower[53] of 112 cases, 32% were cryptogenic, 60% were symptomatic and 18% were doubtful in origin. The cryptogenic group had an apparently normal birth and development until the onset of the spasms. In the symptomatic cases, a large number of different causes was identified. The largest subgroup of these by far (35%), had an abnormal perinatal history.

Jeavons and Bower[53] stated that 14% of their cases started within one week of an immunization. A very interesting debate followed the initial reports that immunization, particularly the pertussis immunization, might precipitate infantile spasms. Baird and Borofsky[56] reported that nine of 24 previously normal children had immunizations shortly before the onset of infantile spasms. The results of the National Childhood Encephalopathy Study in the UK are of particular interest. Two studies[57,58] reported that the pertussis immunization seemed to bring cases of infantile spasms forward in time but did not generally increase the overall risk. They suggested the possibility that the febrile reaction to the vaccine might have been a non-specific triggering factor in a susceptible child but this should not be interpreted as stating that immunization was the cause of the seizures, which would have presented with another precipitant had it not been for the immunization.

The later review by Jeavons and Livet[59] has pointed out that with better investigation facilities, including computed tomography (CT) scanning, magnetic resonance imaging (MRI), single photon emission tomography (SPET) and positron emission tomography (PET), many of the cases which previously would have been classified as cryptogenic can now be identified as being symptomatic. Causes in the symptomatic group include prenatal factors such as infections with cytomegalovirus, toxoplasmosis and rubella, prenatal and perinatal brain insults of various types, brain malformations (including Aicardi syndrome), agenesis of the corpus callosum without the Aicardi syndrome, specific brain malformation such as pachygyrias, lissencephaly, hemimegalencephaly, cortical dysplasias of various types, tuberous sclerosis and metabolic disorders, including phenylketonuria, nonketotic hyperglycinaemia and pyridoxine dependency.

Jeavons and Livet[59] have commented that symptomatic infantile spasms are usually linked to diffuse brain damage but are sometimes associated with focal lesions such as angiomas, tumours and porencephalic cysts. Chugani *et al.*[60] in PET studies using fluorodeoxyglucose found specific regions of hypometabolism in five out of 13 cases of infantile spasms which had previously been thought to be cryptogenic. Four of these infants underwent surgical resection of the lesion. He has recently reported[61] that at least one of the surgically treated infants has developed into a child of above-average intelligence.

Another interesting subcategory of symptomatic infantile spasms is that of tuberous sclerosis. It has recently become clear that this group of infants responds remarkably well to the relatively new antiepileptic drug vigabatrin[62]. It is possible that this treatment will change the outcome of infantile spasms substantially in those cases in which tuberous sclerosis is the underlying cause.

With the exceptions just stated, the treatment of infantile spasms has generally been rather disappointing. Responses to ACTH or steroids is often initially quite good but relapses may occur. Nitrazepam has also been used. A number of other drugs have been tried but without great success.

A recent review[63] has emphasized that a high proportion of children with infantile spasms also exhibit seizures of other types, particularly partial seizures. A prospective study using 24-hour EEG monitoring in 74 patients found that partial seizures occurred in 51% of the symptomatic cases and 33% of the cryptogenic cases[64]. In 14 of the patients the partial seizures were immediately followed by a cluster of spasms. Although the existence of partial seizures was not related to a defined cortical lesion, they seemed frequently to be associated with brain malformation.

Plouin and Dulac[63] specifically discussed the question of myoclonic seizures in association with infantile spasms. Although they agreed with the comment of Kellaway *et al.*[65] that infantile spasms should be differentiated clearly from myoclonic jerks, they also pointed out that myoclonic seizures can occur in association with infantile spasms. The epileptic–myoclonic jerk is a brief muscular contraction preceded by a burst of polyspikes or polyspikes and waves. An infantile spasms is a short tonic contraction accompanied by generalized low amplitude fast activity or by generalized high amplitude slow waves[65]. Dulac *et al*[66] reported four families with both infantile spasms and myoclonic seizures. These families may have had a metabolic disorder. Donat and Wright[67] found myoclonic seizures in 11% of their patients with infantile spasms. Plouin and Dulac[63] have pointed out that it is possible that epileptic and non-epileptic myoclonic jerks may occur in children with infantile spasms.

The outcome of infantile spasms is generally poor. Many of the children will proceed to the Lennox–Gastaut syndrome, already discussed. The specific results of outcome studies depend on the length of follow up. The spasms usually resolve and are said to be rare after the age of 5 years. The EEG generally changes from hypsarrhythmia, either showing other abnormalities or becoming normal. Depending on the length of follow up, around one-half of the children continue to have seizures of other types. Learning disability, which is often severe, is present in 80–91% of cases. The mortality figures are also a cause for concern. Different authors have quoted figures varying from 3–30%. Jeavons and Bower[53] found a mortality of 13% by 3 years 6 months of age in their own series. Most of the deaths were in the symptomatic group and the mortality in the majority of cases probably reflected the severity of the underlying pathology.

Infantile spasms remain a severe, early onset epilepsy of childhood with a poor outlook.

NON-MYOCLONIC ABNORMAL MOVEMENTS IN EPILEPSY AND NON-EPILEPTIC MYOCLONUS IN CHILDREN WITH EPILEPSY

Included in this group are non-myoclonic abnormal movements in epilepsy and non-epileptic myoclonus in children with epilepsy. An indication has been given of the various classifications of the myoclonic epilepsies but many other abnormal movements occur as a manifestation of epilepsy. Most of these would not be confused with myoclonus but some are quite difficult to distinguish from it. The rhythmical movements of a clonic seizure will usually be recognized as such. Some classifications of myoclonus include epilepsia partialis continua but, as already discussed, the consensus suggested by Lance[1] would imply that this should be excluded. The wide variety of odd movements seen in complex partial seizures often cause considerable diagnostic confusion but this arises primarily because they are all too frequently not recognized as being epilepsy at all. They are not, however, likely to be confused with myoclonus. Perhaps the most interesting and confusing situation arises in the child who falls as a result of an epileptic attack. Severe injuries may result from falls in tonic seizures, atonic seizures and massive myoclonic jerks. Although pathophysiologically these seizures are distinct, they may inappropriately be lumped together as 'drop attacks'. In the tonic seizure, the child stiffens, often letting out a cry as the breath is exhaled as a result of the contraction of the chest muscles against the partly-closed larynx. Because there is no saving reactions, the head may fall in a long arc to the ground, causing quite severe injury. The flexor tonic seizure may fling the child to the ground, again causing injury. The atonic seizure is the opposite of a tonic seizure. All muscle tone is suddenly lost and the child falls hard to the ground because there is nothing to support the standing posture. If the atonic attacks are very brief, the child may sag momentarily at the knees but recover in time to prevent a full fall. Some children fall to their knees in brief atonic seizures and may require knee-pads to prevent injury. In other children the fall is complete and a protective helmet, sometimes with a face-guard, may be necessary to prevent severe and repeated injury. Massive myoclonic jerks may also fling the child from the standing position and result in injury. In both atonic seizures and massive myoclonic jerks, the recovery is usually swift. Tonic seizures tend to last a little longer and recovery may not be quite so rapid. To add to the complexity of the situation, the atonic attack may be preceded by a myoclonic jerk. Video telemetry is invaluable for distinguishing these types of seizures.

It has already been pointed out that infantile spasms are clinically and neurophysiologically different from myoclonic jerks: the duration is slightly longer and the EEG pattern is different.

Another area of confusion which can easily lead to mismanagement is the occurrence of non-epileptic myoclonic jerks in someone who has epilepsy. A good example of this is the precipitation of non-epileptic myoclonic jerks by carbamazepine[68]. Addition of sodium valproate to treat these myoclonic jerks, on the assumption that they are part of the epileptic syndrome, would be totally inappropriate. The correct measure is to reduce or withdraw the carbamazepine, if possible.

EXAMINATION AND INVESTIGATION OF THE CHILD WITH MYOCLONUS

A careful and detailed history is undoubtedly one of the most important factors in ensuring that the right diagnosis is made in the child with myoclonus. The presence of a family history may alert the clinician to the possibility of benign familial myoclonus, a childhood variant of Huntington's chorea, Unverricht–Lundborg disease or a metabolic disorder. The history of the progression of the condition in other members of the family may distinguish the benign from the serious. Specific enquiry about seizures may distinguish non-epileptic from epileptic myoclonus. Similarly, when clinicians take a seizure history, it is important to ask specifically about myoclonus. A characteristic history of juvenile myoclonic epilepsy generally implies a good response to sodium valproate and avoids the frustration of trying ineffective management strategies. The parents may not ask for the referral until the associated tonic–clonic seizures cause them concern and they may neglect to tell the doctor about the myoclonic seizures. A careful drug history to exclude drug-induced myoclonus is also important. Similarly a history of anoxic or toxic brain injury may give a strong indication of the cause of the myoclonus.

Physical examination of the child may reveal the stigmata of tuberous sclerosis which has presented with infantile spasms or has proceeded to the Lennox–Gastaut syndrome. The characteristic pale patches on the skin are more obvious if examined using the ultraviolet Wood's light. Adenoma sebaceum, the characteristic facial 'rash' of tuberous sclerosis, tends to appear later in childhood. The shagreen patch of roughened skin, usually in the lumbar area, can also be a useful diagnostic sign indicating tuberous sclerosis. Again, the family history may be invaluable in the diagnosis of the condition, which is transmitted as an autosomal dominant, although a large proportion of cases appear to be new mutations. The diagnosis is important because babies with infantile spasms associated with this condition usually respond well to vigabatrin. Genetic counselling is also an important aspect of the overall management of tuberous sclerosis.

Myoclonus may be exacerbated by anxiety or by asking the child to do something. Observation of the myoclonus by the clinician helps to characterize it. The presence or absence of other neurological signs may also give an indication of the diagnosis; in particular, cerebellar signs should be sought.

The present author always asks the child to hold his or her hands outstretched with eyes closed. This may indicate the presence of brief epileptiform discharges leading to momentary losses of muscle tone. These are not usually true myoclonic movements. However, if the child is having frequent myoclonic movements these will be clearly demonstrated if the hands are held outstretched. Another useful technique is to hold the child's hands whilst engaging in conversation. Sometimes multiple small twitches may be felt rather than seen. Subsequent video/EEG recording will determine whether these movements are directly related to epileptiform discharges or not. Prolonged EEG monitoring may be necessary to characterize myoclonic movements, especially if they are infrequent. Cassette recording of the EEG is invaluable but video/EEG telemetry is a much more powerful technique because the clinical appearance and the EEG abnormality can be correlated exactly in time. The present author has certainly seen examples of young people with abnormal epileptiform discharges in the EEG and series of jerks, but the jerks did not correspond in time to the EEG abnormalities.

If a metabolic disorder is suspected, it is essential to carry out basic biochemical screening together with serum amino acids and urinary organic acids. Some of the rare forms of metabolic disorders require specific biopsies. These investigations are summarized well in standard textbooks of paediatric neurology[69].

CONCLUSION

The causes of myoclonus in childhood vary from the benign to the very serious. Careful characterization of the cause of the myoclonus by taking a detailed history, examining the child and arranging selected neurophysiological and biochemical tests, allows the clinician to provide accurate information to the family and to ensure appropriate management of the child.

ACKNOWLEDGEMENT

The author is deeply indebted to three outstanding colleagues for their help and encouragement: Professors David Marsden, Olivier Dulac and Jean Aicardi.

REFERENCES

1. Lance, J. W. (1986) Concluding remarks, in Myoclonus. *Adv. Neurol.*, **43**, 707–709.
2. Fahn, S., Marsden, C. D. and Van Woert, M. H. (1986) Myoclonus. *Adv. Neurol.*, **43**.
3. Huntington, G. (1872) On chorea. *Med. Surg. Reporter*, **26**, 317–321.
4. Hallett, M. (1986) Early history of myoclonus. *Adv. Neurol.*, **43**, 7–10.
5. Unverricht, H. (1891) *Die Myoklonie*. Franz Deuticke, Leipzig und Wien.
6. Lundborg, H. (1903) *Die Progressive Myoklonus-epilepsie*. Almqvist and Wiksell, Uppsala.
7. Marsden, C. D., Hallett, M. and Fahn, S. (1982) The nosology and pathophysiology of myoclonus. In *Movement Disorders* (C.D. Marsden and S. Fahn, Eds). Butterworth, London, pp. 196–248.
8. Wilson, S. A. K. (1940) In *Neurology* (Bruce A. M. Ed). Williams and Wilkins, Baltimore.
9. Van Woert, M. H. and Chung Hwang, E. (1979) Myoclonus. In *Handbook of Clinical Neurology*, Vol 38 (P.J. Vinken and G.W. Bruyn, Eds). North-Holland, Amsterdam, pp. 575–593.
10. Fahn, S., Marsden, C. D. and Van Woert, M. H. (1986) Definition and classification of myoclonus. *Adv. Neurol.*, **43**, 1–5.
11. Daube, J. and Peters, H. A. (1966) Hereditary essential myoclonus. *Arch. Neurol. (Chicago)*, **15**, 587–594.
12. Bressman, S. and Fahn, S. (1986) Essential myoclonus. *Adv. Neurol.*, **43**, 287–294.
13. Coleman, R. M., Pollack, C. P. and Weitzman, E. D. (1980) Periodic movements in sleep (nocturnal myoclonus): relation to sleep disorders. *Ann. Neurol.*, **8**, 416–421.
14. Korten, J. J., Notermans, S. L. H., Frenken, C. W. G. M., Gabreels, F. J. M. and Joosten, E. M. G. (1974) Familial essential myoclonus. *Brain*, **97**, 131–138.
15. Fahn, S. and Sjaastad, O. (1991) Hereditary essential myoclonus in a large Norwegian family. *Mov. Disord.*, **6**, 237–247.
16. Suhren, O., Bruyn, G. W. and Tuynman, J. A. (1966) Hyperekplexia. A hereditary startle syndrome. *J. Neurol. Sci.*, **3**, 577–605.
17. Gastaut, H. and Villeneuve, A. (1967) The startle disease or hyperekplexia: pathological surprise reaction. *J. Neurol. Sci.*, **5**, 523–542.
18. Kahn, E. and Falcke, H. C. (1956) A syndrome simulating encephalitis affecting children recovering from malnutrition (kwashiorkor). *J. Paediatr.*, **49**, 37–45.

19. Woodd-Walker, R. B. (1970) Kwashi shakes, *Lancet*, **i**, 299.
20. Aicardi, J. (1992) Electrolyte and acid-base metabolism disturbances, nutritional disorders and other systemic diseases. In *Diseases of the Nervous System in Childhood. Clinics in Developmental Medicine*; Nos 115–118. MacKeith Press, London, pp. 1241–1275.
21. Dawson, J. R. (1934) Cellular inclusions in cerebral lesions of epidemic encephalitis. *Arch. Neurol. Psychiatry*, **31**, 685–700.
22. Townsend, J. J., Baringer, J. R., Wolinsky, J. S., Malamud, N., Mednick, J. P., Panitch, H. S., Scott, R. A. T., Oshiro, L. S. and Cremer, N. E. (1975) Progressive rubella panencephalitis: late onset after congenital rubella. *N. Engl. J. Med.*, **292** 990–993.
23. Lebon, P. and Lyon, G. (1974) Non-congenital rubella encephalitis. *Lancet*, **2**, 468.
24. Barakat, A. Y., Bitar, J. and Nassar, V. H. (1973) Whipple's disease in a seven-year-old child: report of a case. *Am. J. Proct.*, **24**, 312–314.
25. Halperin, J. J., Landis, D. M. D and Kleinman, G. M. (1982) Whipple disease of the nervous system. *Neurology*, **32**, 612–617.
26. Kinsbourne, M. (1962) Myoclonic encephalopathy of infants. *J. Neurol. Neurosurg. Psychiatry*, **25**, 271–279.
27. Ichiba, N., Miyake, Y., Sato, K., Oda, M. and Kimoto, N. (1988) Mumps-induced opsoclonus-myoclonus and ataxia. *Pediatr Neurol*,. **4**, 224–227.
28. Roger, J., Bureau, M., Dravet, Ch., Dreifuss, F. E., Perret, A., Wolf, P. (eds). (1992) *Epileptic Syndromes in Infancy, Childhood and Adolescence* (2nd ed). John Libbey, London.
29. Aicardi, J. (1992) Epilepsy and other seizure disorders. In *Diseases of the Nervous System in Childhood. Clinics in Developmental Medicine*; Nos 115–118. MacKeith Press, London, pp. 911–1000.
30. Lombroso, C. T. (1990) Early myoclonic encephalopathy, early infantile epileptic encephalopathy and benign and severe infantile myoclonic epilepsies: a critical review and personal contributions. *J. Clin. Neurophysiol.*, **7**, 380–408.
31. Aicardi, J. (1992) Early myoclonic encephalopathy (neonatal myoclonic encephalopathy). In *Epileptic Syndromes in Infancy, Childhood and Adolescence* (2nd ed) (J. Roger, M. Bureau, Ch. Dravet, F. E. Dreifuss, A. Perret and P. Wolf, Eds). John Libbey, London, pp. 13–23.
32. Schlumberger, E., Dulac, O. and Plouin, P. (1992) Early infantile epileptic syndrome(s) with suppression-burst: nosological considerations. In *Epileptic Syndromes in Infancy, Childhood and Adolescence* (2nd ed) (J. Roger, M. Bureau, Ch. Dravet, F. E. Dreifuss, A. Perret and P. Wolf, Eds). John Libbey, London, pp. 35–42.
33. Dravet, Ch., Bureau, M. and Roger, J. (1992) Benign myoclonic epilepsy in infants. In *Epileptic Syndromes in Infancy, Childhood and Adolescence* (2nd ed) (J. Roger, M. Bureau, Ch. Dravet, F. E. Dreifuss, A. Perret and P. Wolf, Eds). John Libbey, London, pp. 67–74.
34. Dravet, Ch., Bureau, M., Guerrini, R., Giraud, N. and Roger, J. (1992) Severe myoclonic epilepsy in infants. In *Epileptic Syndromes in Infancy, Childhood and Adolescence* (2nd ed) (J. Roger, M. Bureau, Ch. Dravet, F.E. Dreifuss, A. Perret and P. Wolf, Eds). John Libbey, London, pp. 75–88.
35. Dravet, C., Roger, J., Bureau, M. and Dalla Bernardina, B. (1982) Myoclonic epilepsies in childhood. In *Advances in Epileptology, XIIIth Epilepsy International Symposium* (H. Akimoto, H. Kazamatsuri, M. Seino and A. A. Ward, Eds). Raven Press, New York, pp. 135–140.
36. Doose, H. (1992) Myoclonic astatic epilepsy of early childhood. In *Epileptic Syndromes in Infancy, Childhood and Adolescence* (J. Roger, M. Bureau, Ch. Dravet, F. E. Dreifuss, A. Perret and P. Wolf, Eds). John Libbey, London, pp. 103–114.

37. Dulac, O., Plouin, P., Chiron, C., Schlunberger, E. and Jambaque, I. (1995) Non progressive myoclonic epilepsy in childhood. A combination of cryptogenic and idiopathic disorders (in press).
38. Aicardi, J. (1994) Personal communication.
39. Beaumanoir, A. and Dravet, C. (1992) The Lennox–Gastaut syndrome. In *Epileptic Syndromes in Infancy, Childhood and Adolescence* (J. Roger, M. Bureau, Ch. Dravet, F. E. Dreifuss, A. Perret and P. Wolf, Eds). John Libbey, London, pp. 115–134.
40. Chevrie, J. J. and Aicardi, J. (1972) Childhood epileptic encephalopathy with slow spike-wave. A statistical study of 80 cases. *Epilepsia*, **13**, 259–271.
41. Oller, L., Russi, A. and Oller Daurella, L. (1991) Lamotrigine in Lennox-syndrome. *Epilepsia*, **32**, (Suppl 1) 58.
42. Tassinari, C. A., Bureau, M. and Thomas, P. (1992) Epilepsy with myoclonic absences. In *Epileptic Syndromes in Infancy, Childhood and Adolescence* (J. Roger, M. Bureau, Ch. Dravet, F. E. Dreifuss, A. Perret and P. Wolf, Eds). John Libbey, London, pp. 151–160.
43. Jeavons, P .M. (1982) Myoclonic epilepsies: therapy and prognosis. In *Advances in Epileptology, XIIIth Epilepsy International Symposium* (H. Akimoto, H. Kazamatsuri, M. Seino and A. A. Ward, Eds). Raven Press, New York, pp. 141–144.
44. Appleton, R. E., Panayiotopoulos, C. P., Acomb, B. A. and Beirne, M. (1993) Eyelid myoclonia with typical absences: an epilepsy syndrome. *J. Neurol. Neurosurg. Psychiatry*, **56**, 1312–1316.
45. Panayiotopoulos, C. P. (1995) Epilepsies characterized by seizures with specific modes of precipitation (reflex epilepsies). In *Epilepsy in Children* (S. Wallace, Ed). Chapman and Hall, London.
46. Janz, D. and Christian, W. (1957) Impulsiv-petit mal. *J. Neurol.*, **176**, 346–386.
47. Wolf. P (1992) Juvenile myoclonic epilepsy. In *Epileptic Syndromes in Infancy, Childhood and Adolescence* (2nd ed) (J. Roger, M. Bureau, Ch. Dravet, F. E. Dreifuss, A. Perret and P. Wolf, Eds). John Libbey, London, pp. 313–327.
48. Greenberg, D. A., Delgado-Escueta, A. V., Widelitz, H., Sparkes, R. S., Treiman, L., Maldonado, H. M., Park, M. S. and Terasaki, P. I. (1985) Juvenile myoclonic epilepsy (JME) may be linked to the BF and HLA loci on human chromosome 6. *Am. J. Med. Gen.*, **31**, 185–192.
49. Whitehouse, W. P., Rees, M., Curtis, D., Sundqvist, A., Parker, K., Chung, E., Baralle, D. and Gardiner, R. M. (1993) Linkage of idopathic generalized epilepsy (IGE) and marker loci on chromosome 6p in families of patients with juvenile myoclonic epilepsy: no evidence for an epilepsy locus in the HLA region. *Am. J. Hum. Genet.*, **53**, 652–662.
50. Roger, J., Genton, P., Bureau, M. and Dravet, Ch. (1992) Progressive myoclonus epilepsies in childhood and adolescence. In *Epileptic Syndromes in Infancy, Childhood and Adolescence* (2nd ed) (J. Roger, M. Bureau, Ch. Dravet, F. E. Dreifuss, A. Perret and P. Wolf, Eds). John Libbey, London, pp. 381–400.
51. Marseille Consensus Group. (1990) Classification of progressive myoclonus epilepsies and related disorders. *Ann. Neurol.*, **28**, 113–116.
52. Koskiniemi, M. (1990) Progressive myoclonic epilepsy. In *Paediatric Epilepsy* (M. Sillanpää, S. I. Johannessen, G. Blennow and M. Dam, Eds). Wrightson Biomedical, Petersfield, pp. 137–144.
53. Jeavons, P. M. and Bower B. D. (1964) Infantile spasms. *Clin. Develop. Med.*, **15**, 1–82.
54. West, W. J. (1841) On a peculiar form of infantile consulvants. *Lancet*, **1**, 724–725.
55. Gibbs, F. A. and Gibbs, E. L. (1952) Infantile spasms. In *Atlas of electroencephalography in epilepsy* (2nd ed) (Vol 2). Addison-Wesley, MA, pp. 24–30.

56. Baird, H. W. and Borofsky, L. G. (1957) Infantile myoclonic seizures. *J. Paediatri.*, **50**, 332.
57. Bellman, M. H., Ross, E. M. and Miller, D. L. (1983) Infantile spasms and pertussis immunisation. *Lancet*, **i**, 1031–1034.
58. Bellman, M. H. and Ross, E. M. (1985) Pertussis immunisation and fits. In *Paediatric Perspectives on Epilepsy* (E. Ross and E. Reynold, Eds). John Wiley, Chichester, pp. 53–62.
59. Jeavons, P. M. and Livet, M. O. (1992) West syndrome: infantile spasms. In *Epileptic Syndromes in Infancy, Childhood and Adolescence* (2nd ed) (J. Roger, M. Bureau, Ch. Dravet, F. E. Dreifuss, A. Perret and P. Wolf, Eds). John Libbey, London, pp. 53–65.
60. Chugani, H. T., Shields, W. D., Shewmon, D. A., Olson, D. M., Phelps, M. E. and Peacock, W. J. (1990) Infantile spasms: 1. PET identifies focal cortical dysgenesis in cryptogenic cases for surgical treatment. *Ann. Neurol.*, **27**, 406–413.
61. Chugani, H. T. (1994) Personal communication.
62. Chiron, C., Dulac, O., Beaumont, D., Palacios, L., Pagot, N. and Mumford, J. (1991) Therapeutic trial of vigabatrin in refractory infantile spasms. *J. Child Neurol.*, **6** (Suppl), 2S52–2S59.
63. Plouin, P. and Dulac, O. (1994) Personal communication and in press.
64. Plouin, P., Dulac, O., Jalin, C. and Chiron, C. (1993) Twenty-four-hour ambulatory EEG monitoring in infantile spasms. *Epilepsia*, **34**, 686–691.
65. Kellaway, P., Hrachovy, R. A., Frost, J .D. Jr. and Zion, T. (1979) Precise characterization and quantification of infantile spasms. *Ann. Neurol,.* **6**, 214–218.
66. Dulac, O., Feingold, J., Plouin, P., Chiron, C., Pajot, N. and Ponson, G. (1993) Genetic predisposition to West syndrome. *Epilepsia*, **34**, 732–737.
67. Donat, J. F. and Wright, F .S. (1992) Myoclonic seizures and infantile spasms. *Epilepsia*, **33** (Suppl 3), 6.
68. Snead, O. C. and Hosey, L. C. (1985) Exacerbation of seizures in children by carbamazepine. *N. Engl. J. Med.*, **313**, 916–921.
69. Aicardi, J. (1992) *Diseases of the Nervous System in Childhood. Clinics in Developmental Medicine*; Nos 115–118. MacKeith Press, London.

10 Rare Movement Disorders Associated with Metabolic and Neurodegenerative Diseases

MARK STACY
University of Missouri, Columbia, MO, USA
and
JOSEPH JANKOVIC
Baylor College of Medicine, Houston, TX, USA

INTRODUCTION

Movement disorders are often associated with or may be the initial manifestation of a variety of metabolic and neurodegenerative diseases (Tables 10.1 and 10.2). These diseases often affect children and therefore a thorough paediatric neurological assessment is essential in order to derive the correct diagnosis[1]. The recognition of abnormal movements in a paediatric patient may facilitate the diagnostic evaluation and may eventually lead to more effective treatment of the underlying disease process and the movement disorder.

Table 10.1. Rare metabolic disorders associated with movement disorders in children*

Disease	Movement disorder	Other features	Inheritence
Aromatic L-amino acid decarboxylase deficiency[74]	Rubral tremor, chorea	Hypotonia, oculogyric crisis	
Biopterin synthesis defect[75]	Tremor, orofacial dyskinesia	L-dopa response	
Ceroid lipofuscinosis[76–78]	Dystonia, chorea, tremor, parkinsonism	Blindness, seizures, curvilinear bodies	AR
Galactosaemia[21]	Chorea, tremor	MR, hypotonia, ataxia	AR
Glutaric acidaemia I	Choreoathetosis, dystonia,	Seizures, hypotonia	AR
GM-1 gangliosidosis[79]	Myoclonus, dystonia	MR, dysarthria	AR

continued overleaf

Movement and Allied Disorders. Edited by M. M. Robertson and V. Eapen

Table 10.1. *(continued)*

Disease	Movement disorder	Other features	Inheri-tence
GM-2 gangliosidosis	Myoclonus, dystonia	MR, dysarthria	
Leber's disease	Dystonia	Loss of central vision	Mit
Lesch–Nyhan syndrome[23]	Chorea, dystonia, tremor	SIB, non-ambulatory	XL
Leigh's syndrome[12]	Dystonia, chorea, tremor, parkinsonism	Lactic acidosis, recurrent vomiting, striatal lesions	
Maple syrup urine disease	Myoclonus	Opththalmoplegia, respiratory abnormality	AR
Methylmalonic acidaemia[16]	Dystonia, parkinsonism	Leigh's syndrome	AR
Phenylketonuria	Tremor, dystonia, chorea	Dementia	AR
Porphyria	Chorea	Abdominal pain, seizures	AD
Triosephosphate isomerase deficiency	Dystonia, tremor	Anaemia, motor neuron involvement	
Wilson's disease	Dystonia, chorea, tremor, parkinsonism	Caeruloplasmin	AR

AD = autosomal dominant, AR = autosomal recessive, MR = mental retardation, Mit = mitochondrial inheritance, SIB = self-injurious behaviour, XL = X-linked
*Adapted from Jankovic[3] and Swaiman[14]

Table 10.2. Rare degenerative disorders associated with movement disorders in children*

Disease	Movement disorder	Other features	Inheri-tance
Degenerative Alper's disease	Myoclonus	Seizures, MR	
Angelman's syndrome[64]	Stereotypy, chorea, tremor	Autistic, 'happy puppet'	
Asperger syndrome[70]	Tics	Autistic, psychiatric disease, MRI abnormalities	
Ataxia-telangiectasia[80]	Chorea, dystonia	Ocular telangiectasia, immunodeficiency, ataxia	AR

Bassen–Kornzweig disease[41]	Chorea	Ataxia, retinitis pigmentosa, neuropathy	
Bilateral striatal necrosis[15]	Dystonia, chorea	Leigh's syndrome	
Canavan's disease	Choreoathetosis	Megalencephaly, seizures, optic atrophy, urine N-acetylaspartate	
Down's syndrome with Moyamoya disease[81]	Parkinsonism, chorea		
Hallervorden–Spatz disease[49]	Dystonia, chorea, tremor, myoclonus, parkinsonism	Gait disorder, 'Tiger eye' on MRI	AR
Huntington's disease	Dystonia, chorea, myoclonus, parkinsonism	Dementia, depression	AD
Incontinenti pigmenti	Myoclonus, chorea	MR, skin lesions	
Lafora body disease	Myoclonus	Seizures, MR	
Myoclonic epilepsy	Myoclonus, chorea	Seizures	
Neuroacanthocytosis[37]	Chorea, tics, dystonia stereotypy, parkinsonism	SIB, gait disorder	AR, AD, XL
Pelizaeus–Merzbacher disease	Chorea, dystonia, tremor	Ataxia, optic atrophy	XL
Ramsay Hunt syndrome	Myoclonus	Seizures, ataxia	
Rett's syndrome[62]	Stereotypy, dystonia	Dementia, SIB, only girls	
Sturge–Webber	Myoclonus, chorea	Facial port-wine stain, seizures, MR	
Sudanophilic leukodystrophy	Myoclonus	Seizures, MR, visual impairment	XL
Tuberous sclerosis[82]	Myoclonus, chorea	Facial angiofibroma, MR, seizures, skin lesions	AD
Unverricht–Lundberg disease	Myoclonus, chorea	Seizures, MR	
Xeroderma pigmentosum	Choreoathetosis	MR, ataxia, microcephaly	

AD = autosomal dominant, AR = autosomal recessive, MR = mental retardation, Mit = mitochondrial inheritance, SIB = self-injurious behaviour, XL = X-linked

*Adapted from Jankovic[3] and Swaiman[14]

EVALUATION OF MOVEMENT DISORDERS IN CHILDREN

Obtaining an accurate account of pre-, peri-, and postnatal history is essential to the diagnosis of any childhood-onset neurological disorder[2]. The abnormal movements should be characterized by type of involuntary movement, timing, location of onset, duration, severity and progression of symptoms. In addition, the influence of certain activities, stress, sleep and diurnal variations should be noted. Comorbid problems, such as mental retardation, developmental delay, seizures, self-abuse, sleep abnormalities or hyperactivity, may provide helpful clues as to the aetiology of the disorder. Furthermore, a history of psychiatric problems or prior exposure to medications that may cause movement disorders (e.g. dopamine receptor blocking drugs) must be explored. A detailed family history, and whenever possible an examination of relatives, is important in order to categorize properly the pattern of inheritance of the illness as autosomal dominant, recessive, X-linked, or other pattern.

Neurological examination should begin with vital signs and growth chart data, and a general neurological examination. Since neurodegenerative and metabolic disorders are associated with multiple system involvement, careful evaluation should include mental status examination, supplemented by neuropsychological testing. Cranial nerve testing is also important, particularly for ophthalmic and bulbar abnormalities. Assessment of the motor system should detail findings associated with muscle bulk, tone and power, as well as cerebellar function. If weakness is present, it should be categorized into upper or lower motor neuron, proximal or distal, fluctuating, progressive or other patterns. Sensory testing may be helpful in some instances.

Hypokinetic movement disorders, such as parkinsonism, often result from damage to the nigrostriatal pathway, and are characterized by slowness of movement, rigidity, masked facies, and gait abnormality. The gait is slowed, often shuffling, and is associated with reduced armswing. In juvenile Parkinson's disease and other parkinsonian disorders (e.g. Wilson's disease, Hallervorden–Spatz disease) there may be a resting tremor of approximately 6–8 Hz in frequency[3]. This tremor will often diminish with movement.

Hyperkinetic movement disorders include chorea, athetosis, dystonia, stereotypy, ballism, tremor, tic and myoclonus[3–5]. Chorea is a rapid, continuous, flowing, random involuntary movement, while athetosis is a slower, writhing form of 'slow chorea'. Both are thought to be secondary to striatal abnormalities, and typical diseases include Huntington's disease, Sydenham's chorea, Lesch–Nyhan disease, and neuroacanthocytosis. Ballism is a more abrupt and violent form of chorea often unilateral (hemiballism) resulting most often from ischaemic damage to the contralateral subthalamic nucleus or globus pallidus medius. Dystonia consists of sustained involuntary contractions of muscle producing a twisting (e.g. torticollis) or squeezing (e.g. blepharospasm) movement or posture[6]. Tremor is defined as an oscillatory movement about a joint ranging from 3–10 Hz in frequency, and may be present at rest (parkinsonian tremor), with movement (cerebellar or essential tremor), or when holding a sustained posture (essential tremor). Tics are characterized by abrupt involuntary movements or vocalizations that occur out of a background of normal motor activity, and are often suppressible. Tics occur transiently in about 25% of normal children, and when both motor and vocal tics occur are the hallmark of Gilles de la Tourette syndrome (GTS)[7]. Myoclonus is a simple jerk-like movement due to an abrupt and brief muscle contraction (positive myoclonus) or loss of muscle contraction (negative myoclonus). In contrast to tics, myoclonus is not usually suppressible; it is more closely associated with seizures than other movement disorders. Stereotypies are repetitive, purposeless, and seemingly planned involuntary movements. They are frequently encountered in autistic and mentally retarded children; in adults stereotypies are typically associated with the use of dopamine receptor blocking drugs[8]. Laboratory investigation in this population is discussed throughout this review (Table 10.3).

LEIGH'S SYNDROME AND OTHER DISEASES OF OXIDATIVE METABOLISM

The frequency of neurometabolic disorders secondary to inborn errors of metabolism is difficult to assess, but autosomal recessive diseases are estimated to affect 1 in 1000 children world-wide[9]. Saudubray *et al.* in reviewing 326 children referred to a French tertiary care center from 1968–1987 found 102 (31%) patients with aminoacidopathies, 93 (28%) with oxidative metabolism disorders, 88 (27%) with organic acidurias, 68 (21%) with hyperammonaemias, and 15 (5%) peroxisomal disorders[10]. A review of 473 children diagnosed with metabolic disease in Saudi Arabia has found lysosomal storage diseases (32%), chromosomal abnormalities (26%), organic acid disorders (16%), amino acid disorders (14%), and various metabolic diseases (12%)[11]. Ozand *et al.* believe that the differences in relative frequencies of these disorders are most likely due to the high frequency of consanguinity in the Arab population[9]. While it is accepted that the presence of dystonia, choreoathetosis, tremor and other movement disorders is infrequent even in these rare conditions, perhaps movement disorders are simply not well-recognized in metabolic and neuro-degenerative diseases. Macaya *et al.* have reported that movement disorders occur in 22 of 34 patients (64.7%) with Leigh's syndrome (LS), although an average frequency of only 26.4% was previously reported in the literature[12].

Table 10.3. Laboratory investigation in childhood movement disorders

Blood studies
caeruloplasmin
copper
complete blood count
chromosomal analysis
erythrocyte sedimentation rate
antinuclear antibody
protein electrophoresis
biochemistry profile
serology
arterial blood gas
metabolic screen
lactate, pyruvate
urine for organic acids, oligosaccharides, amino acids
serum for acanthocytes, amino acids
Brain MRI
Electroencephalogram
Evoked potentials
Bone marrow biopsy ('sea-blue' histiocytes)
Brain biopsy
Conjunctival biopsy (neuronal inclusions)
Liver biopsy (copper)
Muscle biopsy (mitochondrial abnormalities)
Rectal biopsy (neuronal inclusions)
Skin biopsy (fibroblasts for lysosomal enzymes)
Psychometric testing

Adapted from Stacy and Jankovic[6]

Besides LS, other disorders of oxidative metabolism include diseases of respiratory chain, carbohydrate, and fatty acid metabolism, such as pyruvate dehydrogenase deficiency, glycogen storage diseases, and carnitine deficiency. Oxidative disorders result in reduced energy production, usually by disruption of electron transport, and are associated with myopathy, encephalopathy, and cardiomyopathy[13]. Laboratory studies often demonstrate lactic acidosis, hypoglycaemia and hyperammonaemia[13,14]. If a disorder of oxidative metabolism is suspected clinically, serum lactate, pyruvate, carnitine, ammonia, quantitative amino acids, and urine for organic acids should be obtained[13] (Table 10.3). Muscle biopsy is helpful in both mitochondrial and lipid storage diseases, and cultured fibroblasts from skin biopsy may be assayed for enzymes involved in pyruvate metabolism and electron transport[13]. Liver biopsy is useful for disorders of β-oxidation and gluconeogenesis[13].

The diagnosis of LS or subacute necrotizing encephalitis should be considered in a child with central nervous system disease, ophthalmoplegia, myopathic weakness, nausea, vomiting, respiratory irregularities and episodes of lactic acidosis, who on computed tomography (CT) or magnetic resonance imaging (MRI) demonstrate bilateral striatal lesions[13]. A retrospective analysis of patients with LS found 22 of 34 patients to have at least one movement disorder: dystonia (19), rigidity (four), tremor (two), chorea (two), hypokinesia (two) and myoclonus (one)[12]. At onset the dystonia was multifocal in eight patients, generalized in six, segmental in three, and unilateral in two. In the 75 of 284 LS patients previously reported to have movement disorders, dystonia, myoclonus and hypokinetic rigid syndromes were seen in 45%, 25%, and 24% respectively[12]. Metabolic disorders producing LS include pyruvate dehydrogenase deficiencies, respiratory chain abnormalities (complex I and IV), methylmalonic acidaemia, and hypoxic and toxic encephalopathy. In addition, vasculitis, trauma and infections have also produced striatal abnormalities on MRI scans[15,16]. Various mitochondrial DNA mutations have been reported with LS and there is often a marked clinical heterogeneity within a single kindred[17,18]. In a review of 34 patients with LS secondary to cytochrome oxidase deficiency, three clinical stages have been identified[18]. Stage 1 consists of normal development with diarrhoea, vomiting, and decelerating growth during the first year of life. Stage 2 is associated with neurological decline, and stage 3 is associated with severe hypotonia, dysphagia and malnutrition. Santorelli *et al.* have reported a point mutation at nt8993 in 12 children from 10 different families with LS, while no such mutation was found in over 200 patients with other mitochondrial encephalopathies[19].

DISORDERS OF CARBOHYDRATE METABOLISM

Disorders of carbohydrate metabolism may be subdivided into glycogen storage diseases, galactosaemia, galactokinase deficiency and hereditary fructose intolerance[14]. Glycogen storage diseases are associated mainly with muscle pathology, while fructose intolerance produces nausea, vomiting and mental retardation if not diet restricted; none of these conditions is associated with movement disorders. Galactosaemia, caused by a deficiency in the galactose-1-phosphate uridyltransferase enzyme, and galactokinase deficiency, produces liver impairment and mental retardation if galactose is not removed from the diet. Although the pathological mechanisms of cortical neuronal degeneration are unknown, it is believed to be secondary to accumulation of galactitol, the end-product of galactose reduction by alternate metabolic pathways. These children are normal at birth, but develop jaundice, progressive oedema, hepatomegaly and hepatorenal impairment, often leading to mental retardation, seizures and 'extra-pyramidal symptoms'[20]. In a review of 134 patients with galactosaemia from 102 families, death occurred before 4 weeks of life in 12 children, from

4 to 9 weeks in 10 children, and in one severely retarded child at 3 years[21]. In 78 patients followed by the authors, 49 had normal neurological examinations, 12 had severe clumsiness, 11 had tremor, and six had ataxia[21]. In two siblings recognized to have galactosaemia by neonatal screening and maintained on lactose restricted diet, progression of encephalopathy, cortical atrophy and demyelination still occurred[20]. Fatty acid metabolism disorders include the carnitine and beta-oxidation deficiencies and disorders of lipid storage. Systemic carnitine deficiency may resemble Reye syndrome in presentation, and in these instances may be associated with dystonia.

LESCH–NYHAN SYNDROME

Lesch–Nyhan syndrome (LNS) is an X-linked recessive disorder localized to the q26–q27.2 region of the X-chromosome[22]. LNS is manifested by self-injurious behaviour (SIB), mental retardation, choreoathetosis, dystonia, dysarthria, spasticity and other neurological disturbances progressing to wheelchair and bed confinement[23]. Because LNS is an X-linked recessive disorder, it is nearly always found in boys, but two girls with consanguinous ancestry and a maternally-derived phenotype believed to result from random gene activation have been reported[24,25]. Lip and finger biting begin before the second year of life, and may be controlled by limb restraints and tooth extraction (Figs. 10.1A and 10.1B)[26]. With disease

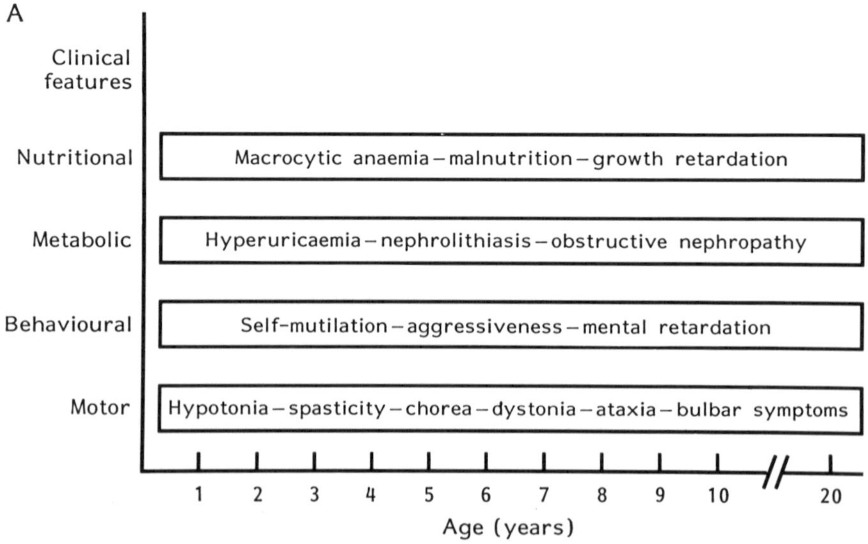

Figure 10.1A. Natural course of Lesch–Nyhan syndrome

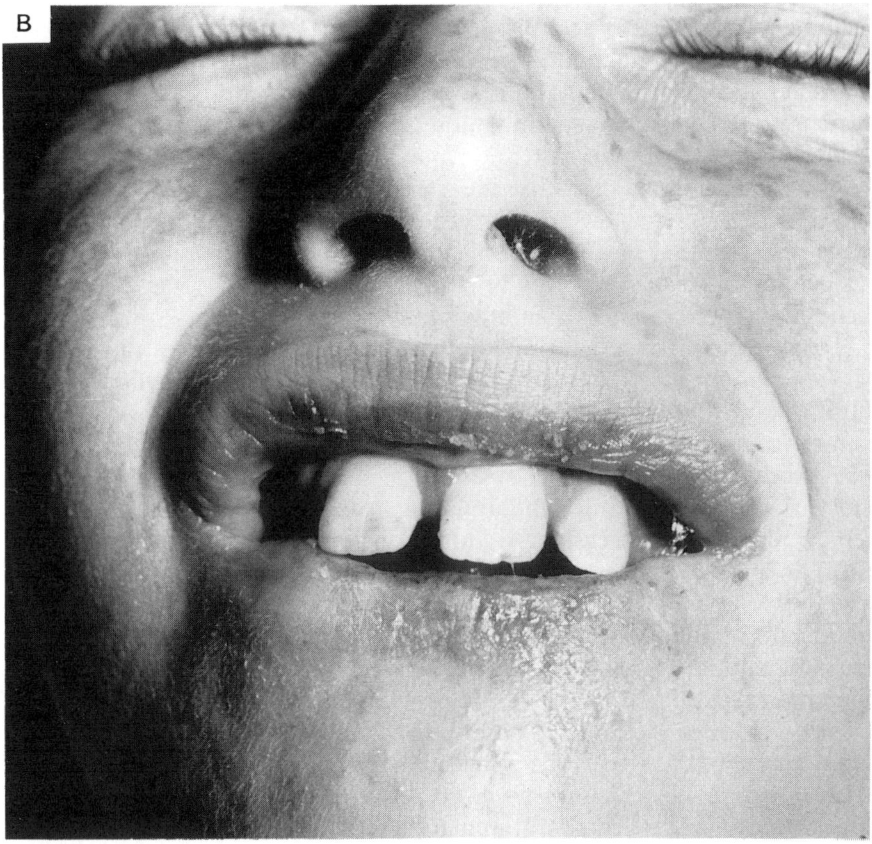

Figure 10.1B. Lip mutilation characteristic of the SIB in Lesch–Nyhan syndrome

progression patients exhibit an increasingly irresistible urge to injure themselves and others, and will often plead with caretakers to maintain four-point restraints to prevent compulsive self-harm.

In a review of five boys, aged 2–10 years, Jankovic *et al.* found hypotonia, poor head control and motor delay to be present by 9 months of age[27]. By 12 months of age hypotonia was replaced by hypertonia producing trunk and limb extension. In three patients SIB was the most distressing symptom; chorea was found in all five boys, while dystonia was noted in four. No correlation was noted between age and severity of SIB or the movement disorders. In all cases choreoathetosis, intermittent dystonia, and ataxia advanced to produce severe motor disability, and prevent ambulation[27].

Mental retardation has been considered a component of this disease, but cognitive impairment may be less severe than originally suspected. Anderson *et al.* believe previously published mean IQ levels of 60 may be falsely low because of testing difficulties and bias associated with motor disability and SIB[28]. Based on questionnaires completed by parents of patients with LNS, all children were found to be oriented to person, place and time, and 41 of 42 had a full range of affect and appropriate emotional response to environmental stimulation[28]. Many of the children were able to recall anecdotes from the past, and 35 of 36 patients over the age of 5 years were able to follow correctly the storylines of films with laughter at appropriate moments. More than 90% of patients could communicate verbally or by other means, and 58% of children over the age of 4 years had some ability to read. Only 38% of patients demonstrated some insight into their SIB or could predict when it would occur[28].

Hyperuricaemia results from a defect in purine metabolism caused by a deficiency in the enzyme hypoxanthine guanine phosphoribosyl transferase (HPRT), and 90% of patients have point mutations in exon 9 of the HPRT gene[22]. The lack of HPRT results in marked overproduction of uric acid, and may produce gout and renal dysfunction. In addition to hyperuricaemia and uricosuria, systemic abnormalities associated with LNS include nephrolithiasis, and occasionally, tophi and arthritis. Cerebrospinal fluid (CSF) analysis in some patients reveals diminished levels of homovanillic acid (HVA) and 3-methoxy-4-hydroxyphenylethylene glycol (MHPG), and increased 5-hydroxy-indole-acetic acid (5-HIAA); this corresponds to neurotransmitter changes found at post-mortem examination[27]. Levels of dopamine (DA), HVA, tyrosine hydroxylase, and dopa-decarboxylase are markedly decreased in the striatum, external pallidum, and nucleus accumbens, but the levels are preserved in the substantia nigra (SN)[26].

Since morphological analysis has failed to demonstrate any specific histological changes, the symptomatology of LNS has been thought to result from biochemical alteration at pre- and postsynaptic terminals in the nigrostriatal synapse[26]. HPRT activity in the brain is normally highest in the basal ganglia, where it is believed necessary for DNA, RNA and protein synthesis. It has been postulated that deficiency in this enzyme results in impaired development of nigral neuronal terminals and striatal synaptogenesis. Pardo *et al.* have demonstrated marked increase in the synthesis of D_1 receptors without significant change in D_2 receptor concentrations during the perinatal period[29]. Because D_1 receptor density is diminished while D_2 receptors are relatively preserved in LNS, SIB has been postulated to result from overstimulation of D_1 receptors[30,31].

SIB has been reproduced in animals exposed to methylxanthines, amphetamines, opiates and clonidine[32]. In addition, pharmacological upregulation of the gamma-amino-butyric acid (GABA) feedback loop in the SN also produces SIB[32]. Administration of D_1, but not D_2, dopamine agonists in animals with lesions in the dopaminergic axis have also produced SIB and stereotypies. Some suggest that altered activity of the D_1 receptors in LNS is an indirect consequence of diminished concentration of DA in the striatum[33].

The reasons for DA depletion in LNS are not known, but may be secondary to the metabolic stress caused by increased purine synthesis or toxic effects of increased purine metabolites[34]. The study of the HPRT-deficient mouse may provide insights into the pathogenesis of LNS, but because of parallel metabolic pathways or different metabolic responses to the genetic abnormality in this model as compared to human LNS, neurotoxic effects of uric acid do not occur in these animals and they are unaffected by the mutations[35]. HPRT-deficient mice, however, have been found to be much more sensitive to amphetamine administration than normal mice, and at high doses seem to exhibit stereotypic activity and SIB[35].

NEUROACANTHOCYTOSIS

Neuroacanthocytosis (NA) is a term that may be used to describe at least five different conditions associated with neurological dysfunction and acanthocytosis (abnormal spike-like projections on erythrocytes)[36]. Neurological abnormalities may start in late childhood but usually not until the third or fourth decades. They include dementia, chorea, orofacial stereotypies, involuntary vocalizations, dystonia, tics, parkinsonism, ataxia, peripheral neuropathy and amyotrophy[36,37]. Although the mechanism of acanthocyte formation in these disorders is unknown, in NA types I, II, III and V abnormal protein/fatty acid ratios have been found, and in NA type IV, an abnormal erythrocyte surface antigen is believed important. Despite normal serum lipoprotein levels, Sakai *et al.* have demonstrated elevated ratios of erythrocyte membrane protein palmitic acid (C16:0) and stearic acid (C18:0) in NA type I[38]. They suggested that this abnormal composition of covalently bound fatty acids in erythrocyte membrane may disrupt normal membrane protein interaction. In NA types II and III, deficiency of β-lipoproteins is seen, and reversal of the phosphatidylcholine-to-sphingomyelin ratio may lead to loss of membrane stability in these disorders[39,40]. Type II NA (hypo-β-lipoproteinaemia) produces a multiple sclerosis-like syndrome[40], while Type III NA (a-β-lipoproteinaemia) or the Bassen–Kornzweig syndrome, is manifested by ataxia, atypical retinitis pigmentosa, and peripheral neuropathy[41]. Type IV NA or McLeod's syndrome is an X-linked abnormality associated with elevated serum creatine kinase, and mild myopathy. In this disorder, acanthocytes are thought to be a result of an abnormal erythrocyte surface antigen protein[26]. Type V NA is associated with deficiencies in the apoprotein α and absent pre-α lipoprotein subcomponents[26]. Hallervorden–Spatz disease (HSD), an autosomal recessive parkinsonian syndrome of children, is sometimes associated with acanthocytes, and hypoprebetalipoproteinaemia, will be discussed later in this chapter[42].

Type I NA is associated with a wide variety of movement disorders, orofacial self-mutilation, areflexia and muscle wasting. This disorder usually begins in the third or fourth decade and has also been termed choreoacanthocytosis, the Levine–Critchley syndrome or familial amyotrophic chorea with acanthocytosis, but because not all patients with this condition demonstrate chorea, 'neuroacanthocytosis' may be a more encompassing term[43]. NA type I occurs in autosomal dominant, recessive and X-linked pedigrees, and has also been seen sporadically. Consanguinity is common, particularly in the autosomal recessive forms. The Huntington's disease gene has been excluded in patients with autosomal dominant and sporadic NA[44].

Neurobehavioural abnormalities of NA type I include cognitive disturbances and personality change; dementia is present in over one-half of reported cases. Seizures occur in one-third of patients, and depression, anxiety and obsessive–compulsive disorder are also seen. In their review of 19 patients, Hardie *et al.* report all patients became 'vague and distractable, ...neglected their personal appearance and social skills, and were no longer able to work'[37]. Psychometric testing in this series suggested frontal lobe dysfunction.

Of the 62 patients well described in the literature, 56 were noted to have chorea at some time in the clinical course[36–43]. Chorea affected 17 of 19 patients in the English series. Dystonia was the predominant movement disorder in four patients, but was also present in five others; in all cases speech was severely limited. Dysarthria was produced by a combination of involuntary movements and pseudobulbar palsy; five patients were anarthric. One of the most distinguishing features of NA type I is an eating dysfunction due to orolingual dystonia manifested by expulsion of food from the mouth by a protruding tongue. Involuntary vocalizations occurred in nine patients and included sniffing, clicking, spitting, grunting, sucking, glowing, gasping, sighing or non-recognizable utterances. Biting lips, tongue and cheek was seen in only three patients. Other neurological abnormalities in these patients included muscle wasting (three cases), areflexia (seven), hyporeflexia (six), and extensor plantar responses (three). Peppard *et al.* have reported two patients with parkinsonism responsive to L-dopa, and associated with L-dopa-related hyperkinesias[45]. Two brothers of consanguinous origin presenting with tongue and lip biting, orofacial hyperkinesias and vocalizations evolving into marked parkinsonism not responsive to dopaminergic therapy have also been reported[43]. Progression of the illness is variable, but death usually occurs within 15 years of diagnosis[37].

In the English series acanthocytes were seen in 17 of 19 patients, the remaining two patients exhibited features of NA, and had a family history of this disease in each instance[37]. Although acanthocytes are considered necessary for this diagnosis, not all patients demonstrate this finding on fresh wet preparations; Feinberg *et al.* report two patients in which acanthocytes were not found until erythrocytes were incubated in normal saline for 3–5 minutes[46]. CT of the head demonstrated cerebral and caudate atrophy in six, cerebral atrophy only in two, and was unremarkable in seven; MRI revealed focal cerebral asymmetry in three of four patients[37]. Single photon emission tomography (SPET) scanning in one woman showed severe hypoperfusion of bifrontal lobes[47], and position emission tomography (PET) in another patient revealed marked bilateral reduction in fluorodopa similar to severe idiopathic parkinsonism[45]. PET scanning in a series of six patients with NA revealed putamenal and caudate fluorodopa uptake reduced to 42% and 54% of normal controls. Using raclopride as a D_2 receptor ligand, PET scans showed 65% and 53% reduction in the D_2 receptor density in the caudate and putamen, respectively[48]. These data suggest the movement disorders seen in NA are partially related to the loss of the axon terminals of the nigral neurons and from decreased postsynaptic D_2 receptors. Biopsy in two patients has revealed decreased myelinated fibres, confirmed by electron microscopy, and the neostriatum is primarily affected[37].

HALLERVORDEN–SPATZ DISEASE

Hallervorden–Spatz disease (HSD) is an autosomal recessive disorder associated with excessive iron deposition in the globus pallidus (GP)[49]. HSD was initially described in a single family of 12 children, three of whom died at birth[50]. Five girls developed symptoms at 7–9 years of life with deterioration until death at 16–27 years. However, three of the four remaining siblings (all boys) later developed athetosis, tremor and visual difficulties similar to the five sisters, and autopsy of the oldest was consistent with the previous studies. Swaiman summarized the clinical features associated with this disorder to include gait disturbance, movement disorders, rigidity, dysarthria, blindness, intellectual decline and seizures with onset usually in the first decade of life[49]. Of 42 patients previously reported in a clinical-pathological study, 24 presented prior to age 10 years, 34 prior to age 15, and 39 by age 22. Gait difficulty was the presenting symptom in 27 patients with others showing mental deterioration or blindness. Movement disorders consisted of dystonia in 23, choreoathetosis in 19, and tremor in 15. In addition, severe dysarthria was seen in all patients, retinitis pigmentosa was present in 11, and seizures in nine. In a series of 11 patients diagnosed by MRI, the average age at onset was 7.6 years[51]. Seven presented with gait disturbance, three with behavioural disturbance and one with a writing dystonia. Affected siblings were identified in eight of these patients and two were products of consanguinous marriage. All these patients developed generalized and oromandibular dystonia, retinal degeneration and mental impairment; nine also exhibited pyramidal signs[51]. Besides these clinical features, parkinsonism may also be present, but it is usually more prominent in late-onset patients[52,53].

Blood laboratory tests are usually not helpful. Cultured fibroblasts have been reported to accumulate radioactive transferrin, and blood platelet monoamine oxidase-B activity may be elevated[49]. Furthermore, increased ceroid-lipofuscin accumulation has been seen in circulating lymphocytes with electron microscopy[49]. A radiographic study using CT has revealed high signal intensity in the medial GP. MRI demonstrates marked hypointensity in the GP on T2-weighted images, sometimes associated with the characteristic 'tiger eye' appearance, produced by local deposition of iron[51]. In some cases, areas of high signal are separated by patchy areas of low signal that may represent calcium deposition[49,50]. In serial MRI examinations in one girl with HSD, the initial examination revealed patchy areas of pallidal hyperintensity that became more homogeneous in the next 18 months. The final study, 3 years later, demonstrated the typical 'tiger eye' appearance[54]. Another case of an 11-year-old girl revealed homogeneous hyperintensities initially with a similar target appearance at 5 year follow-up[55]. These authors reviewed eight other cases reported in the literature and added the MRI findings of two sisters with adult-onset HSD with similar observations[56].

The most striking autopsy finding in HSD patients is the asymmetrical rust-brown pigmentation of the GP and zona reticulata of the SN[49]. The iron pigmentation is both extracellular and intracellular, but it is predominantly found in astrocytes, microglia and neurons. 'Mulberry' concretions are also typically present in the extracellular space. In addition, large *spheroid bodies* identified by myelin stains and surrounded by neuromelanin pigment granules can be found in the medial GP, zona reticulata on the SN, cortex and subthalamic nucleus. The spheroid bodies represent degenerating myelinated axons, and are most abundant in the GP and SN, but may also occur in the cortex[50]. They are similar to structures seen in post-mortem specimens of patients with infantile neuraxonal dystrophy (INAD), a neurodegenerative condition that at times is clinically and pathologically similar to HSD, but in this disorder spheroids are much more prominent than in HSD, and no pigmentary abnormalities are present[49,57]. Although retinal degeneration often accompanies other neurological symptoms, there is poor correlation between brain and eye pathological findings. Tripathi *et al.* have reported a case of an 11-year-old girl with typical spheroid bodies in the brain, degeneration of photoreceptors, thinning of the outer nuclear and plexiform layers, and retinal gliosis[58]. They postulate lipid peroxidation, deficiency of fatty acid membrane components, or increased cyclic guanosine monophosphate as a common mechanism for the pathological brain and retinal changes.

RETT SYNDROME AND OTHER AUTISTIC DISORDERS

Rett syndrome is an autistic disorder most typically manifested by abnormal motor behaviours. Rett syndrome was first described in 1966, and was further clarified by Hagberg *et al.* with the addition of 35 patients to the 22 described in the original series[59]. This disorder occurs only in girls, and is believed to be linked to the X-chromosome, but lethal to hemizygous male children. Some authors have suggested that Rett syndrome is a result of disordered lipid metabolism, while others believe these children have a derangement in neuronal mitochondria[60]. Typically, these children develop normally through the first 6–12 months of life, at which time motor abnormalities emerge, accompanied by cognitive regression[26]. Four clinical stages are accepted with the *early-onset stagnation stage* beginning at 6–18 months and accompanied by developmental arrest, and diminished play[61]. The *rapid destructive stage* is marked by developmental and cognitive deterioration, seizures, stereotypic hand movements and irregular breathing and lasts from 1–4 years. The *pseudostationary stage* is present from 4–10 years and is associated with seizures, stabilization of autism, and prominent truncal and gait ataxia *late motor deterioration* may occur from 5 years to adolescence and is associated with motor and cognitive deterioration and cachexia[61]. In a review of 32 Rett patients, hand stereotypies were seen in all girls and most often consisted of clapping, wringing, clenching, washing, patting and rubbing behaviours (Fig. 10.2)[26,62]. Other hyperkinetic disorders of movement included oromandibular dystonia (with or without bruxism) (31), other dystonias (19), scoliosis (16), myoclonus (11), and athetosis (four). All patients had gait disturbance, and parkinsonian findings were manifested chiefly as hypomimia (20), rigidity (14) and bradykinesia (13)[63]. Routine laboratory data, CSF and chromosomal studies are usually normal[60]. No consistent neurochemical data has been determined. Post-mortem studies reveal microcephaly and mild neuronal loss with diffuse gliosis throughout the cortex and cerebellum. Increased lipofuscin is present in brain, conjunctiva and muscle, and the substantia nigra has reduced pigmentation[61].

Another disorder manifested by stereotypies mainly in girls is the 'happy puppet' syndrome, described by Angelman in 1965[64]. These children have a jerky gait, tendency to exhibit hand flapping stereotypies, and laughter with minimal stimulus. In a review of 46 girls and 36 boys with Angelman's syndrome in the UK, Clayton-Smith found all of these children to have psychomotor and cognitive delay, ataxia, and almost completely absent speech[65]. Seizures were seen in 86%, and 72% had early feeding problems. Eventually, 70% learned to walk, and many were able to help with household chores. The most characteristic movement was of hand flapping with elbow and wrist flexion, but athetosis and tremulousness were also seen[65]. A similar 15q11-13 deletion has been found in boys with

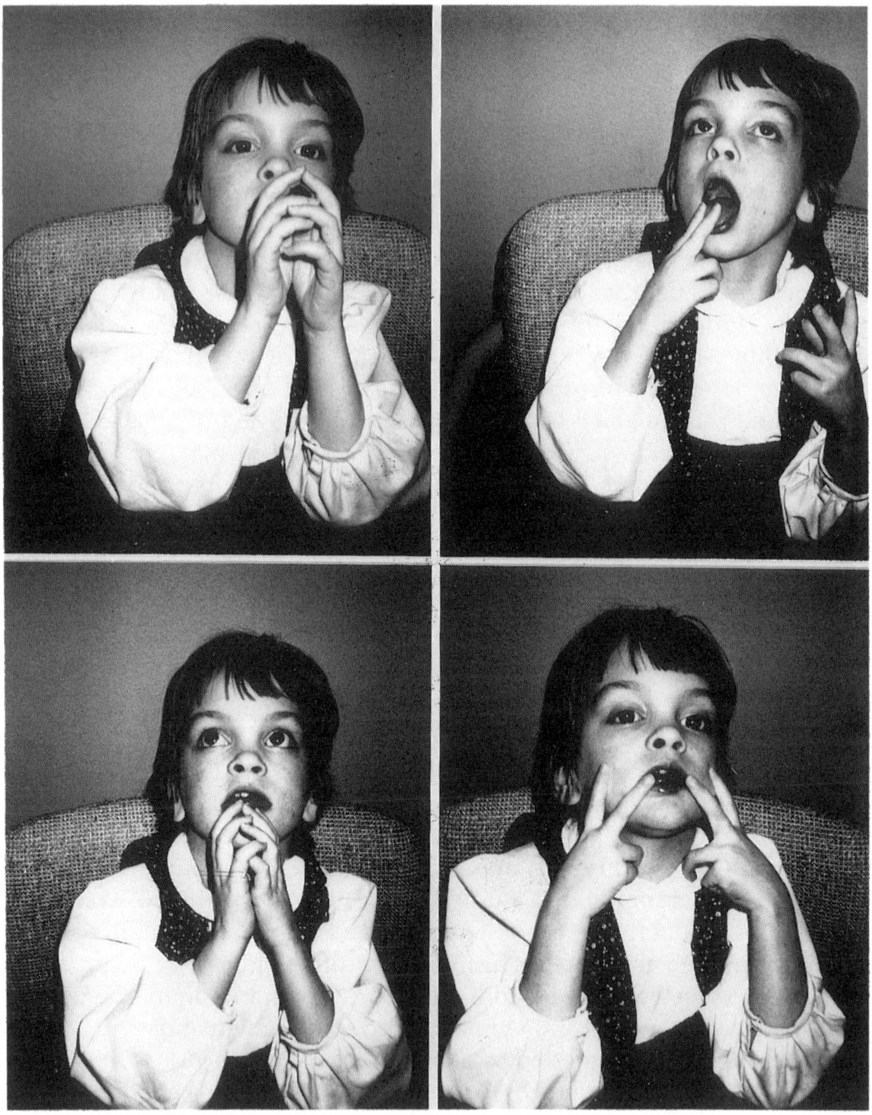

Figure 10.2. Young girl with Rett syndrome exhibiting stereotyped hand movements and mouthing

Prader–Willi syndrome, and parental origin of the chromosomal abnormality has been postulated to play a role[66,67].

Asperger's syndrome (AS), is an autistic disorder manifested by poor reciprocal interaction, inappropriate emotional expression, impaired non-verbal communication, circumscribed interests and repetitive activities.

These children in general function at a higher intellectual level than most patients with developmental disorders[68,69]. Similar to other autistic patients, these children exhibit stereotyped motor behaviour, clumsiness, and a tic disorder ('tourettism')[70]. Berthier *et al.* have recently compared seven patients with coexistent tic disorder and AS to nine age-matched controls with typical GTS and found that AS patients were most likely to have a history of psychiatric hospitalizations, and on average attended school for 2 years less than the GTS only group[71]. Neurological and psychiatric evaluations revealed the AS child to be significantly slower in finger tapping and have diminished grip strength. Furthermore, they were much more likely to exhibit behaviour and school difficulties. Evaluation by MRI revealed abnormalities in five out of seven of the AS children, and only one of the nine GTS group. Abnormalities included cortical atrophy with widened Sylvian fissure anomalies (the opercular sign)[72]. Another AS patient has been found to have a lipoma of the corpus callosum on CT evaluation[73].

In summary, the recognition of movement disorders in children may lead to a diagnosis of a specific metabolic or degenerative disorder. Careful investigation with laboratory and imaging studies may provide additional clues. Although effective therapies are rarely available for the underlying disorder, the abnormal movements may improve with symptomatic treatment discussed elsewhere in this volume.

REFERENCES

1. Dure, L. and Jankovic, J. (1988) Childhood-onset movement disorders. *Curr. Opin. Neurol. Neurosurg.*, **1**, 347–352.
2. Pranzetelli, M. R. (1993) An approach to movement disorders of childhood. *Pediatr. Ann.*, **22**, 13–17.
3. Jankovic, J. (1995) Basal ganglia and neurotransmitter disorders. In *Principles and Practice of Pediatrics* (2nd ed) (F. A. Oski *et al.* Eds). J. B. Lippincott, Philadelphia, pp. 2113–2125.
4. Butler, I. J. (1992) Movement disorders in children. *Pediatr. Neurol.*, **39**, 727–742.
5. Segawa, M. (1993) Extrapyramidal disorders in childhood. *Curr. Opin. Neurol. Neurosurg.*, **6**, 387–392.
6. Stacy, M. and Jankovic, J. (1993) Differential diagnosis and treatment of childhood dystonia. *Pediatri. Ann.*, **22**, 353–358.
7. Jankovic, J. (1993) Tics in other neurological disorders. In *Handbook of Tourette's Syndrome and Related Tic and Behavioural Disorders* (R. Kurlan, Ed). Marcel Dekker, New York, pp. 167–181.
8. Stacy, M., Cardoso, F. and Jankovic, J. (1993) Tardive stereotypy and other movement disorders in tardive dyskinesias. *Neurology*, **43**, 937–941.
9. Ozand, P. T., Devol, E. B. and Gascon, G. G. (1992). Neurometabolic disease at a national referral center: Five years experience at the King Faisal specialist hospital and research center. *J. Child Neurol.*, **7** (Suppl), 4–11.

10. Saudubray, J. M., Ogier, H., Billette de Vilmeur, T., Munnich, A., Lombeo, A., *et al.* (1989) Clinical approach to inherited metabolic diseases in the neonatal period: a 20 year survey. *J. Inherit. Metab. Dis.*, **12** (Suppl), 25–41.
11. Ozand, P. T. and Gascon, G. G. (1992) Treatment of inherited neurometabolic diseases: The future. *J. Child Neurol.*, **7** (Suppl), 132–140.
12. Macaya, A., Munell, F., Burke, R. E. and De Vivo, D. C. (1993) Disorders of movement in Leigh syndrome. *Neuropediatrics*, **24**, 60–67.
13. Breningstall, G. N. (1993) Approach to diagnosis of oxidative metabolism disorders. *Pediatr. Neurol.*, **9**, 81–90.
14. Swaiman, K. F. (1989) Diseases associated with primary abnormalities in carbohydrate and copper metabolism. In *Pediatric Neurology* (K. F. Swaiman, Ed). CV Mosby, St. Louis. pp. 987–1004.
15. Roig, M., Calopa, M., Rovira, A., Macaya, A., Ruidor, E. and Losada, M. (1993) Bilateral striatal lesions in childhood. *Pediatr. Neurol.*, **9**, 349–358.
16. Roodhooft, A. M., Baumgartner, E. R., Martin, J.J., Blom, W. and Van Acker, K. J. (1990) Symmetrical necrosis of the basal ganglia in methylmalonic acidaemia. *Eur. J. Pediatr.*, **149**, 582–584.
17. Crimmins, D., Morris, J. G. L., Walker, G. L., Sue, C. M., Stevens, S. *et al.* (1993) Mitochondrial encephalomyopathy: variable clinical expression within a single kindred. *J. Neurol. Neurosurg. Psychiatry*, **56**, 900–905.
18. Van Coster, R., Lombes, A., DeVivo, D. C., Chi, T. L., Dodson, W. E., *et al.* (1991) Cytochrome c oxidase-associated Leigh syndrome: phenotypic features and pathogenetic speculations. *J. Neurol. Sci.*, **104**, 97–111.
19. Santorelli, F. M., Shanske, S., Macaya, A., DeVivo, D. C. and DiMauro, S. (1993) The mutation at nt8993 of mitochondrial DNA is a common cause of Leigh's syndrome. *Ann. Neurol.*, **34**, 827–844.
20. Koch, T. K., Schmidt, K. A., Wagstaff, J. E., Ng, W. G. and Packman, S. (1992) Neurologic complications of galactosemia. *Pediatr. Neurol.*, **8**, 217–220.
21. Schweitzer, S., Shin, Y., Jakobs, C. and Brodehl, J. (1993) Long-term outcome in 134 patients with galactosaemia. *Eur. J. Pediatr.*, **152**, 36–43.
22. Sculley, D. G., Dawson, P. A., Emmerson, B. T. and Gordon, R. B. (1992) A review of the molecular basis of hypoxanthine-guanine phosphoribosyltransferase (HPRT) deficiency. *Hum. Genetics.*, **90**, 195–207.
23. Nyhan, W. L. (1973) The Lesch-Nyhan syndrome. *Annu. Rev. Med.*, **24**, 41–60.
24. Yukawa, T., Akazawa, H., Miyake, Y., Takahashi, Y., Nagao, H. and Takeda, E. (1992) A female patient with Lesch–Nyhan syndrome. *Dev. Med. Child. Neurol.*, **34**, 543–546.
25. Marcus, S., Steen, A. M., Andersson, B., Lambert, B., Kristoffersson, U. and Francke, U. (1992) Mutation analysis and prenatal diagnosis in a Lesch–Nyhan family showing non-random X-inactivation interfering with carrier detection tests. *Hum. Genetics*, **89**, 395–400.
26. Jankovic, J. (1988) Orofacial and other self-mutilations. *Adv. Neurol,.* **49**, 365–381.
27. Jankovic, J., Caskey, T. C., Stout, J. T. and Butler, I. J. (1988) Lesch–Nyhan Syndrome: A study of motor behavior and cerebrospinal fluid neurotransmitters. *Ann. Neurol.*, **23**, 466–469.
28. Anderson, L. T., Ernst, M. and Davis, S. V. (1992) Cognitive abilities of patients with Lesch–Nyhan disease. *J. Autism Dev. Discord.*, **22**, 189–203.
29. Pardo, J. V., Creese, I., Burt, D. R. and Snyder, S. H. (1977) Autogenesis of dopamine receptor binding in the corpus striatum of the rat. *Brain Res.*, **125**, 376–382.
30. Baumeister, A. A. and Frye, G. D. (1985) The biochemical basis of the behavior disorder in the Lesch–Nyhan syndrome. *Neurosci. Bio. Behav. Rev.*, **9**, 169–178.
31. Goldstein, M., Anderson, L. T., Reuben, R. and Dancis, J. (1985) Self-mutilation

in Lesch–Nyhan disease is caused by dopaminergic and denervation. *Lancet*, **1**, 338–339.

32. Jinnah, H. A., Gage, F. H. and Friedmann, T. (1990) Animal models of Lesch–Nyhan syndrome. *Brain Res. Bull.*, **25**, 467–475.
33. Breese, G. R., Criswell, H. E., Duncan, G. E. and Mueller, R. A. (1990) A dopamine deficiency model of Lesch–Nyhan Disease—the neonatal-6-OHDA-lesioned rat. *Brain Res. Bull.*, **25**, 477–484.
34. Jinnah, H. A., Page, T. and Friedmann, T. (1993) Brain purines in a genetic mouse model of Lesch–Nyhan disease. *J. Neurochem.*, **60**, 2036–2045.
35. Jinnah, H. A., Langlais, P. J. and Friedmann, T. (1992) Functional analysis of brain dopamine systems in a genetic mouse model of Lesch–Nyhan syndrome. *J. Pharmacol. Exp. Ther.*, **263**, 596–607.
36. Hardie, R. J. (1989) Acanthocytes and neurological impairment—a review. *Q.J.Med.*, **71**, 291–306.
37. Hardie, R. J., Pullon, H. W. H., Harding, A. E., Owen, J. S., Pires, M., *et al.* (1990) Neuroacanthocytosis. *Brain*, **114**, 13–49.
38. Sakai, T., Antoku, Y., Iwashita, H., Goto, I., Nagamatsu, K. and Shii, H. (1991) Chorea-acanthocytosis: Abnormal composition of covalently bound fatty acids of erythrocyte membrane proteins. *Ann. Neurol.*, **29**, 664–669.
39. Mars, H., Lewis, L. A., Robertson, A. L., Butkis, A. and Williams, G. H. (1969) Familial hypobetalipoproteinemia. A genetic disorder of lipid metabolism with nervous system involvement. *Am. J. Med.*, **46**, 866–900.
40. Iwakawa, Y., Shimohira, M., Kohvama, J. and Kodama, H. (1993) Sibling cases of a degenerative neurological disease associated with hypocupraemia and hypobetalipoproteinaemia. *Eur. J. Pediatr.*, **152**, 368–371.
41. Bassen, F. A. and Kornzweig, A. L. (1950) Malformation of the erythrocytes in a case of atypical retinitis pigmentosa. *Blood*, **5**, 381–387.
42. Higgins, J. J., Patterson, M. C., Papadopoulos, N. M., Brady, R. O., Pentchev, P. G. and Barton, N. W. (1992) Hypoprebetalipoproteinemia, acanthocytosis, retinitis pigmentosa, and pallidal degeneration (HARP syndrome). *Neurology*, **42**, 194–198.
43. Spitz, M. C., Jankovic, J. and Killian, J. M. (1985) Familial tic disorder, parkinsonism, motor neuron disease, and acanthocytosis: a new syndrome. *Neurology*, **35**, 366–377.
44. Ashizawa, T., Wong, L-J. C., Richards, S. J., Caskey, T. and Jankovic, J. (1994) The CAG repeat size and clinical presentation in Huntington's disease. *Neurology*, **44**, 1137–1143.
45. Peppard, R. F., Lu, C. S., Chu, N-S., Teal, P., Martin, W. R. W. and Calne, D. B. (1990) Parkinsonism with neuroacanthocytosis. *Can. J. Neurol. Sci.*, **17**, 298–301.
46. Feinberg, T. E., Cianci, C. D., Morrow, J. S., Pehta, J. C., Redman, C. M., *et al.* (1991) Diagnostic test for choreoacanthocytosis. *Neurology*, 1000–1006.
47. Delecluse, F., Deleval, J., Gerard, J-M., Michotte, A. and Zegers de Beyl, D. (1991) Frontal impairment of hypoperfusion in neuroacanthocytosis. *Arch. Neurol.*, **48**, 232–234.
48. Brooks, D. J., Ibanez, V., Playford, E. D., Sawle, G. V., Leigh, P. N., *et al.* (1991) Presynaptic and postsynaptic striatal dopaminergic function in neuroacanthocytosis: A positron emission tomographic study. *Ann. Neurol.*, **30**, 166–171.
49. Swaiman, K. F. (1991) Hallervorden–Spatz syndrome and brain iron metabolism. *Arch. Neurol.*, **48**, 1285–1293.
50. Olanow, C. W. (1994) Hallervorden–Spatz syndrome: an iron storage disease. In *Neurodegenerative Diseases* (D. B. Calne, Ed). W. B. Saunders, Philadelphia, pp. 807–823.
51. Angelini, L., Nardocci, N., Rumi, V., Zorzi, C., Strada, L. and Savoiardo, M.

(1992) Hallervorden–Spatz disease: clinical and MRI study in cases diagnosed in life. *J. Neurol.*, **239**, 417–425.

52. Jankovic, J., Kirkpatrick, K. A., Langlais, P. J. and Bird, E. D. (1985) Late-onset Hallervorden–Spatz disease presenting in familial parkinsonism. *Neurology*, **35**, 227–234.
53. Yamamoto, T., Kawamura, J., Hashimoto, S., Nakamura, M., Iwamoto, H., *et al.* (1990) Pallido-nigro-luysian atrophy, progressive supranuclear palsy and adult onset Hallervorden–Spatz disease: a case of akinesia as a predominant feature of parkinsonism. *J. Neurol. Sci.*, **101**, 98–106.
54. Brouwer, O. F., Laboyrie, P. M., Peters, A. C. B. and Vielvoye, G. J. (1992) Follow-up magnetic resonance imaging in Hallervorden–Spatz disease. *Clin. Neurol. Neurosurg.*, **94** (Suppl), 57–60.
55. Gallucci, M., Cardona, F., Arachi, M., Splendiani, A., Bozzao, A. and Passeriello, R. (1989) Follow-up MR studies in Hallervorden–Spatz disease. *J. Comput. Assist. Tomogr.*, **14**, 118–120.
56. Ambrosetto, P., Nonni, R., Bacci, A. and Gobbi, G. (1992) Late onset familial Hallervorden–Spatz disease: MR findings in two sisters. *Am. J. Neurol. Radiol.*, **13**, 394–396.
57. Gaytan-Garcia, S., Kaufman, J. C. E. and Young, G. B. (1990) Adult onset Hallervorden–Spatz syndrome or Seitelberger's disease with late onset: variants of the same entity? A clinico-pathological study. *Clin. Neuropathol.*, **9**, 136–142.
58. Tripathi, R. C., Tripathi, B. J., Bauserman, S. C. and Park, J. K. (1992) Clinicopathologic correlation and pathogenesis of ocular and central nervous system manifestations in Hallervorden–Spatz syndrome. *Acta Neuropathol.*, **83**, 113–119.
59. Hagberg, B., Aicardi, J., Dias, K. and Ramos, O. (1983) A progressive syndrome of autism, dementia, ataxia, and loss of purposeful hand use in girls; Rett's syndrome: report of 35 cases. *Ann. Neurol.*, **14**, 471–479.
60. Hagberg, B. and Witt Engerstrom, I. (1986) Rett syndrome: a suggested staging system for describing impairment profile with increasing age towards adolescence. *Am. J. Med. Genet.*, **24**, 47–59.
61. Jellinger, K. A. (1994) Rare neurodegenerative disorders. In *Neurodegenerative Diseases* (D. B. Calne, Ed). W. B. Saunders, Philadelphia, pp. 909–931.
62. FitzGerald, P. M., Jankovic, J. and Percy, A. K. (1990) Rett syndrome and associated movement disorders. *Mov. Disord.*, **5**(3), 195–202.
63. FitzGerald, P. M., Jankovic, J., Glaze, D. G., Schulz, R. and Percy, A. K. (1990) Extrapyramidal involvement in Rett's syndrome. *Neurology*, **40**, 293–295.
64. Angelman, H. (1965) 'Puppet' children: a report of three cases. *Dev. Med. Child Neurol*,. **7**, 681–688.
65. Clayton-Smith, J. (1993) Clinical research on Angelman syndrome in the United Kingdom: observations on 82 affected individuals. *Am. J. Med. Genet.*, **46**, 12–15.
66. Magenis, R. E., Toth-Fejel, S., Allen, L. J., Black, M., Brown, M. G., *et al.* (1990) Comparison of the 15q deletions in Prader–Willi and Angelman syndromes: specific regions, extent of deletions, parental origin, and clinical consequences. *Am. J. Med. Genet.*, **35**, 333–349.
67. Imaizumi, K., Takada, F., Kuroki, Y., Naritomi, K., Hamabe, J. and Niikawa, N. (1990) Cytogenetic and molecular study of Angelman syndrome. *Am. J. Med. Genet.*, **35**, 314–318.
68. Ghaziuddin, M., Tsai, L. Y. and Ghaziuddin, N. (1992) Brief report: A comparison of the diagnositc criteria for Asperger syndrome. *J. Autism Dev. Disord.*, **22**, 643–649.
69. Ghaziuddin, M., Tsai, L. Y. and Ghaziuddin, N. (1992) Brief report: A reappraisal of clumsiness as a diagnostic feature of Asperger syndrome. *J. Autism Dev. Disord.*, **22**, 651–656.

70. Littlejohns, C. S., Clarke, D. J. and Corbett, J. A. (1990) Tourette-like disorder in Asperger's syndrome. *Br. J. Psychiatry*, **156**, 430–433.
71. Berthier, M. L., Bayes, A. and Tolosa, E. S. (1993) Magnetic resonance imaging in patients with concurrent Tourette's disorder and Asperger's syndrome. *J. Am. Acad. Child. Adolesc. Psychiatry*, **32**, 633–639.
72. Tatum, W. O., Coker, S. B., Ghobrial, M. and Abd-Allah, S. (1989) The opercular sign: diagnosis and significance. *Ann. Neurol.*, **25**, 196–199.
73. David, A. S., Wacharasindhu, A. and Lishman, W. A. (1993) Severe psychiatric disturbance and abnormalities of the corpus callosum. *J. Neurol. Neurosurg. Psychiatry*, **56**, 85–93.
74. Hylund, K., Surtees, A. H., Rodeck, C. and Clayton, P. T. (1992) Aromatic L-amino acid decarboxylase deficiency: clinical features, diagnosis, and treatment of a new inborn error of neurotransmitter amine synthesis. *Neurology*, **42**, 1980–1988.
75. Factor, S. A., Coni, R. J., Cowger, M. and Rosenblum, E. L. (1991) Paroxysmal tremor and orofacial dyskinesia secondary to a biopterin synthesis defect. *Neurology*, **41**, 930–932.
76. Wisniewski, K. E., Kida, E., Connell, F., Elleder, M., Eviatar, L. and Konkol, R. J. (1993) New subform of the late infantile form of neuronal ceroid lipofuscinosis. *Neuropediatrics*, **24**, 155–163.
77. Gospe, S. M. and Jankovic, J. (1986) Drug-induced dystonia in neuronal ceroid lipofuscinosis. *Pediatr. Neurol.*, **2**, 236–237.
78. Jankovic, J., Armstrong, D., Low, N. L. and Rapin, I. (1988) Progressive myoclonic epilepsy, dementia, and blindness in a young girl. *Mov. Disord.*, **3**, 362–369.
79. Nardocci, N., Bertagnolio, B., Rumi, V., Combi, M., Bardelli, P. and Angelini, L. (1993) Chronic GM1 gangliosidosis presenting as dystonia: clinical and biochemical studies in a new case. *Neuropediatrics*, **24**, 164–166.
80. Leuzzi, V., Ellis, R., Antonelli, A., Chessa, L., Cardona, F., *et al.* (1993) Neurological and cytogenetic study in early-onset ataxia-telangiectasia patients. *Eur. J. Pediatri.*, **152**, 609–612.
81. Takanashi, J-I, Sugita, K., Honda, A. and Niimi, H. (1993) Moyamoya syndrome in a patient with Down's syndrome presenting with chorea. *Pediatr. Neurol.*, **9**, 396–398.
82. Evans, B. K. and Jankovic, J. (1983) Tuberous scleroris and chorea. *Ann. Neurol.*, **13**, 106–107.

11 Drug-related Movement Disorders

DAVID G. CUNNINGHAM-OWENS
University of Edinburgh, UK

INTRODUCTION

Nowadays, if one wishes to observe the range of extrapyramidally-mediated motor disturbance to which the human brain may fall victim, one need go no further than the local psychiatric hospital. While the association between major psychiatric illness and disorders of movement can be traced from Haslam and Griesinger to the present, the veracity of this statement has its roots in different soil.

In 1955, Jean Delay coined the term 'neuroleptic' in recognition of the frequency, if not the inevitability, of motor signs developing in the course of treatment with chlorpromazine. Briefly, the theory prevailed that such signs were a necessary herald of antipsychotic efficacy, although the blow of a few incompatible facts soon laid that one to rest. For most clinicians, these were simply side effects, and to a generation emerging from therapeutic impotence, were seen as an inconvenience rather than a source of concern. This complacent view was to be eroded and eventually swept away by acceptance of the concept of tardive dyskinesia—although it might be said that in day-to-day practice a certain amount of complacency, or perhaps ignorance, still abounds.

If drug-related movement disorders have been a major focus of the research literature in adult psychiatry in the past two decades, the same cannot be said of that pertaining to child and adolescent psychiatry or other potentially 'at risk' groups, especially those with learning disability. The role of psychopharmacology in treatment of these groups has traditionally been founded on less sure ground than in adults, but in recent years clinical trials have substantiated a number of specific indications for psychotropic drugs, including antipsychotics[1,2]. Thus the issue of movement disorders associated with exposure to these compounds *is* pertinent in such populations. Whatever the justifications for the glaring neglect, irrelevancy is not, as will become clear, one that can be substantiated.

In this chapter the extrapyramidal syndromes associated with psychotropic drug use will be reviewed. As far as the frame of reference is concerned, a bias towards the adult literature will be evident. The reasons for this are firstly the

Movement and Allied Disorders. Edited by M. M. Robertson and V. Eapen

superior knowledge and descriptive power within this literature, and secondly the assumption of a fundamental similarity between adults and 'others' with regard to drug-related movement disorders. Points on which this assumption is contradicted by the literature or seems intuitively unsound will be highlighted. Although a number of studies have looked at populations with learning disability, especially with regard to tardive movement disorders, these have frequently included a high proportion of adult subjects, who probably differ little from adults with psychiatric illness. The comparisons and contrasts where appropriate will therefore be on the basis of age, i.e. children and adolescents. Finally, a brief overview of some standardized techniques for recording disorders of this type will be presented.

CLASSIFICATION

There is no entirely satisfactory way of classifying drug-related movement disorders. 'Acute' and 'chronic' (or tardive) is the simplest, although to refer to disorders, some of which may not become evident for weeks or months, as 'acute' seems perverse.

The terms 'hyperkinetic' and 'bradykinetic' have been used, both tightly and loosely defined. Tightly defined, they are the 'positive' and 'negative' symptomatology of the motor system. This attempt at simplicity bears the seeds of confusion. Clinically, chorea and tremor are both 'hyperkinetic', but while the former is an integral part of tardive dyskinesia, the latter is specifically excluded, being predominantly classified with the major bradykinetic syndrome, parkinsonism. A number of similar examples could be quoted, and this use of the terminology is probably best laid to rest. Loosely defined, 'hyperkinetic' is synonymous with tardive dyskinesia and 'bradykinetic' with parkinsonism. The problem with this is that it is restrictive and underplays major clinical issues (e.g. acute dystonias).

The most useful way to classify drug-related movement disorder is on the basis of the relationship of its onset to the duration of exposure to the offending agent. This defines syndromes of clinical relevance in terms of symptom/sign profiles and treatment options and probably has pathophysiological merit.

DRUGS ASSOCIATED WITH THE DEVELOPMENT OF MOVEMENT DISORDERS

An extensive range of drugs of different classes has been implicated in the development of movement disorders. This diversity is particularly evident in relation to tardive dyskinesia, where tricyclic antidepressants (TCAs)[3] and even benzodiazepines[4] have been drawn into the debate. In relation to the frequency with which these drugs have been prescribed over the years, especially traditional TCAs, reports of an association have been very few—in fact no more than isolated case reports, and it is likely that with a couple of caveats (see below) these were examples of incidental or possibly state-dependent spontaneous disorder.

The common thread linking the major compounds implicated is their essential anti-dopamine action. Thus with regard to all the syndromes discussed here, antipsychotics are top of the list—the exception (thus far) probably being clozapine. It must be remembered, however, that drugs with other clinical uses may also have significant anti-dopaminergic actions. The antiemetic metoclopramide can, for example, be associated with the development of the range of extrapyramidal disorders including tardive dyskinesia. The caveat mentioned above refers to the TCA amoxapine, a drug with potent antidopaminergic activity and one which has been implicated in the development of movement disorder. Clomipramine also possesses more potent dopamine-blocking ability than traditional TCAs, and its use may indeed be associated with galactorrhoea, although the risk of disordered movement may be more theoretical. Of distinct practical importance, however, are the non-antipsychotic antihistamines, a number of which possess antidopaminergic actions and have been reported as being associated with the development of movement disorder, especially acute dystonias[5–7]. This is a particular point of note for those dealing with children. One only has to browse cursorily through the relevant pages of the *British National Formulary* to see the range of paediatric formulations, mainly for respiratory ailments, that contain these compounds.

Other compounds have been associated with other movement disorders, mostly hyperkinetic in type, which bear an undetermined relationship, or at most only a superficial resemblance, to tardive dyskinesia. The commonest is undoubtedly the hyperkinetic disturbance associated with long-term L-dopa administration to patients with Parkinson's disease. Others include involuntary movements during treatment with antiepileptic drugs (AEDs), especially phenytoin[8] and carbamazepine[9], psychostimulant use, particularly amphetamines[10,11] and methylphenidate[12], and excessive recreational use of cocaine. The antimalarial chloroquin[13] and the anticancer drug vincristine[14] have also rarely been implicated.

Overwhelmingly the following discussion concerns movement disorders associated with antipsychotic (neuroleptic) drug use.

ACUTE DYSTONIAS

INTRODUCTION

Dystonia is the sign produced by relatively slow involuntary muscle activity that is either sustained and recurrent or maintained for prolonged periods. The former, kinetic type, presents as constant, writhing movement while the latter, myostatic type, results in abnormal posture or attitude. Acute dystonias are overwhelmingly myostatic, and develop significantly earlier in exposure than the other drug-related extrapyramidal syndromes[15].

This type of disorder is still appallingly under-recognized. In one study, only 33% of the disorder evident to specialist researchers was detected by clinicians[16], which is probably not unrepresentative of routine practice. Such a degree of oversight is however, increasingly indefensible.

CLINICAL FEATURES

Objective dystonia is often preceded by a purely subjective phase where the patient may complain of stiffness, discomfort or pain in the affected part, or may describe clumsiness or impaired function. Affective disturbances, such a prominent feature of acute dystonic disorder, is evident even in this early, mild stage. Patients are invariably anxious and distressed, with behaviour that is restless and importuning. In the absence of objective signs, language can seem histrionically extravagant. It is all too easy to interpret such a predominantly behavioural disturbance as an extension of the illness for which the drug treatment was initiated in the first place, a particular trap in those unable to articulate subjective complaints.

This mild stage may be traversed too rapidly to be brought to medical attention, and the first indication of disorder will then be frank dystonia. Any voluntary muscle or muscle group may be affected, but in general, abnormality in adults tends to be more circumscribed with a head/neck emphasis, while in younger age groups disorder is more likely to be generalized. By 'younger age groups' one certainly means adolescents, but extension of this statement to children is dependent on the analogy with idiopathic dystonia, since the paediatric psychiatry literature provides no guidance.

The commonest presentation in adults, and probably younger patients also, is torticollis or any of its variants (retro-/antero-/laterocollis). Extraocular dystonia is by contrast relatively uncommon, accounting for only about 6% of incidents[17]. Rare cases have been reported where oculogyrus has been associated with concurrent psychiatric symptomatology, especially auditory hallucinations[18], but, as has been pointed out, the classical oculogyric *crises* of encephalitis lethargica were polysymptomatic neuropsychiatric states to which simple drug-related ocular deviations bear little resemblance[19].

The tongue may rotate or elevate within the mouth, affecting speech and swallowing, or may be forcibly protruded, a particular problem if associated with forced jaw closure (trismus) rather than opening. This combination can result in severe trauma, and the author has been apprised of one complete and one partial amputation of the tongue in this situation, although is unaware of such reports in the literature.

Neck spasms may overflow to axial antigravity muscles, producing oposthotonos, from bilateral involvement, or unilateral truncal leans. Upper limbs, if affected, tend to adopt an attitude between hyperpronation on elbow extension with wrist and metacarpalphalangeal flexion, and hypersupination on elbow flexion, while for lower limbs an attitude between foot inversion with extension of the knee and eversion with knee flexion may be found. Spasm of leg adductors can result in a 'scissor' gait, making independent walking impossible.

The silence with which such patients often present may be explained by the terror frequently registered on their faces, but involvement of tongue, pharynx and intrinsic laryngeal muscles is another potential explanation that must not be overlooked.

PREVALENCE/INCIDENCE

The widely quoted prevalence figure of 2.3%[20] is a gross underestimate and an artefact of the method of calculation in the review in which it was published[19]. Recent retrospective[21] and prospective[15,22] studies provide a more realistic figure in the range 25–36%.

The consensus is that 90% occur within the first five days of exposure[23], although a delay of more than six weeks has been reported in 10% of adult, first episode schizophrenic patients[22].

PREDISPOSING FACTORS

As a general rule all 'acute' drug-related extrapyramidal syndromes are more likely with:

1. high as opposed to low potency compounds;
2. higher dose regimes;
3. rapid as opposed to gradual dose increments, and these are pertinent to acute dystonias.

There is, in addition, general agreement that the risk of acute dystonias is inversely related to age. Addonizio and Alexopoulos found a rate of 36% in younger patients (mean age 26 years) but only 2% in the elderly (mean age 67 years)[21]. It is also widely held that males are affected about twice as often as females, although this entrenched view is not supported by prospective data. Singh *et al.*[15] found a comparable *incidence* in both genders when *all* other variables were accounted for, while Chakos *et al.*[22] actually found a 2:1 *female* excess. These two reports are not necessarily incompatible. Thus, one predictor noted in the former study was antipsychotic dose in terms of mg/kg body weight. In research, as in routine practice, dosages are rarely modified for the lower average weight of females, who in the latter study may have received a greater mg/kg dose than males. At present it must be concluded that accounting for all other variables, especially age and mg/kg drug dose, the risk of acute dystonias is equal in both genders.

COURSE/OUTCOME

Untreated, the course of acute dystonic episodes conforms to one of three main patterns. A full-blown but rarely extending disorder may recur and remit completely in cycles over hours to days, or may fluctuate in intensity but with core abnormality evident throughout. Alternatively, once present, signs may persist without change until spontaneous resolution gradually takes place, again usually over hours to days.

Isolated reports have described catastrophic neurological disorder after exposure to antipsychotics in children[24], some, though not all, following a presumed overdose[25,26]. These are likely to represent idiosyncratic or toxic reactions to antipsychotic ingestion rather than acute dystonias as described here, which although severely distressing, are *usually* medically benign. Such reports do not amount to a sufficient body of data to suggest the situation is otherwise in children.

PATHOPHYSIOLOGY

The pathophysiology of acute dystonias is unknown and somewhat controversial. The simple view is that dopamine blockade promotes a cholinergic preponderance in the normal cholinergic–dopaminergic balance in the striatum. A more complex hypothesis involves the different acute and chronic mechanisms dopaminergic systems develop to overcome receptor blockade. Developing postsynaptic receptor supersensitivity (the chronic mechanism) renders striatal systems vulnerable to excess transmitter coming from increased dopamine turnover (the acute mechanism) which has not quite returned to baseline[27]. Hence this theory infers dopaminergic excess. The simple theory is probably too simple and the complex one, although intriguing, remains somewhat speculative.

CHILDREN/ADOLESCENTS

The position regarding many aspects of acute dystonia in young populations must be surmised, as published data are very sparse and of generally poor quality (Table 11.1). Certainly such an abnormality does occur. One could postulate that by extending the age association back, children might be at even greater risk than young adults, although this does not appear to be the case. Clearly, high doses of high potency compounds produce high incidence figures[31] as would be expected in adults, but the

Table 11.1. Acute dystonia in children and adolescents

Author	Diagnosis	Age	*N*	Acute dystonia	%	Comment
Cunningham *et al.* (1968)[28]	(?) (Not psychotic)	Mean 10.25	12	?3	?25	'transient muscle pains or spasms'
Barker and Fraser (1968)[29]	Multiple	4–15	16	0	0	Coincidental benzhexol
Polizos and Engelhardt (1978)[30]	Schizophrenia with autistic features	Mean 8.8	95*	?	5.75	'25% of children who developed extrapyramidal symptoms' i.e. of 23%
Chiles (1978)[31]	Acutely psychotic	13–18	11	7	63.6	Treatment with high dose, high potency drugs
Campbell *et al.* (1984)[32]	Aggressive/ conduct disorder	5–13	61	10	16.4	
Spencer *et al.* (1992)[33]	Schizophrenia	Mean 8.78	12	2 (?+2)	17.5 (35)	Prospective study 'acute dystonia' 2 ('Tongue discomfort' 2)

*95 individuals participated in 284 treatment episodes

consistent rates over an 8-year period reported by the New York group using more modest dose regimens are striking[32,33].

At present it is not possible to explore any other correlates or peculiarities of acute dystonic reactions in children, and the need for further work is evident.

TREATMENT

Patients with acute dystonias can find themselves catapulted in one of two opposite directions. Such patients have found themselves the victims of intensive and unnecessary investigations, while others have been considered 'hysterical' and denied simple and effective treatment[19], both of which are nowadays unacceptable. The sudden onset and bizarre, affectively laden presentation should be pointers *to* the diagnosis, not away from it. Those working with children must be especially alert to the problem and to the dazzling array of proprietary preparations containing antihistamines and non-antipsychotic phenothiazines, a number of which have been implicated in acute, childhood dystonia[7].

A range of preparations has been used to treat acute dystonias in the past, but these have largely been superseded by anticholinergics, which are safe and effective both orally (after 15–20 minutes) and by slow intravenous (IV) injection (after 1–2 minutes). In the UK, procyclidine is the most widely used, on the basis of habit rather than proven superiority. The average dose of 10 mg in adults should be titrated downwards in pre-adolescent children. Some authors, especially American, still recommend the antihistamine diphenhydramine (25 mg intramuscularly (IM) or orally) for use in children.

There is no management consensus on what to do thereafter. It is prudent to maintain antipsychotic doses stable for several days and then increase (if required) gradually, but regular oral anticholinergics are probably only helpful if acute dystonia recurs, and then should not be necessary for more than 5–7 days.

Routine prophylaxis has been much debated, but practice continues to vary. However, it would seem best to avoid the automatic prescription of an anticholinergic from the start of antipsychotic treatment. The majority of patients will not develop acute neurological reactions, and anticholinergics have practical as well as theoretical problems associated with their use, including, in children, the possibility of impairment of learning. It is therefore wise to avoid unnecessarily complicating pharmacology in this way.

PARKINSONISM

INTRODUCTION

In the study of Weiden *et al.*[16] referred to earlier, clinicians did best with parkinsonism recognizing 60% of that identified by the researchers. In the early adult literature the term 'Parkinson-like syndrome' was often used to highlight a difference in the presentation of drug-related disorder from idiopathic disease. In fact it is now clear that any of the features of Parkinson's disease (PD) can be found in drug-related parkinsonism. The emphasis, however, is strongly towards *bradykinesia* with the other 'core' features of tremor (especially resting) and rigidity playing in general a subsidiary role. Poor recognition may thus be explained—though not justified—by the superficial resemblance of some manifestations of bradykinesia to certain mental state disorders, especially the psychomotor retardation of depression, the affective flattening of schizophrenia and other neuropsychiatric disorders.

Bradykinesia results in slowing of voluntary movement, loss of background motor activity and, in severe cases, interruption of the flow of consecutive movements. As in other forms of parkinsonism this, along with other 'core' features, may present unilaterally.

CLINICAL FEATURES

It is often forgotten that parkinsonism of whatever type is associated with *symptoms*, and any assessment of a drug-related disorder should begin with a symptomatic enquiry. Patients may experience weakness or stiffness, especially of the proximal muscles and in the early part of the day. The pillow may be moist on wakening, from nocturnal drooling. Movement may feel subjectively slowed and they may be aware of clumsiness from impaired dexterity. They may also be embarrassed by their immobile walk or feel unstable, or may even have fallen, both of which can exaggerate social isolation.

Hypomimia, or facial mask, tends to produce a slightly open-mouthed expression with a wide-eyed, staring quality from decreased blink frequency. Glabellar tap may be positive (Myerson's sign) although, especially in psychiatric patients, this is a somewhat non-specific finding. Seborrhoea may produce a greasy, scaly quality to the skin and the mouth may be moist with pooling of saliva and possibly drooling. Sialorrhoea probably results from bradykinesia of the swallowing musculature rather than from production of excess saliva (although the sometimes prominent sialorrhoea with clozapine may spring from the latter mechanism).

Posture is often stiff and statuesque with loss of interactive gesture. Classical 'triple flexion' is—or ought to be—uncommon, the more characteristic appearance being of an erect, slightly hyperextended spine. Arms tend to be held slightly flexed at the elbow and abducted, and most typically of all there is a reduction in pendular arm swing on walking, perhaps *the* most sensitive sign of antipsychotic exposure. Gait itself is also infrequently affected, and by the time length and height of step decline and festination is evident, treatment plans are in need of review. Postural instability is rarely sought but is not uncommon, and can decrease independence and result in injury.

Rigidity tends to be slight in drug-related disorders and often needs reinforcement to elicit. Both cogwheel *and* lead-pipe varieties carry equal diagnostic importance. Likewise the typical, slow resting tremor of paralysis agitans tends to be a relatively infrequent and late feature in drug-related parkinsonism. Postural or action tremor, best seen in the outstretched hand is, by contrast, an early and common feature.

It is easy to see how the withdrawn, expressionless appearance of bradykinetic parkinsonism could be confused with depression, and indeed depressed mood is common in such patients, a situation sometimes referred to as 'akinetic depression'[34]. It is unclear, however, whether this represents a separate nosological entity.

PREVALENCE/INCIDENCE

Figures for the prevalence of drug-related parkinsonism vary, with 15–40% most widely quoted. It is essential to appreciate that such inconsistency is an understandable consequence of the variables that influence the development of the disorder, and not merely a reflection of professional incompetence. Most important of these is how one defines the disorder, whether broadly in terms of any clinical abnormality no matter how slight, or tightly in terms of syndromal criteria. Also of importance are drug variables (as noted) and the phase of treatment in which the assessment is made.

In a recent prospective study an incidence of 35% was found over an 8-week treatment period[22]. This figure was based on rigidity criteria from a rating scale heavily biased towards this sign (Simpson–Angus Scale—see below), and on the basis of the clinical comments above, is probably an underestimate. It is likely that the great majority of adequately treated adult patients followed closely enough will show at least some mild features of parkinsonism at some time.

The majority of diagnosed cases are evident in the first 2–3 months of treatment. In Ayd's study 90% occurred within the first 72 days[20] and 72% of those identified prospectively were diagnosed within six weeks[22].

PREDISPOSING FACTORS

The drug variables of potency, dose and rate of increase are relevant here as in all 'acute' extrapyramidal syndromes.

It has in addition been reported that the age distribution of drug-related parkinsonism parallels that of idiopathic disease[23]. This is certainly logical and is compatible with the known age-related decline in several major neurochemical constituents of the striatum, including dopamine[35]. However, it must be remembered that individuals vary greatly in their intrinsic striatal dopaminergic reserve, and hence some patients may be constitutionally predisposed, regardless of the effects of age.

It is also widely believed that females are approximately twice as commonly affected as males. This again arose from the large retrospective analysis conducted many years ago by Ayd[20]. When drug variables are accounted for, and examination thorough and ongoing, it is unclear whether primary gender differences would be sustained.

COURSE/OUTCOME

The course of untreated drug-related parkinsonism is poorly described. In general it tends to fluctuate. On stable regimes, the majority of cases will tend to a plateau in both extent and severity of features, around which a degree of variation is likely to occur, perhaps relating in some degree to mental state. However, an undetermined proportion of cases will spontaneously remit, usually after 2–3 months on stable drug doses.

It is accepted wisdom that the condition automatically resolves on discontinuing the offending agent. This is probably reasonable, but has never been scientifically proved in adequate discontinuation studies. There are certainly some, usually older, patients in whom it cannot be taken as axiomatic. Even in those where resolution does occur, features may persist for 12–18 months.

PATHOPHYSIOLOGY

By analogy with PD, the pathophysiology is seen to be a straightforward consequence of decreased nigrostriatal dopaminergic transmission resulting from postsynaptic receptor blockade.

CHILDREN/ADOLESCENTS

The account provided here relates to the position as described in adults for over 40 years. A reasonable comparative literature in children and adolescents, amazingly, does not exist.

The proposal that, by extending backwards the inverse age-relationship reported in adults, children and adolescents may not be at risk of developing drug-related parkinsonism is clearly untenable. The very young exposed to the same provoking agents as adults can and *do* develop features of parkinsonism. What is not clear however, is whether the risk is greater or less than in adults. Richardson *et al.*[36] found a *prevalence* of 34% in a sample of children and adolescents (mean age 14.9 years) with learning disability. This is precisely the figure for *incidence* reported in first-episode schizophrenics by Chakos *et al.*[22] (see above) using the same recording instrument. Richardson and colleagues noted the wide age range in their sample, from children through to adolescents, but did not find age to be a specific determinant in their population[36]. At present it must therefore be assumed that the risk of drug-related parkinsonism developing in children and adolescents is probably similar to that of younger adults.

A further unresolved issue is whether the presentation is different in the young compared to adults. In a prospective study[33], four parkinsonian features were recorded—facial mask, rigidity, decreased arm-swing and drooling—but this sample was small ($N = 12$)—and data were not presented for individual patients. Drooling was recorded in four instances while the others were only noted in one instance each. Engelhardt and Polizos[37] also found hypersalivation to be the most common neurological side effect. Whether this means that sialorrhoea is a more prominent sign in children, or merely that their less refined social behaviour allows it to be more evident, is unclear.

With indications for long-term antipsychotic use in children now being more clearly defined, the need for further studies in this field is pressing.

TREATMENT

If there is one therapeutic fact known to even the most junior trainee, it is that treatment of drug-related parkinsonism is with anticholinergics. This fact is so ingrained that one might suppose it is supported by a wealth of scientific data. This is not the case! This treatment strategy was introduced largely on the basis of analogy with PD, in which it was itself established empirically. As Mindham has pointed out, the scientific evidence that anticholinergics are effective in drug-related disorder is much less than their widespread use would imply[38]. This certainly accords with clinical experience—that despite frequent improvements in well-being, objective signs often persist.

Anticholinergics should *always* be used sparingly and *never* routinely. They can have serious side effects (e.g. paralytic ileus, impaired learning), are frequently abused, and may exacerbate productive psychiatric symptomatology.

Emergence of parkinsonian features is not in itself an indication for intervention, which should depend on an objective assessment of severity, incapacitation *and* on the patient's subjective awareness/distress. Should management be required, one should consider the feasibility of a slight reduction (e.g. 25%) in antipsychotic dose first, which is usually practicable. Change to a lower potency compound may also be an option.

If indicated, anticholinergics should be used conservatively. In the UK, procyclidine is most widely used for reasons that are unclear. In adults an initial dose of 5 mg twice daily is reasonable, although if symptoms are severe or distressing, the relatively short half-life of most anticholinergics may demand a thrice daily regimen. Doses in the evening should be avoided, as the stimulant effects of these drugs may disrupt sleep.

In evaluating each of these steps it is important to allow adequate time for benefits to filter through—e.g. at least one week. If using anticholinergics, it is also important not to push to high levels. If benefits are not evident with 20 mg procyclidine per day or its equivalent, they are unlikely to occur with higher doses and the risks of inadvertently straying into the toxic range, associated with anticholinergic psychosis, is not insubstantial.

Practice with regard to prophylaxis is also varied. Evidence from studies of the course of drug-related parkinsonism and from discontinuation studies indicate that the majority of patients will not require long-term prophylaxis. Hence an attempt to discontinue anticholinergics should be made after 2–3 months of stability. If this is unsuccessful, further attempts should be made at a later stage. The point is that long-term use of anticholinergics must be *justified*.

Psychiatrists have been remarkably timorous in evaluating other compounds used in idiopathic PD. Reserve about L-dopa is largely based on the negative predictions of the dopamine hypothesis of schizophrenia, but it is clear that the effects of dopamine agonists in this situation are not as clear-cut as the hypothesis would suggest[39]. Clinical trials with L-dopa in adults have been equivocal but the issue is worthy of further consideration. Amantadine was ineffective in one study—but so was an anticholinergic[40]. Early reports of a favourable response to selegiline[41] are encouraging but must await confirmation.

In children, the same general treatment plan outlined above is relevant. However, the need to consider antipsychotic dose reduction as *the* essential element is all the greater, as is the requirement for anticholinergic use to be conservative and repeatedly justified. Evidence that might allay fears about the detrimental effects of anticholinergics on learning does not as yet exist.

AKATHISIA

INTRODUCTION

Akathisia has been described for almost a century in association with PD, yet despite being recognized early on in the history of antipsychotic drug use, and despite being common and a frequent source of non-compliance and rarely of violence and suicide, it remains relatively under-researched and certainly under-recognized. In the study of Weiden *et al.* clinicians acknowledged only about one-quarter of this type of disorder[16].

Akathisia literally means 'an inability to sit still' (tasikinesia—an inability to stand still—is probably a clinical variant of the same problem). As classically conceptualized, akathisia is essentially a dysphoric affective state. Movement is excessive and purposeless in the sense of being non-goal directed, but is not 'involuntary' as in the other drug-related extra-pyramidal syndromes. However, although movement is under 'willed' control, the subjective distress it is designed to alleviate is often such that sufferers feel they have no choice but to move.

CLINICAL FEATURES

The syndrome has two main characteristics—an extremely unpleasant inner restlessness and a desire to move in an attempt (usually in vain) to ease the distress. This would of course stand as a definition of psychomotor agitation and clinically the two can be indistinguishable, although the 'driven' quality of akathisia and a tendency to localization to the lower limbs may help.

On examination, sufferers look tense. Facial expression, in the absence of coincidental parkinsonism (see below) shows the wide-eyed apprehension of the hyper-aroused. Patients tend to sit forward, erect and tense in posture but fidgety in movement. They may rock or, characteristically, cross and uncross their legs or swing their crossed leg back and forwards constantly. These leg movements in particular have a 'hectic', ill-modulated and graceless quality. In more severe cases, patients may be unable to sit for any length of time, and conversation, however brief, may be punctuated by them standing suddenly and without warning. In the standing position, patients may shift weight constantly from one foot to the other, like 'walking on the spot', a sign which if not evident spontaneously may emerge when they are asked to perform some cognitive task such as simple arithmetic.

As the level of activity progresses with severity, so the repertoire becomes impoverished and more and more of the day is spent simply pacing up and down the same seemingly predetermined path, to the extent that the feet may become traumatized and blistered.

Upper limbs are not immune and patients may be seen to fidget or finger fillip or rub hands and arms. Rubbing behaviour—such as rubbing the side of the head or face and rubbing the eyes, or running the hand through the hair or over the scalp—is also frequently seen, but whether this is 'akathisic' or manneristic, or indeed whether such a distinction can be validly made, is unclear.

PREVALENCE/INCIDENCE

The early studies of drug-related akathisia reported a prevalence between 21%[20] and 32%[42] and figures over the years have tended to fall within this range. Two prospective studies of incidence over 6–7 week treatment intervals with fluphenazine have however reported quite wide diversity, from 18%[22] to 43%[43].

As with parkinsonism, 80–90% of cases are evident in the first 6–10 weeks of treatment.

PREDISPOSING FACTORS

Dose, potency and rate of increase of medication are again of relevance, and females have again been traditionally considered at greater risk. This has not been confirmed prospectively[22], and, as with parkinsonism, such differences may reflect differing treatment practices rather than fundamental differences relating to gender *per se*.

As will be evident, the demographics of akathisia are very similar to those of parkinsonism, and akathisia was of course first described as the 'paradoxical restlessness' of PD. This raises the question as to whether the two drug-related syndromes should be more accurately considered as a single entity. Information to address this issue is not as yet available, although it has been found that while anticholinergics may bring about improvement in both parkinsonism and akathisia in some patients, in others the latter may persist[44], suggesting that in terms of treatment characteristics at least, the distinction does have validity.

COURSE/OUTCOME

Unlike parkinsonism, akathisia does not appear to undergo spontaneous resolution, and the course seems more closely linked to dose regimen–stability on stable regimens, exacerbation and amelioration with increments and decrements respectively.

Over time, many patients appear to lose the affective distress that is the cornerstone of 'classical' akathisia, while an outwardly restless, fidgety appearance persists. This situation has been referred to as tardive or pseudo-akathisia and raises important conceptual and practical questions (see below). The risk of such a development is unknown.

PATHOPHYSIOLOGY

This has not been elucidated. However, the association with PD and antidopaminergic medication would clearly implicate inhibition of central dopamine transmission. Nonetheless the emergence of excessive motor activity in the context of profound motor poverty suggests a different site for the two pathophysiologies. Mesocortical dopamine systems appear to exert some inhibitory functions on certain aspects of the higher control of motor functions, and have been suggested as a possible site for the disturbances[27].

CHILDREN/ADOLESCENTS

The literature on akathisia in children and adolescents is rudimentary, although in relation to the volume of the adult literature the void is probably proportionate (Table 11.2). No studies to date have been specifically devoted to this topic, and even authors in the field of drug-related movement disorders in children have made only passing reference to it. While this could mean that akathisia did not emerge in their samples, such a conclusion cannot be assumed.

There is nonetheless evidence that children and adolescents are not immune to developing akathisia. The risk, however is in effect a 'guestimate', as it is hard to interpret published data. Engelhardt and

Table 11.2. Akathisia in children and adolescents

		With akathisia	
	N	*N*	%
Barker and Fraser (1968)[29]	16	0	0
Engelhardt and Polizos (1978)[37]	95 (284)	2	2 (0.7)
Chiles (1978)[31]	11	1	9
Stone *et al.* (1988)[45]	1282		13
Bruun (1988)[46]	208	9	4.8
Richardson *et al.* (1991)[36]	104	2	2

Polizos[37], noted akathisia 'in only two children' but these data are based on 95 *children* who participated in a total of 284 treatment *periods*, with a resultant prevalence that is either low (2%) or ultra-low (0.7%), while the study of Bruun[46] is an essentially anecdotal account of her experience with Gilles da la Tourette syndrome (GTS) patients. Overall, the reported prevalence of akathisia in the young does appear to be lower than that for adults. This conclusion may to some extent be an erroneous consequence of the inadequate data on which it is based, but if justified, is likely to be a reflection of differing treatment practices rather than any specific 'protective' effect of age *per se*.

Children do present particular problems for the diagnosis of akathisia. Their lack of linguistic sophistication for describing essentially subjective disturbances of affect, their relatively less organized patterns of behaviour and the clinical features of disorders from which they tend to suffer, especially hyperactivity, all make evaluation problematic. These very facts, however, make it incumbent on the psychiatrist to be particularly alert to the possibility of akathisia in 'at risk' patients in this age group.

TREATMENT

It seems to have become accepted practice that akathisia is to be treated with additional medication and that this should be anticholinergics. This probably sprang from the association with parkinsonism, but as was stated above, is at best probably only partly true. Any semi-keen clinical eye will certainly appreciate the inadequacy of anticholinergics for many patients with akathisia.

The first treatment option following emergence of akathisia should involve, where possible, manipulation of the primary causative agent rather than a rush to additional medications. Antipsychotic doses should be stabilized for one week, since early in treatment, restlessness may ease following a moratorium on regular dose increments. If the situation does not improve, doses should be slightly reduced (e.g. 25% or so), a strategy that is only likely to be impractical in the most disturbed patients. Switching to a lower potency drug may be a useful additional or alternative measure.

The additional treatment of proven efficacy in akathisia is β-blockers, and propranolol should be the drug of choice[47]. In relatively low doses (20–60 mg per day) propranolol has been shown to produce improvement within a few days, by a mechanism probably involving blockade of central rather than peripheral β-adrenergic receptors[48]. If this fails, then anticholinergics may be tried, and benzodiazepines may help both by non-specific anxiolysis and perhaps more specific GABA-ergic facilitation, but their use in this situation is of course subject to the usual limitations.

TARDIVE DYSKINESIA

If the finding that clinicians in routine psychiatric practice recognize only 10% of the tardive dyskinesia (TD) present in their patients[16], is at all representative, then one is forced to ponder what aspects of the specialist literature they have been reading in the past 10–15 years, for this has been one of the major focuses of published research in adult psychiatry. Much of this work came from the USA and was fuelled less by the clinical than by the medico-legal issues of a potentially common, progressive, incurable and disfiguring condition that was potentially iatrogenic. The legal position has in fact been restrained, especially in the UK, perhaps in acknowledgement of the dilemma posed by a serious side effect to what is nonetheless the primary and necessary treatment for a serious disorder. It would be an error to assume that such restraint will continue. Professional vulnerability has mainly lain thus far in a mode of practice which, it has been argued, reflected either ignorance or indifference. It is now incumbent on all psychiatrists to be aware of the issue and to express that awareness *tangibly*.

Several preliminary points are worth emphasizing. Firstly, TD is an epidemiological concept whose boundaries, even now, are unclear. While the term implies that any type of involuntary movement might be included, tremor is specifically excluded[49]—largely, one assumes, on theoretical grounds. The relationship of a 'tardive' disorder to motor abnormalities long known to be a feature of major psychiatric disorders, especially schizophrenia, is unknown and although the question of what can legitimately be attributed to illness and what to treatment has been relatively little considered in the adult literature, it is one that has been considered in detail by some paediatric authors[50]. While there is no clear relationship in the literature between TD and most drug variables, 'tardive' movements can clearly be suppressed by increasing doses of the implicated drug or may be temporarily exacerbated—or may even first emerge—with dose reduction. The distinction between the 'treatment-emergent' and the 'withdrawal-emergent' disorder has also not received great emphasis in the adult literature, perhaps because discontinuation of the major offending agents (antipsychotics) in their major target population (schizophrenics) is a luxury that seldom arises. This distinction has, however, clearly influenced paediatric psychiatrists, in whose constituency withdrawal-emergent dyskinesias appear to have greater relevance.

Finally, the term TD allows one inference, and one only—an involvement of drugs in causation. One need not argue about the precise nature of this involvement, but this general principle is intrinsic to the concept. It therefore follows that to speak of 'spontaneous' TD is to betray a more than trifling ignorance.

CLINICAL FEATURES

Involuntary tongue activity is usually cited as the earliest manifestation of the disorder, although whether there is an orderly progression from this to other sites is unknown. Tongue movements of uncertain significance are certainly likely to become significant after only 6 months, so any untoward activity here is worthy of note. Movements tend to be described as 'vermicular' or worm-like in the first instance, to be followed by longitudinal or horizontal displacement within the dental margin. Overflow beyond the dental margin gives rise to sweeping of the inner buccal surface ('bon-bon' sign) or rigid, jerky protrusion usually to one side ('fly-catcher' sign). Jaw movements may result in antero-posterior or lateral displacement, or combined movements simulating chewing or grinding, or the mouth may forcibly open. Lips may pucker or purse, cheeks balloon and the lateral angles of the mouth extend ('bridling'), any of which may occur silently or with rudimentary clicks, smacks or puffing noises. This bucco-linguo-masticatory or BLM triad is the commonest presentation, affecting some 80% of cases.

Spread to the general muscles of facial expression can give rise to grimacing, blepharospasm or blepharoclonus, jerky eyebrow elevation and furrowing of the forehead. Axial movement can lead to all varieties of head/neck displacement, to unilateral truncal leans of the so-called 'Pisa' syndrome, and to irregular, thrusting pelvic activity resembling copulation. Limbs may develop rotational and non-rotational movements with or without outsplaying or flexion/extension ('piano playing') actions in the digits.

Grunting or breathless sounds may result from extension to diaphragmatic and intercostal muscles and swallowing may become impaired from oropharyngeal involvement, as may speech from involvement of the intrinsic muscles of the larynx.

The symptomatology of TD is dependent on the level of arousal, and hence is exacerbated by anxiety and diminished by composure and sedation. It disappears during sleep. Sometimes movements may only emerge when the patient is performing some voluntary action in a distant body part and this is often recommended as a procedure to elicit early or mild signs—so-called 'activation'. Results from such manoeuvres can, however, be variable because of the unpredictable effect of the degree of concentration needed to execute them.

Descriptively, any type of involuntary movement can be considered 'tardive', with the exception of tremor. Thus the syndrome can embrace chorea, athetosis/dystonia, tics, myoclonus, myokymia or any combination of these. Some clinical situations where a particular type of movement predominates have, however, been singled out for special consideration, examples being tardive multifocal motor and vocal tics (GTS) and tardive dystonia. The latter is especially worthy of note. Although much less common than the 'classical' choreiform syndrome (probably only about 5% of tardive disorders or less) it tends to affect a younger age group, to be much more functionally incapacitating and to have possibly different treatment characteristics (see below). It certainly can be associated with serious complications, such as speech disorder[19], asphyxia[51] and rib fractures[52].

While these 'sub-syndromes' are varieties of the same basic problem, the position of so-called tardive akathisia is conceptually less clear. In this situation the dysphoric effect that is the cardinal feature of 'classical' akathisia, is lost, and movement, although excessive and non-goal directed, is no longer 'driven', and indeed frequently appears automatic, with patients unaware of their activity. Whether such patients have indeed progressed to truly involuntary motor disorder or whether this situation is more akin to manneristic/stereotyped activity is unclear and until questions of this sort can be answered, tardive or pseudo-akathisia is probably best considered separately.

PREVALENCE/INCIDENCE

The published figures for the prevalence of TD do not represent an exercise in professional consensus. Rates have varied from 0.5% to over 60%! There are, however, explanations for this discrepancy—such as definition of boundaries, heterogeneity of study samples, the influence of severity on caseness, and the gradual introduction of standardization of assessment. Two large reviews from the early 1980s[53,54] concluded that the prevalence of involuntary movement disorder in psychiatric patients was about 20% overall, with approximately 5% attributable to spontaneous disorder. This left a figure of 13–15% for drug-related disorder. Later studies have found higher prevalences in the range 30–40% or more, probably mainly a reflection of increased recognition of mild cases associated with the widespread use of standardized recording instruments.

Incidence data have been sparse, with only some seven studies reported to date. Follow-ups have ranged from 2 to 7 years but the data pool remains at just over 1500 patients world wide. Average rates per year vary between 0.0385 and 0.1093. The two largest studies have produced comparable figures. Kane *et al.*[55], studying younger patients, found an incidence rate of 0.04/year—i.e. four new cases per 100 person-years of follow-up. The risk of developing TD after 5 years of cumulative antipsychotic exposure—i.e. the cumulative incidence—was 17.8%. In the Yale Study, encompassing the spectrum of the adult age range, the incidence was found to be 0.053 per year with a 5-year risk of 20%[56].

Using the 5-year data from the Yale Study, Glazer *et al.*[57] have calculated an extended risk of persistent TD based on the net years of exposure at first contact during which TD did *not* develop, and the additional years of antipsychotics (Table 11.3). These are troubling figures, but should come as no surprise. The estimate of almost two-thirds affected with at least mild disorder after 25 years' exposure are comparable to *prevalence* figures found using the same recording instrument, the abnormal involuntary movement scale (AIMS) and the same criteria in middle-aged and elderly institutionalized schizophrenics[58].

The minimum period of exposure to a provoking agent that is necessary for associated movements to be called 'tardive' has not been specified. The concept only requires that these features post-date other extrapyramidal manifestations. Originally 2 years was proposed, although movements have been called 'tardive' after just a few months of exposure. A 6–12 month minimum would seem a prudent if arbitrary period, the former especially for chronic dystonia which may have an earlier onset than choreoathetoid disorder.

PREDISPOSING FACTORS

The journey towards identifying factors predisposing to the development of

Table 11.3. Estimated risk (%) of persistent TD by years of previous antipsychotic exposure without abnormality and additional years of antipsychotic exposure

Years of previous antipsychotic use without TD developing	Additional years on antipsychotics				
	5	10	15	20	25
0	32.7	45.8	53.8	60.2	64.7
5	19.4	31.3	40.9	47.6	
10	14.7	26.7	35.0		
15	14.0	23.7			
20	11.3				

From Glazer *et al.*, 1993[57], with permission

TD has been along a barren road. Retrospective studies have failed to produce a consensus on the role of drug variables, such as antipsychotic potency, maximal daily dose, cumulative intake, duration of exposure, polypharmacy and the like, or anticholinergics. A possible predisposing effect of multiple drug-free intervals of longer than 1–3 months[59,60] remains to be confirmed prospectively, but is a potential source of concern.

Of the non-drug-related variables explored, neither gross organic brain damage nor past physical treatments such as electroconvulsive therapy (ECT) can be confirmed, and associations with cognitive impairment and 'negative' schizophrenic deficits, although intriguing, remain controversial. Likewise, associations with late-onset psychosis and a primary affective diagnosis look less secure than at one time.

This group of non-drug-related variables, evaluated in retrospective studies, has however provided one strong association, one that is widely accepted but questionable, and two 'probables'. The strong association is that TD clearly increases with age. This may apply to severity as well as prevalence, and also to the likelihood of movements being irreversible once established, but these latter two points are less clear in prospective studies than retrospective ones. The questionable one is gender. It is widely believed that females are at greater risk (F:M = 1.6:1) but this has consistently been an inconsistent finding, and when evident might well have reflected the influence of interposing variables. The 'possibles' are firstly, a history of acute extrapyramidal side effects in the early phase of exposure[61], and secondly, diabetes mellitus[62].

The Yale Study has prospectively confirmed the positive association with age[56]. In addition it has reported higher rates in non-white (mainly African American) patients, a finding not previously reported. Most importantly this study has found a positive relationship between TD development and antipsychotic drug dose. This clearly requires replication, but as it has the authority of emerging from a prospective design and is certainly logical, it would seem prudent to consider it a cautionary signal for routine clinical practice.

COURSE/OUTCOME

The early concern, widely articulated in the USA, was that TD might be endowed with inexorable progression. Long-term follow-up does not however, suggest that this is the case, an observation that has had a major impact in quelling some of the more hysterical pronouncements on the subject.

A fundamental question relates to the definition of 'course'—whether this refers to the untreated condition following antipsychotic withdrawal, or to the behaviour of the disorder under 'naturalistic' (i.e. routine clinical) conditions. In adult psychiatry the former is probably unattainable, besides which it could be argued that the 'natural history' of a disorder associated with the administration of a necessary drug ought to be considered in the context of continued administration of that drug. More recent work has accepted this argument.

At this stage the literature is not such that clear percentages for categories of outcome can be extracted. Partly this is a consequence of the populations comprising study samples. As Gardos *et al.*[63] have pointed out, studies of antipsychotic-treated populations comprising differing proportions of patients with a clear disorder and some with none, tend to show *increasing* abnormality over time. A proportion of patients in these studies did remit, but this was more than offset by new patients developing the disorder for the first time. However when cohorts of patients, all of whom already have the disorder, are followed, the finding is of overall *improvement*. This appears to be due to the fact that the majority of patients plateau in terms of severity and possibly extent, while the small number who progress (perhaps less than 20%) are more than compensated for by those who remit to varying degrees.

These data are clearly 'soft', but do emphasize the variable and fluctuating natural history of the disorder. The outcome is not inevitably gloomy. The problem remains, however, that there are no clear predictors at first contact of who will end up in what category.

PATHOPHYSIOLOGY

Theories on the pathophysiological mechanisms underlying TD have been dominated by the phenomenon of supersensitivity and constrained by our ignorance of the neurochemical jungle that is the striatum.

Postsynaptic receptor supersensitivity is the major long-term adaptive response to chronic blockade of dopaminergic systems by antidopamine drugs. Although a 'long-term' response to 'chronic' administration, it is actually a process which can be demonstrated in animals, very early in exposure, even after the first dose[64]. Such changes in the striatum are seen as increasing the responsivity of the system to an available transmitter, thereby tipping the normal acetylcholine–dopamine balance in favour of the latter, thus promoting hyperkinesis. By this model, therefore TD is the pathophysiological 'opposite' of parkinsonism.

The fact that this theory has reached maturity almost untouched by the hand of change reflects its sterility rather than its robustness. It does accommodate some of the clinical observations, most notably the suppression-withdrawal phenomena mentioned above. However, supersensitivity develops long before tardive symptoms in general become evident, and is of course an event which follows on from blockade. It would therefore seem logical to expect that tardive movements would emerge in the distribution previously exhibiting parkinsonism, or at least would have the more peripheral distribution of that disorder, as for example do the hyperkinesias associated with L-dopa administration[65], which is clearly not the case. It is also puzzling how parkinsonism and TD could co-exist, as they frequently do, when they are conceived of as pathophysiological striatal 'opposites'. These, and a number of other objections, make it likely that the postsynaptic dopamine receptor supersensitivity hypothesis of TD is at best an over-simplification.

A degree of heterogeneity has been reported in the response of patients to various pharmacological probes[66,67]. In addition to being inconsistent with the straightforward supersensitivity hypothesis, it has been proposed that this speaks of pathophysiological heterogeneity which may in future be a way of characterizing the disorder more precisely in individual patients, although this approach has as yet no place in routine assessment and management.

It may be that striatal postsynaptic dopamine receptor supersensitivity has some—perhaps even necessary—role in the development of TDs, but it is also likely that other players share the stage. A disruption of the normal GABA-mediated inhibition of striatal dopamine systems is an obvious contender, although support for this, and for disturbance focused primarily on the cholinergic side of the acetylcholine–dopamine equation, remains weak. Understanding of the issue will most probably have to await a clearer resolution of the complexities of striatal function.

CHILDREN/ADOLESCENTS

Although the first reports of a hyperkinetic movement disorder in children treated with long-term antipsychotics appeared in the early 1970s, the literature in this field remains disconcertingly slim (Table 11.4). As in the adult literature, early studies were retrospective, and involved diagnostically heterogeneous samples assessed by unstandardized techniques. Most significantly for this age group, pre-treatment baseline measures were not possible. The more recent literature is dominated by the New York group (Campbell and colleagues), who are also the only group to undertake prospective investigation.

As with the other extrapyramidal syndromes associated with antipsychotic drug use, children and adolescents are clearly not immune to developing a 'tardive' type movement disorder. Prevalence figures are not dissimilar to those reported for adults (Table 11.4). While this must be a source of concern to those working with the very young, several points of contrast with the adult literature may permit a ray of optimism.

Firstly there is a sound consensus that 'tardive' type movements in the young are overwhelmingly withdrawal-emergent in type. In the largest sample to date from the New York group 80% of the disorder was of this type, with only six patients—or 5.8% of the total sample—showing

Table 11.4. 'Tardive' dyskinesia in children and adolescents

	N	Age (Yr)	Dyskinesias (%)	Type*	Distribution	Course
McAndrew *et al.* (1972)[68]	125	8–15	8	W/E	Peripheral (upper limbs)	Reversible (3–12 m)
Polizos *et al.* (1973)[69]	34	6–12	41	W/E	Axial/ peripheral orofacial: (1 case)	Reversible—spontaneous and after reintro- duction
Engelhardt *et al.* (1975)[71]	141	5–14	45	W/E	Orofacial: 10 cases (16%)	Reversible—spontaneous and after reintro- duction
Paulson *et al.* (1975)[71]	103	11–16	20	T/E		
Engelhardt and Polizos (1978)[37]	184**	Mean 8.8	46 ('over 90%' of 51%)	W/E	Orofacial <20%	Reversible—spontaneous and after reintro- duction
Winsberg *et al.* (1978)[72]	11	7.5–12.25	45	W/E		
Campbell *et al.* (1982)[73+]	33	2.3–7.9	12	T/E+W/E		
Campbell *et al.* (1983)[74+]	36	2.8–7.8	22	T/E+W/E 3+5		
Gualtieri *et al.* (1984)[75]	41	3–21	37	T/E+W/E 3+9 (+3?)		
Perry *et al.* (1985)[76+]	58	3.6–7.8	22	T/E+ W/E 4+9	Buccal 10 tongue 4	Reversible—spontaneous and after reintro- duction
Campbell *et al.* (1988)[77+]	82	2.7–11	29	T/E+ W/E 5+19	Orofacial alone 37.5% OFD + other 83.3%	Reversible—spontaneous and after reintro- duction

continued

	N	Age (Yr)	Dyskinesias (%)	Type*	Distribution	Course
Malone *et al.* (1991)[78+]	104	2.32–8.22	28	T/E+ W/E 6+23	Orofacial alone 20% OFD + other 50%	Reversible—spontaneous and after reintroduction
Locascio *et al.* (1991)[79+]	(125)73[++]	2.3–8.2	29			
Richardson *et al.* (1991)[36]	41	14–17	12	T/E		

* W/E = Withdrawal-emergent
T/E = Treatment-emergent
** Expanded sample of Engelhardt and Polizos (1975)
\+ New York Group prospective study reported sequentially
++ 'Long-term treatment' group

treatment-emergent movements[78]. Furthermore, this group has also reported that some of this disorder represented an exacerbation of pre-existing stereotyped abnormality rather than involuntary movements emerging *de novo*[73].

Typical orofacial dyskinesia is represented in children, although with this as the sole abnormality in only about 16–40%, the impression is that movement may have a more peripheral distribution than in adults.

A second point of consistency—and one that may not be unrelated to the above—is that these movement disorders seem to be largely reversible on discontinuation of the offending agent. In those patients in whom drugs can be stopped, resolution within 3–12 months appears to be the rule. Where the psychiatric condition does not allow prolonged cessation of medication, movements are usually readily suppressed with its reintroduction.

Slightly higher prevalences of treatment-emergent disorder were reported by Paulson *et al.*[71] and Richardson *et al.*[36] in slightly older (adolescent) patients, the sample reported by the former group also having learning disability. The study of Richardson *et al.* is particularly worthy of note, as it used methodology directly comparable with that applied in adult studies. Although they reported an overall prevalence of 12%, only 7% conformed to the standardized Schooler–Kane criteria for TD widely used in adult studies[80].

Incidence studies in children are severely lacking. Only Campbell *et al*[77], have addressed this issue, reporting an 85% risk over 4 years. This exceptionally high figure is undoubtedly inflated by a study design which encouraged a diagnosis of TD by incorporating repeated periods 'off' medication. Hence the question of incidence in children is still open.

The search for predictors in children has been no more fruitful to date than it has been in adults. In particular, diagnosis and level of intellectual functioning have not emerged as consistent predisposing factors. In one study of patients with learning disability, those with phenylketonuria appeared to be at particular risk[81]. This has echoes of another metabolic disorder recently implicated in adults, namely diabetes[63], but the numbers were small (six affected out of a total of seven) and this must await confirmation. As in the adult literature, drug variables have not as yet clearly emerged as consistent risk factors.

If the total 'pool' of tardive movement disorder in children is indeed comparable to that in adults, but with the balance strikingly against treatment-emergent abnormality, this raises the question as to whether this syndrome is presenting in 'milder' form in the very young—and hence that there may be some protective effect of age—or whether this difference merely reflects different prescribing practices in children. Despite the absence of a clear relationship with drug variables at this stage, the latter would seem the more likely—and more prudent—conclusion.

One further point to emerge from the paediatric literature, that is only indirectly related to the above, is nonetheless worth comment. Several of the workers in this field have observed withdrawal symptoms in children coming off antipsychotics[69,82,83]. This includes the spectrum of symptomatology such as restlessness, irritability, insomnia, nausea, vomiting and, in particular, ataxia. Withdrawal symptoms similar to the above have been documented in adult samples and may be a particular problem with compounds of higher intrinsic anticholinergic activity[84]. The impression is, however, that this represents a relatively infrequent or minor clinical issue in adults. The relative frequency with which this has been commented on in what is a rather small literature is in striking contrast to the infrequency with which it has been raised in the voluminous adult literature, raising the issue of whether the immature brain is more liable to physiological dependency and subsequent withdrawal. This may, however, reflect simply the greater use in children of low potency drugs such as thioridazine, which have substantial anticholinergic activity.

There is a pressing need for further work on the long-term consequences of psychotropic, and in particular antipsychotic, drug use in the young. The message for the clinician, however, is clear—that even in childhood conditions where the use of these compounds is indicated, discontinuation to assess both the need for ongoing treatment *and* side effects is mandatory and, medical conditions permitting, should ideally be a *regular* part of the management plan. This would seem to be an even stronger recommendation to those in paediatric practice than for their adult counterparts.

TREATMENT

There is *no* clearly established treatment for TD, so the emphasis must be on primary prevention, something which can only follow from a *high* index of suspicion, and a conservative approach to the use of, especially, antipsychotic drugs.

The essential management point is that the need for antipsychotics, and dose regimens, *must* be justified. Crucial in this exercise is the clear separation of decisions about maintenance from those bearing on acute treatment. In adults this process may involve a trial period off medication, and in children it probably always should. The same exercise in justification should apply to coincidentally administered anticholinergics.

There is no evidence that any of the traditional antipsychotics is 'safer' than any other, although in light of the possible association between early and late extrapyramidal features (see above), a low potency compound may be preferred. By the same rationale, substituted benzamides have a somewhat more favourable reputation but are not immune to long-term risk. Risperidone is associated with lower rates of acute/intermediate extrapyramidal side effects than haloperidol[85], so may similarly have an edge, but has not been available long enough to evaluate its dyskinetic/antidyskinetic liability directly.

In a review of the early literature on specific treatments, Jeste and Wyatt[86] found that the most successful medication for TD was antipsychotics! One hopes that this is merely a reflection of the suppression phenomenon noted earlier. However, with the theoretical risk of later 'breakthrough' this can only be recommended in serious, probably life-threatening, cases where all else has failed. The early optimism engendered by cholinergic agonists such as choline, lecithin and Deanol, has not been borne out and attempts to 'desensitize' dopaminergic systems with exogenous agonists such as L-dopa have not sustained in practice what in theory was rather a smart idea.

The role of GABA-ergic treatment is unclear, but can be effective and can be simple and safe. Benzodiazepines may therefore be a useful first line, with sodium valproate as an alternative. Likewise, noradrenergic antagonists may have benefit for some patients. Jeste *et al.*[87] reported overall improvement rates with drugs of this type that were comparable to those with antipsychotics, although this was based on only 62 patients. These drugs do need to be used with more care, however. Clonidine (0.15–0.45 mg/day) may have the added bonus of improving the mental state, but is an effective antihypertensive in its own right, and doses of propranolol reported as helpful have been high (up to 800 mg/day) with benefits slow to accrue.

Where dystonia predominates a trial of *gradually* escalating anticholinergics is reasonable, although this is based on the reported benefits of high dose benzhexol in idiopathic dystonia[88]. A careful watch must be kept for choreiform disorder, which may be promoted or exacerbated by anticholinergics.

Of the wide range of miscellaneous compounds tried, recent interest has focused on α-tocopherol or vitamin E. This is in line with a wider interest in the pathogenic effects of free radicals, including their potential neurotoxicity. Vitamin E, an antioxidant, functions as a free radical scavenger and has been reported as effective in treating TD[89–91], although results of larger trials are awaited.

Persistent TD that is deforming, disabling or life-threatening, progressive or afflicting patients early in long-term management, are indications for clozapine, the benefits of which may result from either a specific antidyskinetic action or merely from the fact that it may hold the mental state stable long enough for detrimental effects of earlier treatments to resolve. Whether clozapine can itself be associated with the development of tardive disorder remains unclear, although even if it is, the risk would seem to be substantially less than with standard antipsychotics[92].

ASSESSMENT OF DRUG-RELATED EXTRAPYRAMIDAL DISORDERS

EXAMINATION

All drug-related extrapyramidal syndromes can be assessed in a single, comprehensive examination which, with experience, can be performed in a few minutes. Children and those with learning disability do present special problems since, like most clinical examination, thorough evaluation of extrapyramidal status does require a degree of patient compliance. Akathisia is based largely on the subjective account of the sufferer, as is mild acute dystonia, although the full-blown disorder should be largely a 'spot' diagnosis. The crucial consideration in diagnosing acute dystonia is the sign-time graph, illustrating a sudden onset of gross, distorting neurological disorder. Few other nonvascular conditions give rise to this presentation.

The first step in examination is unobtrusive observation. Posture, fluidity of movement, facial expression and any hyperkinetic movements should be observed without the patient's awareness. Following a symptomatic enquiry if this is possible, formal examination should begin with the patient sitting quietly in a chair with no armrests, and with their shoes removed and mouth empty. Tongue should be assessed in the resting position and on forced protrusion, both with and without reinforcement (e.g. rapid opening and closing of fists). Pooling of saliva can also be sought at this point. Rigidity around all limb joints should be assessed passively and with reinforcement, noting any increased tone, cogwheel *or* lead-pipe. Dexterity in a repetitive task such as rapid alternating supination/pronation should also be examined. With the patient standing, truncal rigidity is evaluated by shaking the shoulders, and postural tremor by asking the patient to stretch out the hands and close the eyes. 'Walking on the spot' may also be seen. Tremor can in addition be demonstrated by asking the patient to copy a spiral drawn first by the examiner. Postural stability, examined by tapping firmly the lateral aspect of each upper arm, then upper spine and sternum, may be more important in adults than children, as may handwriting. A thorough assessment of walking is essential. Posture, ease of movement, length and height of step and speed of walking, and most of all, pendular arm swing, can all be observed. During each of these stages, regular, complete scans of the body should be conducted to note hyperkinetic disorder only evident intermittently. Examination should conclude with unobtrusive observation as the patient leaves.

STANDARDIZED RECORDING

It is beyond the scope of this chapter to review in detail the many proposals for standardized recording of drug-related extrapyramidal disorders put forward over the past 20–30 years. Only the major examples will be outlined.

Scales tend to be of two main types.

1. Global impression: where any relevant disorder in a given body part, or in the whole body, is rated—e.g. any type of tardive movement in say, the upper limbs.
2. Multi-item: where specific, defined disorders are recorded separately—e.g. limb rigidity, puckering of lips.

Ratings have to be placed on a severity continuum, usually numerical, representing no disorder or increasing degrees of disorder. The number of anchor points most frequently varies from 4 to 7. Such scales, although ordinal, are not proportionate. A rating of '4' need only represent more severe disorder than one of '2', but not twice as much. Most scales allow a point on the continuum ('1') for movement that, although present, is not considered pathological in either type or degree. Care must be taken when analysing scales whose total scores comprise a significant number of '1' ratings. In this situation those with clearly abnormal signs may be considered together with those whose ratings were based on the judgement that they had no *abnormal* signs (e.g. one '4' versus four '1s').

Despite many of the scales for both idiopathic and drug-related disorders being long established and widely used, it is important to appreciate that many have poorly established or unknown psychometric properties.

The major emphasis in scale development has been on standardization of recording for parkinsonism and TD. Separate scales for each have traditionally been the rule, but in recent years more combined scales comprehensively covering extrapyramidal features have become available.

SINGLE SYNDROME SCALES

Parkinsonism

Most rating scales for parkinsonian symptomatology were devised by neurologists in order to record accurately and reproducibly response to treatment interventions in idiopathic disease. These are highly variable in content, some being exclusively devoted to objective signs, others to subjective disability in terms of the so-called activities of daily living (ADL), while others are hybrids of the two. These scales were often devised for specific projects and then, having acquired the name of the institution of their birth, were fixed in aspic thereafter. Few were subjected to psychometric evaluation and where this was subsequently undertaken, it frequently demonstrated inadequacies[93]. Most of these scales are therefore best avoided in psychiatric practice, though the 10-item Webster Scale may be an exception worth considering[94].

The most widely used scale devised for rating specifically drug-related parkinsonism is the Simpson–Angus Scale[95]. It was also the first—and it shows it! In a condition dominated by bradykinesia, this scale devotes six of its 10 items to rigidity! Only one item relates to bradykinesia, and this is a compound one. Its examination procedure seems guaranteed to encourage the patient to bolt for the door (parkinsonism permitting!). The Simpson–Angus Scale continues to flourish largely on the patronage of drug regulatory authorities, especially in the USA, and perhaps also because it has become an 'old friend'. It has, however, the wrong emphasis for its target population and diagnoses based on criteria derived from its items are likely to underestimate significantly the presence of disorder (cf. above). Furthermore, its statistical properties are not so impressive as to offset this major disadvantage. Old friends pass on, and by any logical appraisal this scale should have been helped on its way years ago!

The Scale for Targeting Abnormal Kinetic Effects (TAKE) was introduced to complement the AIMS (see below) in format and content[96]. It rates the three 'core' features of bradykinesia, rigidity and tremor, plus autonomic disturbance and akathisia. The objection to incorporating akathisia within parkinsonism has already been alluded to, and although all 'core' features are represented, by allocating each a single item, the scale in effect de-emphasizes the most prominent (i.e. bradykinesia). Nonetheless the AIMS–TAKE package is quick to perform, and is a useful recording method to consider for routine or large-scale work.

Tardive dyskinesia

Scales for the standardized recording of TD arose out of *epidemiological*, not treatment, necessities. The need was to establish prevalence, and later incidence, with reliability and if possible to define the boundaries of this apparently new disorder.

The AIMS is by far the most widely used instrument for dyskinetic disorder[97]. It is a seven-item global impression scale with an orofacial bias (four items) and includes items on overall severity, incapacitation and patient awareness, plus an opportunity to record the patient's dental status, a throw-back to a topical issue at the time of its development. The AIMS has an extensive track record, is easy to gain familiarity with and has good psychometric properties.

The most frequently used multi-item scale is the Simpson (or Rockland) Dyskinesia Rating Scale (SDRS)[98]. This comprises 34 specified movements, arranged regionally, and in addition has nine items for recording any other relevant but unspecified disorder. Its constituent items were derived from clinical observation and hence to theoretical purists it may seem contaminated, including for example a number of tremor items and akathisia. It is nonetheless an extremely comprehensive instrument, although in this may lie its major limitations. The SDRS requires considerable experience to use confidently, and much of its information may have to remain locked within it to make analysis manageable. A simple, abbreviated version, containing some global impression items, has found greater favour.

Akathisia

Scales dedicated to the standardized rating of akathisia are a relatively recent development. The Barnes Akathisia Scale[99] has no regional emphasis, but rather adopts a global approach, rigidly distinguishing between the subjective and objective components of the disorder. The Hillside Akathisia Scale (HAS)[100] is more 'molecular', with a regional breakdown and separate evaluations for the patient sitting, standing and lying.

A number of scales for parkinsonism (e.g. TAKE), and most combined scales, include akathisia items. They betray their authors' orientation to the relationship between akathisia and parkinsonism by either including the former within the latter or maintaining the separation.

A number of other scales for recording a range of movement disorders have been devised—e.g. for Huntington's disease, myoclonus and various manifestations of idiopathic dystonia, but are beyond the scope of this review (see also Marsden and Schachter, 1981[101]).

COMBINED SCALES

The Extrapyramidal Symptoms Rating Scale (ESRS) is the most comprehensive of all the standardized rating schedules for drug-related disorders[102]. Uniquely, this scale incorporates an initial patient questionnaire to record subjective symptoms. This is followed by eight items devoted to parkinsonism (which includes akathisia), seven for choreo-arthetoid dyskinesias and provision for the separate rating of dystonia, although this area seems somewhat confused. A further unique characteristic of this scale is the rating of hyperkinetic disorder, including tremor, on the dual axes of frequency and amplitude. This is a complex instrument to use routinely and although it appears to have good statistical properties, these have not been extensively examined.

The St. Hans Scale[103], on the other hand, has evolved through a number of refinements and has probably had greater attention paid to its psychometric properties than almost any other scale. It rates eight parkinsonian features and divides dyskinesias into eight regional manifestations, thereby providing statistical 'balance'. Movements rated only on activation can be separately accounted for and both dystonia and akathisia are likewise kept discrete. The St. Hans Scale is also a rather complex instrument whose use has been mainly confined to Scandinavia.

The particular problems of rating extrapyramidal disorder in those with learning disability, and the poor psychometric properties of most available scales, prompted Sprague and colleagues to develop the 15 item Dyskinesia Identification System—Condensed User Scale (DISCUS)[104]. This has several novel attributes, including a recording of subject co-operation and provision for noting when items could not be assessed. This was distilled from the 34 item 'DISCO' and both are symptoms—as opposed to syndrome—orientated. It certainly has been developed on sound psychometric principles and may have value in monitoring difficult populations. It may however lack the syndrome specificity required for a wider application.

THE CHOICE OF SCALE

It will be clear that the range of available recording instruments is considerable, with differences evident in the extent of clinical disorder they cover, the focus of symptomatology in any area and the quality of their construction as reflected in their statistical properties. The selection of a scale should not be by happenstance. It should depend on the use to which the recorded information is to be put. This applies as much in routine clinical as in research contexts.

In research projects, scale selection should be an essential part of the initial planning stage and should depend on the questions being posed. In general, large epidemiological studies demand small, manageable recording instruments, whereas investigations of new compounds, or studies of novel treatment agents for extrapyramidal disorders, may require more comprehensive data.

Clinicians in routine practice should not consider the rating scales they read of in the research literature as something detached from their own work. Comprehensive patient assessment should include an assessment of extrapyramidal side effects to recommended medication. It should always have been so, but this is now even more important in view of the potential and unresolved legal issues and the likely demands of health care purchasers that specific quality of care targets be met. A simple rating package such as the AIMS–TAKE or the AIMS/Webster/Barnes can provide more information and allow for much more accurate comparisons than a page of written notes.

REFERENCES

1. Campbell, M. and Spencer, E. K. (1988) Psychopharmacology in child and adolescent psychiatry: a review of the past five years. *J. Am. Acad. Child Adolesc. Psychiatry*, **27**, 269–279.
2. Mirza, K. A. H., Michael, A. and Dinan, T. G. (1994) Recent advances in paediatric psychopharmacology: a brief overview. *Hum. Psychopharmacol.*, **9**, 13–24.
3. Fann, W. E., Sullivan, J. L. and Richman, B. W. (1967) Dyskinesias associated with tricyclic antidepressants. *Br. J. Psychiatry*, **128**, 490–493.
4. Kaplan, S. R. and Murkovsky, C. (1978) Oro-buccal dyskinesia symptoms associated with low dose benzodiazepine treatment. *Am. J. Psychiatry*, **135**, 1558–1559.
5. Lavenstein, B. L. and Cantor, F. K. (1976) Acute dystonia: an unusual reaction to diphenhydramine. *JAMA*, **236**, 291.
6. Sovner, R. (1977) Antihistamine-induced extrapyramidal reactions. *N. Eng. J. Med.*, **296**, 633–634.
7. Rainier-Pope, C. R. (1979) Treatment with diazepam of children with drug-induced extrapyramidal symptoms. *S. Afr. Med. J.*, **55**, 328–330.
8. Chadwick, D., Reynolds, E. H. and Marsden, C. D. (1976) Anticonvulsant induced dyskinesias: a comparison with dyskinesia induced by neuroleptics. *J. Neurol. Neurosurg. Psychiatry*, **39**, 1210–1218.
9. Crosley, C. J. and Swender, P. T. (1979) Dystonia associated with carbamazepine administration: experience in brain-damaged children. *Paediatrics*, **63**, 612–615.
10. Mattson, R. H. and Calverley, J. R. (1968) Dextroamphetamine-sulphate-induced dyskinesias. *JAMA*, **204**, 400–402.
11. McAndrew, J. B. (1974) Dexedrine dyskinesia: an unusual iatrogenic tic. *Clin. Pediatr.*, **13**, 69–72.
12. Denckla, M. B., Bemporad, J. R. and Mackay, M. C. (1976) Tics following methylphnidate adminstration. *JAMA*, **235**, 1349–1351.
13. Singhi, S., Singhi, P. and Singh, M. (1977) Chloroquin-induced involuntary movements. *BMJ*, **2**, 520.
14. Carpentieri, U. and Lockhart, L. H. (1978) Ataxia and athetosis as side-effects of chemotherapy with vincristine in non-Hodgkin's lymphoma. *Cancer Treatment Reports*, **62**, 561–562.
15. Singh, H., Levinson, D. F., Simpson, G. M., Lo, E. S. and Friedman, E. (1990) Acute dystonia during fixed-dose neuroleptic treatment. *J. Clin. Psychopharmacol.*, **10**, 389–396.
16. Weiden, P. J., Mann, J. J., Haas, G., Mattson, M. and Frances, A. (1987) Clinical

non-recognition of neuroleptic induced movement disorders: a cautionary study. *Am. J. Psychiatry*, **144**, 1148–1153.
17. Swett, C. (1975) Drug-induced dystonias. *Am. J. Psychiatry*, **132**, 532–534.
18. Thornton, A. and McKenna, P. J. (1994) Acute dystonic reactions complicated by psychotic phenomena. *Br. J. Psychiatry*, **164**, 115–118.
19. Owens, D. G. C. (1990) Dystonia—a potential psychiatric pitfall. *Br. J. Psychiatry*, **156**, 620–634.
20. Ayd, F. (1961) A survey of drug-induced extrapyramidal reactions. *JAMA*, **175**, 1054–1060.
21. Addonizio, G. and Alexopoulos, G. S. (1988) Drug-induced dystonia in young and elderly patients. *Am. J. Psychiatry*, **145**, 869–871.
22. Chakos, M. H., Mayerhoff, D. I., Loebel, A. D., Alvir, J. M. J. and Lieberman, J. A. (1992) Incidence and correlates of acute extrapyramidal symptoms in first episode of schizophrenia. *Psychopharmacol. Bull.*, **28**, 81–86.
23. Marsden, C. D., Mindham, R. H. S. and Mackay, A. V. P. (1986) Extrapyramidal movement disorders produced by antipsychotic drugs. In *The Psychopharmacology and Drug Treatment in Schizophrenia* (P. B. Bradley and S. R. Hirsch, Eds). Oxford University Press, Oxford, pp. 340–402.
24. Shields, W. E. and Bray, P. F. (1976) A danger of haloperidol therapy in children. *J. Paediatr.*, **88**, 301–303.
25. Angle, C. R. and McIntire, M.S. (1973) Persistent dystonia in a brain-damaged child after ingestion of phenothiazine. *J. Paediatr.*, **73**, 124–126.
26. Dabbous, I. A. and Bergman, A. B. (1966) Neurologic damage associated with phenothiazine. *Am. J. Dis. Child.*, **3**, 291–296.
27. Marsden, C. D. and Jenner, P. (1980) The pathophysiology of extrapyramidal side-effects of neuroleptic drugs. *Psychol. Med.*, **10**, 55–72.
28. Cunningham, M. A., Pillai, V. and Rogers, J. B. (1968) Haloperidol in the treatment of children with severe behaviour disorders. *Br. J. Psychiatry*, **114**, 845–854.
29. Barker, P. and Fraser, I. A. (1968) A controlled trial of haloperidol in children. *Br. J. Psychiatry*, **114**, 855–857.
30. Polizos, P. and Engelhardt, D. M. (1978) Dyskinetic phenomena in children treated with psychotropic medication. *Psychopharmacol. Bull.*, **14**, 65–70.
31. Chiles, J. A. (1978) Extrapyramidal reactions in adolescents treated with high-potency antipsychotics. *Am. J. Psychiatry*, **135**, 239–240.
32. Campbell, M., Small, A. M., Green, W. H., Jennings, S. J., Perry, R., Bennet, W. G. and Anderson, L. (1984) Behavioural efficacy of haloperidol and lithium carbonate: a comparison in hospitalised aggressive children with conduct disorders. *Arch. Gen. Psychiatry*, **41**, 650–656.
33. Spencer, E. K., Kafantaris, V., Padron-Gayol, M. V., Rosenberg, C. R. and Campbell, M. (1992) Haloperidol and schizophrenic children: early findings from a study in progress. *Psychopharmacol. Bull.*, **28**, 183–186.
34. Van Putten, T. and May, P. R. A. (1978) 'Akinetic depression' in schizophrenia. *Arch. Gen. Psychiatry*, **35**, 1101–1107.
35. McGeer, P. L. and McGeer, E. G. (1977) Aging and extrapyramidal function. *Arch. Neurol.*, **34**, 33–35.
36. Richardson, M. A., Haugland, G. and Craig, T. J. (1991) Neuroleptic use, parkinsonian symptoms, tardive dyskinesia, and associated factors in child and adolescent psychiatric patients. *Am. J. Psychiatry*, **148**, 1322–1328.
37. Engelhardt, D. M. and Polizos, P. (1978) Adverse effects of pharmacotherapy in childhood psychosis. In *Psychopharmacology: a Generation of Progress.* (M. A. Lipton, A. Dimascio and K. F. Killam, Eds). Raven Press, New York, pp. 1463–1469.

38. Mindham, R. H. S. (1976) Assessment of drug-induced extrapyramidal reactions and of drugs given for their control. *Br. J. Clin. Pharmacol.*, **3**, 395–400.
39. Lieberman, J. A., Kane, J. M. and Alvir, J. (1987) Provocative tests with psychostimulant drugs in schizophrenia. *Psychopharmacology*, **91**, 415–433.
40. Mindham, R. H. S., Gaind, R., Anstee, B. H. and Rimmer, L. (1972) Comparison of amantadine, orphenadrine and placebo in the control of phenothiazine induced parkinsonism. *Psychol. Med.*, **2**, 406–413.
41. Gewirtz, G. R., Sharif, Z., Cadet, J. L., Sarti, P. and Gorman, J. M. (1993) Selegiline for neuroleptic-induced parkinsonism. *Pharmacopsychiatry*, **26**, 128–129.
42. Kennedy, P. S., Hershon, H. I. and McGuire, R. J. (1971) Extrapyramidal disorders after prolonged phenothiazine therapy. *Br. J. Psychiatry*, **118**, 509–518.
43. Levinson, D. F., Simpson, G. M., Singh, H., Yadalam, K., Jain, A., Stephanos, J. and Silver, P. (1990) Fluphenazine dose, clinical response and extrapyramidal symptoms during acute treatment. *Arch. Gen. Psychiatry*, **47**, 761–768.
44. Braude, W. N., Barnes, T. R. E. and Gore, S. M. (1983) Clinical characteristics of akathisia—the systematic investigation of acute psychiatric in-patient admissions. *Br. J. Psychiatry*, **143**, 139–150.
45. Stone, R. K., Alvarez, W. F. and May, J. E. (1988) Dyskinesia, antipsychotic-drug exposure and risk factors in a developmentally-disabled population. *Pharmacol. Biochem. Behav.*, **29**, 45–51.
46. Bruun, R. D. (1988) Subtle and under-recognised side effects of neuroleptic treatment in children with Tourette's disorder. *Am. J. Psychiatry*, **145**, 621–624.
47. Adler, L., Angrist, B. Y., Peselow, E., Corwin, J., Maslansky, R. and Rotrosen J. (1986) A controlled assessment of propranolol in the treatment of neuroleptic induced akathisia. *Br. J. Psychiatry*, **149**, 42–45.
48. Adler, L. A., Angrist, B., Weinreb, H. and Rotrosen, J. (1991) Studies on the time course and efficiacy of β-blockers in neuroleptic-induced akathisia and the akathisia of idopathic Parkinson's Disease. *Psychopharmacol. Bull.*, **27**, 107–111.
49. Marsden, C. D., Tarsy, D. and Baldessavini, R. J. (1975) Spontaneous and drug-induced movement disorders in psychotic patients. In *Psychatric Aspects of Neurological disease* (D. F. Benson and D. Blumer, Eds). Grune and Stratton, New York, pp. 219–226.
50. Meiselas, K. D., Spencer, E. K., Oberfield, R., Peselow, E. D., Angrist, B. and Campbell, M. (1989) Differentiation of stereotypies from neuroleptic-related dyskinesias in autistic children *J. Clin. Psychopharmacol.*, **9**, 207–209.
51. Flaherty, J. A. and Lohmeyer, H. W. (1978) Largyngeal pharyngeal dystonia as a possible cause of asphyxia with haloperidol treatment. *Am. J. Psychiatry*, **135**, 1414–1415.
52. Szymanski, S., Lieberman, J. A., Safferman, A. and Galkowski, B. (1993) Rib fractures as an unusual complication of severe tardive dyskinesia. *J. Clin. Psychiatry*, **54**, 160.
53. Jeste, D. V. and Wyatt, R. J. (1981) Changing epidemiology of tardive dyskinesia—an overview. *Am. J. Psychiatry*, **138**, 297–309.
54. Kane, J. M. and Smith, J. M. (1982) Tardive dyskinesia: prevalence and risk factors 1959–1979. *Arch. Gen. Psychiatry*, **39**, 473–481.
55. Kane, J. M., Woerner, M., Weinhold, P., Wegner, J. and Kinon, B. (1982) A prospective study of tardive dyskinesia development: preliminary results. *J. Clin. Psychopharmacol.*, **2**, 345–349.
56. Morgenstern, H. and Glazer, W. M. (1993) Identifying risk factors for tardive dyskinesia among long-term outpatients maintained with neuroleptic medications. *Arch. Gen. Psychiatry*, **50**, 723–733.

57. Glazer, W. M., Morgenstern, H. and Doucette, J. J. (1993) Predicting the long-term risk of tardive dyskinesia in outpatients maintained on neuroleptic medications. *J. Clin. Psychiatry*, **54**, 133–139.
58. Owens, D. G. C., Johnstone, E. C. and Frith, C. D. (1982) Spontaneous involuntary disorders of movement: their prevalence, severity and distribution in chronic schizophrenics with and without treatment with neuroleptics. *Arch. Gen. Psychiatry*, **39**, 452–461.
59. Jeste, D. V., Potkin, S. G., Sinha, S., Feder, S. and Wyatt, R. J. (1979) Tardive dyskinesia: reversible and persistent. *Arch. Gen. Psychiatry*, **36**, 585–590.
60. Branchey, M. and Branchey, L. (1984) Patterns of psychotropic drug use and tardive dyskinesia. *J. Clin. Psychopharmacol.*, **4**, 41–45.
61. Jeste, D. V. and Caligiuri, M. P. (1993) Tardive dyskinesia. *Schizophrenia Bull.*, **19**, 303–315.
62. Ganzini, L., Heintz, R. T., Hoffman, W. F. and Casey, D. E. (1991) The prevalence of tardive dyskinesia in neuroleptic-treated diabetics. *Arch. Gen. Psychiatry*, **48**, 259–263.
63. Gardos, G., Cole, J. O., Haskell, D., Marby, D., Paine, S. S. and Moore, P. (1988) The natural history of tardive dyskinesia. *J. Clin. Psychopharmacol. Suppl.*, **8**, 31S–37S.
64. Christensen, A. V., Fjalland, B. and Moller-Nielsen, I. (1976) On the supersensitivity of dopamine receptors induced by neuroleptics. *Psychopharmacology*, **48**, 1–6.
65. Gerlach, J. (1977) Relationship between tardive dyskinesia, L-dopa induced hyperkinesia and Parkinsonism. *Psychopharmacology*, **51**, 259–263.
66. Casey, D. E. and Denney, D. (1977) Pharmacological characterisation of tardive dyskinesia. *Psychopharmacology*, **54**, 1–8.
67. Lieberman, J., Pollack, S., Lesser, M. and Kane, J. (1988) Pharmacological characterization of tardive dyskinesia. *J. Clin. Psychopharmacol.*, **8**, 254–260.
68. McAndrew, J. B., Case, Q. and Treffert, D. A. (1972) Effects of prolonged phenothiazine intake on psychotic and other hospitalized children. *J. Autism Childhood Schizophrenia*, **2**, 75–91.
69. Polizos, P., Engelhardt, D. M., Hoffman, S. P. and Waizer, J. (1973) Neurological consequences of psychotropic drug withdrawal in schizophrenic children. *J. Autism Childhood Schizophrenia*, **3**, 247–253.
70. Engelhardt, D. M., Polizos, P. and Waizer, J. (1975) CNS consequences of psychotropic drug withdrawal in autistic children: a follow-up report. *Psychopharmacol. Bull.*, **11**, 6–7.
71. Paulson, G. W., Rizvi, C. A. and Crane, G. E. (1975) Tardive dyskinesia as a possible sequel of long-term therapy with phenothiazines. *Clinical Paediatr. (Philadelphia)*, **14**, 953–955.
72. Winsberg, B. G., Hurwic, M. J., Sverd, J. and Klutch, A. (1978) Neurochemistry of withdrawal emergent symptoms in children. *Psychopharmacology*, **56**, 157–161.
73. Campbell, M., Anderson, L. T., Cohen, I. R., Perry, R., Small, A. M., Green, W. H., Anderson, L. and McCandless, W. (1982) Haloperidol in autistic children: effects on learning, behaviour, and abnormal involuntary movements. *Psychopharmacol. Bull.*, **18**, 110–112.
74. Campbell, M., Perry, R., Bennett, W. G., Small, A. M., Green, W. H., Grega, D., Schwartz, W. and Anderson, L. (1983) Long-term therapeutic efficacy and drug-related abnormal movements: a prospective study of haloperidol in autistic children. *Psychopharmacol. Bull.*, **19**, 80–83.
75. Gualtieri, C. T., Quade, D., Hicks, R. E., Mayo, J. P. and Schroeder, S. R. (1984) Tardive dyskinesia and other clinical consequences of neuroleptic treatment in children and adolescents. *Am. J. Psychiatry*, **141**, 20–23.

76. Perry, R., Campbell, M., Green, W. H., Small, A. M., Die Trill, M., Meiselas, K., Golden, R. R. and Deutsch, S. I. (1985) Neuroleptic-related dyskinesias in autistic children: a prospective study. *Psychopharmacol. Bull.*, **21**, 140–143.
77. Campbell, M., Adams, P., Perry, R., Spencer, E. K. and Overall, J. E. (1988) Tardive and withdrawal dyskinesia in autistic children: a prospective study. *Psychopharmacol. Bull.*, **24**, 251–255.
78. Malone, R. P., Ernst, M., Godfrey, K. A., Locascio, J. J. and Campbell, M. (1991) Repeated episodes of neuroleptic-related dyskinesias in autistic children. *Psychopharmacol. Bull.*, **27**, 113–117.
79. Locascio, J. J., Malone, R. P., Small, A. M., Kafantaris, V., Ernst, M., Lynch, N. S., Overall, J. E. and Campbell, M. (1991) Factors related to haloperidol response and dyskinesias in autistic children. *Psychopharmacol. Bull.*, **27**, 119–125.
80. Schooler, N. R. and Kane, J. M. (1982) Research diagnosis for tardive dyskinsia. *Arch. Gen. Psychiatry*, **39**, 486–487.
81. Richardson, M. A., Haugland, M. A., Pass, R. and Craig, T.J. (1986) The prevalence of tardive dyskinesia in a mentally retarded population. *Psychopharmacol. Bull.*, **22**, 243–249.
82. Gualtieri, C. T., Barnhill, J., McGimsey, J. and Schell, D. (1980) Tardive dyskinesia and other movement disorders in children treated with psychotropic drugs. *J. Am. Acad. Child Psychiatry*, **19**, 491–510.
83. Gualtieri, C. T. and Guimond, M. (1981) Tardive dyskinesia and the behavioural consequences of chronic neuroleptic treatment. *Dev. Med. Child Neurol.*, **23**, 255–259.
84. Luchins, D. J., Freed, W. J. and Wyatt, R. J. (1980) The role of cholinergic supersensitivity in the medical symptoms associated with withdrawal of antipsychotic drugs. *Am. J. Psychiatry*, **137**, 1395–1398.
85. Owens, D. G. C. (1994) Extrapyramidal side-effects and tolerability of risperidone: a review. *J. Clin. Psychiatry*, **55**, (5 Suppl), 29–35.
86. Jeste, D. V. and Wyatt, R. J. (1979) In search of treatment for tardive dyskinesia: a review of the literature. *Schizophrenia Bull.*, **5**, 251–293.
87. Jeste, D. V., Lohr, J. B., Clark, K. and Wyatt, R. J. (1988) Pharmacological treatments of tardive dyskinesia in the 1980s. *J. Clin. Psychopharmacol.*, **8**, 38S–48S.
88. Burke, R. E., Fahn, S. and Marsden, C. D. (1986) Torsion dystonia: a double-blind prospective trial of high dosage trihexyphenidyl. *Neurology*, **36**, 160–164.
89. Lohr, J. B., Cadet, J. L., Lohr, M. A., Jeste, D. V. and Wyatt, R. J. (1987) Alpha-tocopherol in tardive dyskinesia. *Lancet*, **1**, 913–914.
90. Egan, M. F., Hyde, T. M., Albers, G. W., Elkashef, A., Alexander, R. C., Reeve, A., Blum, A., Saenz, R. E. and Wyatt, R. J. (1992) Treatment of tardive dyskinesia with Vitamin E. *Am. J. Psychiatry*, **149**, 773–777.
91. Adler, L. A., Peselow, E., Rotrosen, J., Duncan, E., Lee, M., Rosenthal, M. and Angrist, B. (1993) Vitamin E treatment of tardive dyskinesia. *Am. J. Psychiatry*, **150**, 1405–1407.
92. Kane, J. M., Woerner, M. G., Pollack, S., Safferman, A. Z. and Lieberman, J. A. (1993) Does clozapine cause tardive dyskinesia? *J. Clin. Psychiatry*, **54**, 327–330.
93. Diamond, S. G. and Markham, C. H. (1983) Evaluating the evaluations: or how to weigh the scales of Parkinsonian disability. *Neurology (Cleveland)*, **33**, 1098–1099.
94. Webster, D. D. (1968) Critical analysis of the disability in Parkinson's disease. *Mod. Treatment*, **5**, 257–282.
95. Simpson, G. M. and Angus, J. W. S. (1970) A rating scale for extrapyramidal side-effects. *Acta Psychiatr. Scand.*, **212** (Suppl), 11–19.

96. Wojcik, J. D., Gelenberg, A. J., LaBrie, R. A. and Mieske, M. (1980) Prevalence of tardive dyskinesia in an outpatient population. *Compr. Psychiatry*, **21**, 370–379.
97. Guy, W. (1976) *ECDEU Assessment Manual for Psychopharmacology*. Department of Health Education and Welfare, Washington D.C.
98. Simpson, G. M., Lee, J. H., Zoubok, B. and Gardos, G. (1979) A rating scale for tardive dyskinesia. *Psychopharmacology*, **64**, 171–179.
99. Barnes, T. R. E. (1989) A rating scale for drug-induced akathisia. *Br. J. Psychiatry*, **154**, 672–676.
100. Fleischhacker, W. W., Bergmann, K. J., Perovich, R., Pestreich, L. K., Borenstein, M., Lieberman, J. A. and Kane, J.M. (1989) The Hillside Akathisia Scale: a new rating instrument for neuroleptic-induced akathisia. *Psychopharmacol. Bull.*, **25**, 222–226.
101. Marsden, C. D. and Schachter, M. (1981) Assessment of extrapyramidal disorders. In *Methods in Clinical Pharmacology—Central Nervous System* (M. H. Lader and A. Richens, Eds). Macmillan, London, pp. 89–111.
102. Chouinard, G., Ross-Chouinard, A., Annable, L. and Jones, B. D. (1980) The extrapyramidal symptom rating scale. *Can. J. Neurol. Sci.*, **7**, 233.
103. Gerlach, J., Korsgaard, S., Clemmesen, P., Lund Lauersen, A-M., Magelund, G., Noring, U., Povlsen, U. J., Bech, P. and Casey, D. E. (1993) The St. Hans rating scale for extrapyramidal syndromes: reliability and validity. *Acta Psychiatr. Scand.*, **87**, 244–252.
104. Sprague, R. L. Kalachnik, J. E. and Shaw, K. M. (1989) Psychometric properties of the dyskinesia identification system: condensed user scale DISCUS. *Ment. Retard.*, **27**, 141–148.

12 Genetics of Movement Disorders: Dystonia, Dopa-responsive Dystonia and Huntington's Disease

SUSAN B. BRESSMAN
Columbia Presbyterian Medical Center, New York, USA
and
NEIL J. RISCH
Yale University School of Medicine, New Haven, CT, USA

IDIOPATHIC TORSION DYSTONIA (ITD)

Dystonia is a syndrome of sustained muscle contractions that produce twisting and repetitive movements and abnormal postures[1–2]. The extent and severity of muscle involvement are remarkably variable, ranging from intermittent contractions limited to single body region (focal dystonia) to generalized dystonia involving the limbs and axial muscles[1].

Dystonia may be due to many different causes. Two broad aetiological categories have been proposed: idiopathic (or primary) torsion dystonia (ITD) and symptomatic (or secondary) dystonia. The symptomatic dystonias encompass a host of disorders that are either inherited (e.g. Wilson's disease, Huntington's disease and the gangliosidoses), or due to exogenous factors (e.g. perinatal injury, neuroleptic medications and infection). In symptomatic dystonia, examination abnormalities other than dystonia (e.g. dementia, weakness and visual abnormalities) are frequently present: often there are pathological changes involving the basal ganglia, and laboratory findings usually help in diagnosis. In contrast, in ITD the only abnormality found on examination is dystonia; there are no consistent pathological changes, and diagnostic studies are unrevealing.

The prevalence of ITD is difficult to estimate because of the variation in expression and tendency for mild cases to go undiagnosed. In one study from Rochester, Minnesota, prevalence was calculated to be 29.5 per 100 000 for focal dystonia and 3.4 per 100 000 for generalized dystonia[3]. There are also ethnic differences in frequency; childhood and adolescent-onset ITD appear to be more common in Jews of eastern European ancestry.

One of the first reports of ITD, published over 85 years ago[4], described affected family members. Although the inherited nature of the condition

Movement and Allied Disorders. Edited by M. M. Robertson and V. Eapen

was suspected, it is only in recent years, particularly with advances in molecular genetic techniques, that inheritance patterns and specific gene loci have been identified. These genetic studies of ITD are reviewed in this chapter.

CLINICAL HETEROGENEITY

As mentioned above, the clinical range of ITD is remarkably variable. Studies over the years have described the clustering of certain clinical features with more or less distinct subtypes emerging. However, the categorization of ITD into clinical subtypes is complicated by the inclusion of rare 'variant' dystonic disorders that do not strictly meet the definition of ITD; namely, those disorders which typically manifest clinical features other than dystonia, such as parkinsonism, hyperreflexia and myoclonus (see Table 12.1). The 'variant ITD' disorders include dopa-responsive dystonia (also known as dystonia with diurnal variation and Segawa's disease)[5–6], myoclonic dystonia[7], rapid-onset dystonia-parkinsonism[8], X-linked dystonia-parkinsonism found in the Filipino population[9–11], dystonia

Table 12.1. Clinical-genetic subtypes of ITD

1. Classic (dystonia is the only neurological abnormality)

A. Childhood and adolescent onset

Ashkenazi

Autosomal dominant (penetrance = 0.3), most due to single mutation event in DYT1

Non-Jewish:

Autosomal dominant (penetrance = 0.4), many due to (different) events in DYT1

B. Adult onset

?Autosomal dominant, extent of DYT1 involvement unknown; not DYT1 in some non-Jewish families and not due to common early onset mutation in Ashkenazim

2. Variant (dystonia plus other neurological abnormalities or dystonia paroxysmal)

A. Childhood and adolescent onset

Dopa-responsive (DRD), autosomal dominant (sex influenced reduced penetrance), 14-q

Myoclonic, autosomal dominant

Paroxysmal kinesigenic, autosomal dominant

Paroxysmal non-kinesigenic, autosomal dominant

Rapid-onset dystonia–parkinsonism, autosomal dominant, not DYT1

B. Adult onset

X-linked Filipino (XPD), Xq13

Whispering dysphonia and Wilson's disease, autosomal dominant, not DYT1 with whispering dysphonia, and Wilson's disease[12]. With the exception of Filipino dystonia-parkinsonism, which is X-linked recessive, the 'variant ITD' disorders are inherited in an autosomal dominant fashion.

Based on their unique clinical features, the 'variant ITD' disorders are each suspected to be due to a different gene. To date, linkage studies confirm this; the gene for dopa-responsive dystonia (DRD) maps to chromosomes 14q, Filipino dystonia-parkinsonism maps to Xq21 and genes for the other variant subtypes, although not mapped, have been excluded from the known ITD locus, DYT1 (see below). Of the 'variant' dystonias, DRD is the most common cause of dystonia in children, constituting about 5–10% of childhood-onset ITD. It is a very important disorder to recognize because it responds dramatically to L-dopa therapy and is discussed below.

Clinical studies of non-variant (or classic) ITD have long noted a relationship between the age at onset of symptoms, the body region first affected and the progression of disease. There is a bimodal distribution in the age at onset with modes at ages 9 (early-onset) years and a nadir at age 27[13].

Early onset ITD usually first involves a limb. An arm or leg are about equally likely to be affected first, with leg-onset cases having an earlier age at onset (8–9 years) compared to those with initial involvement of arm muscles (12–14 years)[14]. Most patients progress to involve more than one limb and over one-half generalize to involve the legs and arms. In contrast, late-onset ITD usually starts in the neck or cranial muscles and signs remain localized. The relationship between early and late onset ITD, and specifically whether these two forms are genetically related, has been debated for over 25 years. Family studies and recent linkage studies address this question and are discussed next.

INHERITANCE PATTERN OF ITD

Early reports of ITD described families with affected siblings, parents, and second and third-degree relatives[4, 15–21]. Most families had early-onset dystonia and many were of Eastern European Jewish ancestry. Nevertheless, the genetic basis of ITD was largely neglected until the detailed report of Zeman and Dyken in 1967[22]. They reviewed the pathology and clinical and genetic aspects of 253 cases of ITD (they used the term 'dystonia musculorum deformans', the name originally coined by Oppenheim in 1911 to describe childhood-onset dystonia). The cases included 217 previously reported and 36 newly described patients. One hundred and forty-eight patients from 31 families (19 Jewish and 12 non-Jewish) were categorized as familial and the remaining 105 (50 Jewish and 55 non-Jewish) were considered sporadic. The median age at onset of the affected individuals was 10 years and over 90% were affected by age 21 years. The authors concluded that ITD is inherited in both Jewish and non-Jewish populations as an autosomal dominant trait with a reduced penetrance of 52%. They also estimated a gene frequency among American Jews of 1 in 38 000, considerably higher than 1 in 200 000 gene frequency they calculated for the general population of the state of Indiana. They did not construe different inheritance patterns or propose the presence of two or more genes based on the difference in disease frequency between Jews and non-Jews.

Three years later, Eldridge presented a detailed report of 156 cases representing 96 families (41 families were Ashkenazi Jewish) and came to a different conclusion[23]. He proposed that ITD is inherited in an autosomal recessive fashion in Jews and in an autosomal dominant fashion in most non-Jewish families. He based his argument of recessive inheritance on three findings.

1. The analysis of sibling risk was consistent with recessive inheritance.
2. The frequency of ITD in Jews is increased over non-Jews, and other disorders that are similarly increased in Jews, such as Tay–Sachs, are autosomal recessive.
3. Clinical differences between Jews and non-Jews were noted. Jews were more likely to have progressive childhood-onset disease with first symptoms in a limb compared to non-Jews who had somewhat later onset, less clinical progression and greater likelihood of initial axial involvement.

Only the first of these points supports directly autosomal recessive inheritance. This point was first challenged by Korczyn and colleagues[24]. They argued that Eldridge miscalculated the recurrence risk to siblings; also the consanguinity rate is too low and there are too many instances of parent and child being affected for an autosomal recessive pattern of inheritance, unless a very high gene frequency is assumed. Eldridge's third point, that there are clinical differences between non-Jewish and Jewish ITD cases, was also challenged[25]. Burke and colleagues reanalysed the clinical features in Eldridge's families as well as their own series of families and found no significant differences in the ages and sites of onset or progression of signs[25].

Subsequently, in the 1980s, Jewish ITD families in Israel and the USA were systematically studied and analyses indicated autosomal dominant inheritance with reduced penetrance; recessive inheritance was rejected. In the Israeli study, Zilber and colleagues[26] analysed the families of 47 ITD patients ascertained from a nationwide survey. Most cases were drawn from a registry of hospital discharge diagnoses, and those with focal dystonia were excluded. The frequency of ITD was found to be highest among Jews of Eastern European ancestry (1 : 15 000) compared to European Jews generally (1 : 23 000) and African–Asian Jews (1 : 117 000). Analyses of family data were not consistent with an autosomal recessive pattern; consanguinity was infrequent, the rates of affected parents, offspring, aunts, uncles and cousins were too high and the observed rate of affected siblings from presumed heterozygous parents was lower than expected. The authors concluded that ITD is inherited in an autosomal dominant fashion with penetrance of 51%. In this study the paternal age of isolated cases was increased over familial cases suggesting that some were the result of new mutations.

In the American study of Ashkenazi ITD, Bressman *et al.* systematically studied the families of 43 probands with early-onset (<28 years) ITD[13]; this included 'blinded' review of videotaped examinations of 90% of living first-degree relatives (FDRs). Late-onset cases were excluded as probands based on the hypothesis that clinical differences between early and late-onset ITD represent differences in aetiologies. However, there are no restrictions in the ages and sites of onset of ITD in relatives diagnosed as affected. The age-adjusted risk to all FDRs was 15.5%; the risk to second-degree relatives was 6.5% and there were no significant sex differences. The risks for parents, offspring and siblings were similar, as expected for an autosomal dominant disorder. The penetrance was calculated at 30%. These results were confirmed in rigorous segregation analysis of the same data[27]. Also, there was no evidence for sporadic cases or new mutations in these families and the higher frequency of the disorder in Ashkenazim was postulated to be due to a founder mutation and genetic drift.

An interesting finding in this study was the range of clinical features observed in affected relatives. Although relatives had milder disease (only one-half were aware they had dystonia), most were affected by the age of 30 years. There were no relatives with onset over 44 years, although over 60% of the examined relatives were at least aged 45 years. Also, none had onset in cranial muscles. These findings are consistent with the hypothesis that early and late-onset ITD have different causes.

These studies demonstrate that early-onset ITD is an autosomal dominant, not recessive, trait in Jews. Furthermore, Pauls and Korczyn[28] performed complex segregation analysis on Eldridge's previously reported Ashkenazi families. The analysis demonstrated that the trait is inherited in an autosomal dominant fashion with reduced penetrance.

In almost all studies of non-Jewish ITD families the disorder is found to be inherited as an autosomal dominant trait[19–22] with penetrance ranging from near complete to about 30%. A recent systematic analysis[29] of 96 non-Jewish probands with generalized, multi-focal and segmental involvement concluded that approximately 85% of cases are inherited as an autosomal dominant trait with reduced penetrance of 40%; the remaining 15% are likely to be non-genetic phenocopies. Increased paternal age of singleton cases was found, and about 14% of genetic cases were thought to be new mutations. As in the study of Ashkenazi families, there was variable and often milder expression in affected relatives, although, unlike that population, a larger proportion (10–15%) of non-Jewish affected family members had late onset (>44 years).

There are few systematic studies of adult-onset or focal dystonia. In an Italian study of 29 patients with cranial-cervical dystonia, four of 58 (0.069) parents and five of 120 (0.042) siblings were affected, whereas no spouse controls were affected[30]. The authors concluded that the findings are consistent with either autosomal dominant transmission with reduced penetrance, or polygenic inheritance. A British study[31] assessed 40 non-Jewish index cases with either torticollis (N=14), cranial dystonia (N=16) or writer's cramp (N=10); the average age of onset was 55 years. There were nine affected out of 153 examined FDRs; none had generalized signs and there was a tendency for the relative to have the same type of dystonia as the proband. The authors concluded that there is autosomal dominant inheritance with reduced penetrance. They also argued that, although there were no affected relatives with childhood-onset among these focal ITD families, early- and late-onset ITD may still be due to the same gene mutation; childhood-onset ITD is about one-tenth as common as the adult focal dystonia, so that one would not expect to find many cases in these focal ITD families; also, because families with childhood-onset generalized ITD would be expected to be ascertained through the most severely affected member, they would not have been included in a family study of focal ITD probands. Despite these arguments, there is limited overlap of clinical features between the families of childhood and adult onset ITD probands. This suggests that perhaps different mutations of the same or different genes may be responsible for these clinical subtypes. Also, recent linkage and linkage disequilibrium findings, described next, lend support to separating these clinical subtypes genetically.

GENETIC LINKAGE STUDIES

Ozelius *et al.*[32] mapped the first ITD locus (DYT1) in 1989. They studied a large North American non-Jewish family of French-Canadian ancestry, first reported by Johnson *et al.*[20], and localized the gene to the 9q32-34 region. Subsequently, Kramer and colleagues found linkage with markers in the same region in 12 Ashkenazi families[33]. Clinical features were similar in the non-Jewish and 12 Jewish families; onset was early in both (average, 14.4 ± 3 and 13.2 ± 1 years respectively) and symptoms usually began in a limb (86% and 90%, respectively) in both. In the study of Kramer *et al.*[33] tightest linkage was found with the gene encoding arginosuccinate synthetase (ASS); subsequent multipoint analysis with markers in the 9q region revealed a similar location for the disease gene in both the Jewish and non-Jewish groups[34], and the same gene is thought to cause dystonia in both. Because the locus for dopamine beta hydroxylase (DBH) maps to the 9q32-34 region, and because this enzyme was implicated in several studies of ITD, this candidate locus was evaluated and excluded soon after DYT1 was localized[35].

Since the initial linkage findings, studies of European[36], non-Jewish North American[37] and Ashkenazi[38,39] families have confirmed that DYT1 is a common cause of early-onset ITD; however, it is not the only gene for ITD[36,40,41].

In a European study of 27 small families (three Jewish and 24 non-Jewish), there was evidence for linkage to the chromosomal region containing DYT1, with a combined lod score of 3.4 at ASS calculated for 24 families. However, tight linkage to ASS was excluded in three non-Jewish families[36]. One of the excluded families was thought to have Dopa-responsive Dystonia (DRD), but otherwise clinical differences between 'DYT1' and 'non-DYT1' families were not noted.

Evidence implicating DYT1 was also provided in a study of six non-Jewish North American families of European descent[37]. The clinical features of affected members in these six families were similar to each other and similar to the non-Jewish and Jewish families first linked to 9q34; age at onset was typically between 6 and 18 years, but could occur in the 30s to mid-40s. Symptoms usually started in an arm or leg, and often dystonia spread to involve other limbs and axial muscles. Occasionally the neck or larynx was affected first, but facial muscles were not commonly involved, and speech was usually normal except in those treated with thalamotomy. Analyses of haplotypes in these non-Jewish families did not suggest linkage disequilibrium and it is presumed that most early-onset ITD in the non-Jewish population results from different mutation events in the DYT1 gene.

In two large North American non-Jewish families the DYT1 locus was excluded[40,41]. These families differed clinically from DYT1 families. In one of these non-DYT1 families, symptom-onset was later (average, 28.4 ± 14.8 years), and most affected family members had first symptoms in the neck or cranial muscles rather than a limb[40]. Clinical features in the second 'non-DYT1 family' were more similar to the typical DYT1 phenotype in that the onset was early, and in many, the dystonia began in the limb[41]. The family differed in that, unlike typical ITD due to DYT1, most affected individuals had significant disability due to laryngeal and other cranial muscle involvement.

Although most affected DYT1 gene carriers have early limb-onset dystonia, there is still a wide range of disease severity, and most gene carriers never express the gene. The cause of low penetrance and variable expression is unknown; possible mechanisms include genomic imprinting, anticipation, modifying genes and environmental factors. Only a few studies have assessed families for these factors. LaBuda *et al.* analysed the pedigrees of four previously published series of early-onset or generalized and segmental families for evidence of genomic imprinting or anticipation[42]. They found that the gender of the transmitting parent did not influence the site of onset, age of onset, or distribution of dystonia, except that there was maternal transmission in almost all later-onset cases. The data were also consistent with anticipation; however, sampling bias could not be ruled out. A similar trend towards later onset of maternally transmitted ITD was noted by deLeon *et al.* in affected Ashkenazi DYT1 gene carriers, but this did not reach statistical significance[43]. Intrafamilial correlations of the clinical features such as age at onset and severity have also been assessed for evidence of genetic heterogeneity or the presence of modifying genes. A very low correlation for age at onset between 23 FDR pairs was found in one British study of generalized and segmental probands; the authors concluded that there was no evidence of genetic heterogeneity or non-allelic modifying genes; they suggested that ITD was due to a single gene and that the expression was influenced by environmental factors or an allelic modifying gene[44]. The same group found that 16.4% of generalized and segmental ITD cases gave a history of trauma exacerbating or precipitating the dystonia[45] with the dystonic movements either worsening or beginning in the same region of the body that was injured. They concluded that peripheral trauma may be a precipitant of dystonia in gene carriers.

LINKAGE DISEQUILIBRIUM OF DYT1 WITH 9Q MARKERS IN ASHKENAZI JEWS

Soon after finding linkage of ITD with 9q markers in Ashkenazi families, it became apparent that these families share a common haplotype 9q alleles. Very strong allelic association or linkage disequilibrium between the DYT1 gene and a haplotype at the 9q marker loci ABL and ASS was found[38]. For markers that are tightly linked to the disease gene, such an association of linked alleles and the disease gene is consistent with the idea that the disease is largely due to a single mutation and equilibrium has not yet been achieved. The presence of very strong linkage disequilibrium at the relatively large genetic distance of at least a few centiMorgans (CM) also suggest that the mutation is recent; Risch *et al.* have calculated that it first appeared around 350 years ago and probably originated in Lithuania or Byelorussia[46].

A recent study of 157 Ashkenazi individuals affected with both early- and late-onset ITD used additional closely linked microsatellite markers and confirmed that the vast majority of both familial and isolated early-onset ITD cases carry the associated haplotype of 9q markers[39]. This study demonstrated that the clinical features of

1. first symptom in a limb,
2. involvement of a leg in the course of disease, and
3. early-onset,

discriminate between those who have the associated haplotype from those who do not, with about 90% accuracy. Conversely, Ashkenazi ITD cases with adult cervical- and cranial-onset ITD very rarely carry the associated haplotype. This implies that a single founder mutation accounts for most early limb-onset ITD among Ashkenazim but this mutation event is not responsible for adult cervical- and cranial-onset ITD. The clinical-genetic difference suggests either a different DYT1 mutation or another dystonia gene.

SUMMARY AND COUNSELLING RECOMMENDATIONS

In summary, ITD is inherited as an autosomal dominant trait with markedly reduced penetrance. Because of this, and also because of the variable expression of ITD with mild cases being undiagnosed, it is not uncommon for a patient to be the only known affected member of a family. In most Ashkenazim and in many non-Jews with early limb-onset symptoms, ITD is due to mutations in the DYT1 gene on chromosome 9q34. The role of the gene in late-onset and cranial-cervical ITD is not clear; evidence suggests that DYT1 is not involved in several families with these clinical subtypes, and other ITD genes are being sought.

In Ashkenazi Jews with early-onset ITD, there is a very strong linkage disequilibrium between DYT1 and a haplotype of 9q34 alleles, implying the presence of a founder mutation in this population. As a practical application of this finding, it is possible to perform carrier testing in Ashkenazi families, including those in which only one member is affected with ITD; diagnosis in an affected member can be confirmed, gene carrier status in an unaffected individual or fetus can be determined, and more accurate counselling provided. In non-Jewish families, carrier testing for the DYT1 gene remains restricted to large families that show linkage to the locus.

DOPA-RESPONSIVE DYSTONIA (DRD)

DRD is a 'variant' form of childhood-onset ITD in which dystonia, although usually predominant, is often combined with parkinsonism and hyperreflexia. The typical clinical picture is that of a child, 4–8 years of age, who develops an abnormal gait that worsens as the day progresses. The gait is frequently stiff-legged and there may be plantar flexion or eversion. Dystonia may also involve the trunk, arms and less commonly the neck. Parkinsonian features include postural instability, hypomimia, bradykinesia with progressive slowing, decrementing amplitude, and rigidity as rapid successive or alternating movements are attempted[6,47]. There may also be hyperreflexia, particularly in the legs, and plantar extensor signs; because of the hyperreflexia and also the stiff-legged scissoring gait, children with DRD are not uncommonly misdiagnosed as having spastic diplegic cerebral palsy[47].

The diagnosis of this condition depends on both the examination findings and a dramatic response to low dose L-dopa therapy. Total daily dosages of as little as 50–200 mg of L-dopa (together with a dopa decarboxylase inhibitor) usually result in complete or near complete reversal of all signs and symptoms. Furthermore, unlike juvenile Parkinson's disease, with which the disorder may be confused, these patients do not develop fluctuations and maintain an excellent response to L-dopa.

The pathogenesis of this condition is thought to involve either the synthesis of dopamine or arborization of dopamine terminals. Evidence for this comes from cerebrospinal fluid (CSF), positron emission tomography (PET) and pathological studies. Specifically, CSF homovanillic acid (a major metabolite of dopamine) and tetrahydrobiopterin (a cofactor for tyrosine hydroxylase) levels are reduced suggesting a defect in dopamine production[48,49]. Fluorodopa uptake PET scans, however, are normal or close to normal indicating a structurally intact nigrostriatal pathway[50]. These two pieces of evidence are consistent with a functional defect in synthesis, possibly at a level prior to formation of dopa, e.g., at the level of tyrosine hydroxylation. Most recently, in a detailed post-mortem study there was a normal number of nigra dopamine neurons with normal nigral tyrosine hydroxylase activity and protein. The nigra dopamine cells, however, were hypopigmented; there was decreased dopamine in the nigra and striatum, and tyrosine hydroxylase protein and activity was diminished in the striatum[51]. One explanation posited for these findings is that there is a developmental disturbance with insufficient terminal arborization of dopamine cells.

DRD is inherited as an autosomal dominant trait with sex-related reduced penetrance. There is a 3:1 female:male ratio, and a penetrance of 45% in women and 15% in men has been estimated[52]. There also appears to be an increased frequency of adult-onset 'pure' parkinsonism without childhood dystonia among family members[53]. This parkinsonism is distinguished from Parkinson's disease by its excellent long-term L-dopa response and normal fluorodopa PET scanning; it may represent an alternate phenotype in some DRD gene carriers. DRD occurs world wide and, unlike ITD, there is no evidence of an increased frequency in any ethnic group.

Nygaard *et al.* recently mapped the gene for DRD to chromosome 14q in three North American families[54] and the locus was confirmed in English, French-Canadian and Japanese families. Further, in a study of Japanese DRD families different mutations in the 14q gene, GTP cyclohydrolase 1, were identified.[55] Also, GTP cyclohydrolase 1 enzyme activity was decreased in the DRD patients, consistent with the hypothesis that this gene, and specifically impaired dopamine synthesis due to diminished activity of the enzyme, is causative in DRD.

HUNTINGTON'S DISEASE

Huntington's disease (HD) is a neurodegenerative disorder characterized by a progressive cognitive loss, psychological changes, and, in particular, involuntary choreic movements. The course of disease is invariably deteriorating, with an inexorable progression to death within 10–15 years of onset. The motor abnormalities in HD usually begin in mild involuntary movements involving the entire body. Brain histological changes in patients are widespread, but the caudate nucleus appears to experience the greatest amount of neuronal loss. As yet, there are no effective treatments to delay the onset of, or ameliorate, the symptoms of this disease[56,57].

HD has long been known to be an autosomal dominant disease with complete or nearly complete penetrance by late age. While there is some variability in the frequency of HD across ethnic groups, there is general agreement that the prevalence ranges from 5–10 per 100 000 in Caucasians[58].

Although the age of onset of symptoms is variable, typically, HD is an adult-onset disorder, with most patients experiencing first symptoms in the fourth decade of life or later. However, the age at onset distribution is roughly normal, with a mean in the 40s, so that both very young and old onset also occur[58]. Juvenile HD is defined by an age at onset prior to 20 years. It is estimated that 1–10% of HD patients are juvenile onset[56]. In a recently reported series of patients from a large clinic, 42 out of 1050, or 4% of HD patients were said to have onset prior to the age of 20 years[59].

There are several clinical distinctions when the disease presents early. The motor disturbances in juvenile HD are more typically parkinsonian with marked rigidity and bradykinesia, as opposed to the chorea in adults; also, myoclonus is more common in juvenile HD, dementia and ataxia are more severe and seizures may be present. Typically, school performance is poor, both intellectually and behaviourally, and the downward course is generally more rapidly progressive than in the adult form of the disease[56]. Pathological studies have documented a strong inverse relationship between age at onset and severity of striatal degeneration[60].

Although HD has always been considered a prototypic autosomal dominant disease, it was noted early that juvenile cases present a discrepancy from the usual mendelian prediction of equal transmission from affected fathers and mothers in that they preferentially occur when the disease is inherited from the father rather than the mother[61,62]. It is estimated that of all juvenile cases, 80% descend from an affected father[56]. When juvenile cases are broken down into childhood (onset before age 10 years) and adolescent (onset between ages 11 and 20 years) forms, the effect is more dramatic. For childhood-onset cases, approximately 90% have an affected father, while only 75% of adolescent-onset cases do[59]. Thus, it appears that the predilection for paternal inheritance increases with decreasing age the onset of the case. This once mysterious observation has now been clarified, since identification of the HD gene, as described below.

MAPPING THE HD GENE

The HD gene was the first disease gene mapped using modern DNA technology. After screening a small collection of restriction fragment length polymorphism (RFLPs), Gusella and colleagues discovered linkage with a DNA probe, G8, located near the telomere of chromosome 4p[63]. This probe was estimated to lie 4 cM (or 4% recombination) away from the HD locus. Further, there was no evidence of non-allelic heterogeneity; in other words, that any families were not linked to this same chromosomal region[64]. Hence, although non-allelic heterogeneity is characteristic of many autosomal dominant disorders, this did not appear to be the case for HD.

Subsequent studies led to the identification of additional DNA markers in the region, flanking the HD gene in about a 2 cM interval[65]. However, precise localization of the HD gene was stymied by conflicting evidence from a small collection of critical recombinants. As is sometimes the case, individuals considered to be affected with a disease may actually have a mimicking disease, leading to genetic misclassification. Even if such individuals are extremely few, they can lead to contradictions in the precise location of a disease gene. Furthermore, the telomeric nature of the gene location made it difficult to identify distal flanking markers. Based on linkage data, two candidate locations were identified, one telomeric and one more proximal, with little assurance as to the exact location.

IDENTIFICATION OF HUNTINGTIN

Ultimately, linkage disequilibrium data provided additional support for the more proximal location of the HD gene. Although a number of different haplotypes are carried by HD patients, the disequilibrium results suggested a 500 kb region within chromosome band 5p16.3 as the site of the HD locus[66]. Expressed sequences of DNA from this 500 kb region were studied for evidence of mutations. One such gene, called IT15, was found to have a trinucleotide $(CAG)^n$ repeat in the proposed open reading frame near its 5′ end. This repeat is polymorphic, and was found to be expanded in HD patients compared to normal controls. Unstable and expanded trinucleotide repeats had been identified as the cause of several other neurological disorders, suggesting that the same mechanism was operating in HD.

The identified gene for HD was named huntingtin. The entire gene is about 210 kb, and gives rise to a 10 366 nucleotide transcript. The derived protein is large (about 348 kd) and of unknown function[67].

In the initial study identifying the huntingtin gene[67], there was no overlap in the size distribution (number of repeats) from normal and HD chromosomes. The number of repeats on normal chromosomes ranged from 11 to 34, while on HD chromosomes the range was from 42 to 100.

Since the initial study identifying huntingtin, numerous other studies have examined the allele size distribution on normal and HD chromosomes. The results generally confirm the initial reports, except that some studies show overlap in the two distributions. The overlap is primarily due to presumed HD patients having allele sizes in the normal range. In many, but not all of these cases, the patients have been re-examined and reclassified as having a disease other than HD. There remains an open question as to whether some small number of HD patients have a cause (or mutation) other than an expanded $(CAG)^n$ repeat of the huntingtin gene. Considering all of the studies to date, it appears that the allele size distribution on normal chromosomes is in the range 6–34, with a median around 20. In fact, most of these distributions are bimodal, with two peaks, one around 17 repeats and the other around 20 repeats. For HD chromosomes, the size ranges from 35–121 repeats (excluding the questionable cases with shorter repeats), although few cases have fewer than 40 repeats. Hence, there is a small region of ambiguity around 35–36 repeats in terms of whether such an individual will be affected or not, but in general the two distributions are non-overlapping.

CORRELATION BETWEEN REPEAT SIZE AND AGE AT ONSET

The initial study identifying the gene huntingtin also reported a negative correlation between the expanded repeat size and age at onset in HD carriers[67]. This observation has now been replicated in numerous other studies[59, 68–77]. The correlation appears to be most dramatic in the range of larger repeat sizes (>50), and much less so in the shorter repeat range (37–50). Thus, as one would predict, juvenile cases tend to have remarkably long repeats. We have pulled together data on age at onset and repeat size for juvenile onset cases from six different studies, Duyao *et al.*[68] (N=22), Snell *et al.*[69] (N=3), Norremolle *et al.*[72] (N=1), Zuhlke *et al.*[71] (N=4), Telenius *et al.*[59] (N=42), Stine *et al.*[73] (N=14), and DeRooij *et al.*[75] (N=6), for a total of 92 juvenile-onset cases (age at onset <20). The age at onset is plotted against number of trinucleotide repeats in Fig. 12.1, along with a fitted linear regression line. The negative correlation is quite striking. It is noteworthy that no child with onset before the age of 10 years has fewer than 60 repeats. From the linear regression we estimated that 52% of the variance in age at onset for this juvenile-onset group could be attributed to repeat size.

As it turns out, the negative correlation between repeat number and age at onset also explains the predominance of paternal inheritance for juvenile cases. The reason is that expanded repeats are unstable when transmitted in meiosis, particularly in males. In male meiosis, there is a strong tendency for the repeats to become larger, while in maternal meiosis the repeat size is more stable. Several studies have examined repeat size in parent–child pairs and documented the change in repeat size[59,68,75,76]. These results are listed in Table 12.2. In general, changes in maternal transmissions are small, with only a slight overall average increase of around 0.4 repeats. By contrast, paternal transmissions are characterized by size increases; these increases, in some cases, can be quite dramatic—up to 70 repeat units. The one study that focused on juvenile onset cases[59] showed the largest

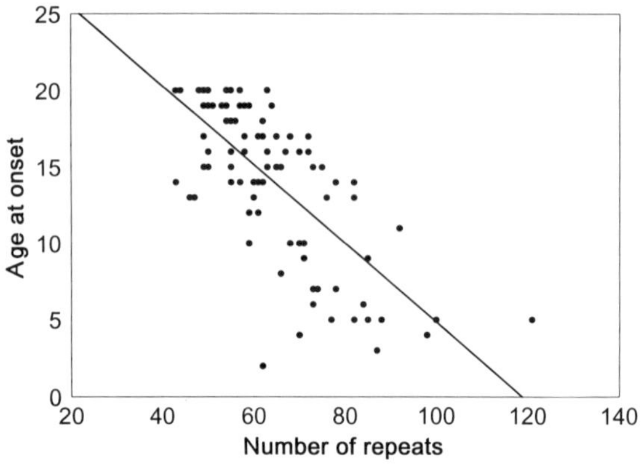

Figure 12.1. Negative correlation between $(CAG)^n$ repeat size and age at onset

increases; for maternal transmissions the average increase was 3.7 units, while for paternal transmissions the average increase was 36.0 units.

Another way of demonstrating the differential expansions in male versus female meioses is to compare repeat sizes on maternally versus paternally inherited chromosomes. We have compiled all such chromosomes from a number of studies[59,68,69] and present the results in Fig. 12.2. We restricted this analysis to repeat sizes of 50 or larger. As can be seen in the Figure, paternally inherited chromosomes have larger repeat sizes, particularly in the upper tail. In fact, for repeat sizes of 60 or greater, 76% are of paternal origin; for repeat sizes of 70 or greater, 100% are of paternal origin.

The results provide an explanation for the paternal excess of juvenile-onset cases. Large expansions occur preferentially on paternally inherited chromosomes, leading to early onset. While one study found that repeat size did not fully explain the effect of sex of transmitting parent on a child's age at onset[68], two other studies found no residual effect of sex of transmitting parent on child's age at onset in a multivariate regression

Table 12.2. Average repeat size increases from parent to child by parental sex

	Maternal inheritance		Paternal inheritance	
Study	*N*	Average change	*N*	Average change
Duyao *et al.*[68]	25	+0.4	37	+19.0
De Rooij *et al.*[75]	13	+0.4	16	+8.0
Barron *et al.*[76]	35	+0.5	31	+2.4
Telenius *et al.*[59*]	6	+3.7	12	+36.0

*In this study, all offspring were juvenile onset cases

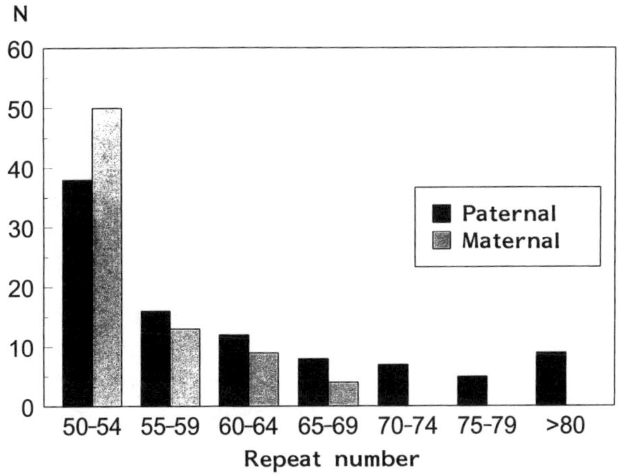

Figure 12.2. Repeat sizes on paternally inherited versus maternally inherited chromosomes

analysis once repeat size was included in the equation[59,73]. The latter study was based solely on juvenile-onset cases. Thus, preferential expansion in male meiosis is the likely explanation for the paternal excess of juvenile-onset cases. Also, these studies demonstrate no effect of the repeat size of the normal allele on age at onset, although some prior evidence had suggested this possibility[78].

CARRIER TESTING

With the discovery of the gene huntingtin, presymptomatic and fetal carrier testing in HD are entering a new era. For the last decade, such testing has been based on linked markers, so that other affected family members were needed to set phase and determine the carrier probability of the at-risk individual. It is now possible to assay directly the gene for HD, and to measure the repeat sizes for the testee. In general, as described above, the distributions for normal and abnormal alleles are well separated except for a small region of possible overlap around 35–36 repeat units. Thus, most individuals will be able to receive a clear result as to their carrier status, with the number of residual ambiguous cases being minimal. The fact that few presumed HD cases do not have expanded repeats may also suggest a small false negative rate by this test, but again the expected number of such cases is small.

The negative correlation between the repeat size and age at onset allows for a prediction of the likely age at onset for a carrier, as well as prediction of carrier status. In the repeat range of 37–50, the correlation appears to be modest and hence a broad range of onset ages is possible, although the probability of juvenile onset for this group is relatively low. For repeat sizes greater than 50, the correlation is stronger, and hence a better prediction of age at onset can be given. In particular, for repeat sizes of 70 or larger, juvenile onset is highly likely, as shown in Fig.12.1

Despite the now widespread availability of direct testing for the repeat size, and the elimination of many of the technical problems with the previous testing methods, the ethical, legal and social problems associated with testing remain. It is still imperative that counselling be provided both to the testee and to other at-risk family members. The social and psychological impact of this diagnosis, particularly to presymptomatic carriers, cannot be overestimated. For asymptomatic at-risk individuals who are under the age of majority, carrier testing is not recommended, and parents are usually counselled to leave the decision regarding testing to the child upon reaching the age of majority.

REFERENCES

1. Fahn, S., Marsden, C. D. and Calne, D. B. (1987) Classification and investigation of dystonia. In *Movement Disorders 2* (C. D. Marsden and S. Fahn, Eds). Butterworth, London, pp. 332–358.
2. Fahn, S. (1988) Concept and classification of dystonia. *Adv. Neurol.*, **50**, 1–8.
3. Nutt, J. G., Muenter, M. D., Aronson, A., Kurland, L. T. and Melton, L. J. (1988) Epidemiology of focal and generalized dystonia in Rochester. Minnesota. *Mov. Disord.*, **3**, 188–194.
4. Schwalbe, W. (1908) *Eine Eigentumliche Tonische Krampfform mit Hysterischen Symptomen. Medicin und Chirugie.* Universitats-Buchdrukerei von Gustav Schade, Berlin.
5. Segawa, M., Hosaka, A., Miyagawa, F., *et al.* (1976) Hereditary progressive dystonia with marked diurnal fluctuation. *Adv. Neurol.*, **14**, 215–233.
6. Nygaard, T. G., Marsden, C. D. and Duvoisin, R. C. (1988) Dopa-responsive dystonia. *Adv. Neurol.*, **50**, 377–384.
7. Quinn, N. P., Rothwell, J. C., Thompson, P. D. and Marsden, C. D. (1988) Hereditary myoclonic dystonia, hereditary torsion dystonia and hereditary essential myoclonus: an area of confusion. *Adv. Neurol.*, **50**, 391–401.
8. Dobyns, W. B., Ozelius, L. J., Kramer, P. L., Braskear, A., Farlow, M. R., Perry, T. R. *et al.* (1993) Rapid-onset dystonia-parkinsonism. *Neurology*, **43**, 2596–2602.
9. Lee, W. H., Pascasoi, F. M., Fuintes, F. D. and Viterbo, G. H. (1976) Torsion dystonia in Panay Philippines. *Adv. Neurol.*, **14**, 137–151.
10. Wilhelmsen, K. C., Weeks, D. E., Nygaard, T. G., Moskowitz, C., Rosales, R. L., de la Paz, D. C. *et al.* (1991) Genetic mapping of 'Lubag' (X-linked dystonia-parkinsonism) in a Filipino kindred to the pericentromeric region of the X chromosome. *Ann. Neurol.*, **29**, 124–131.
11. Kupke, K. G., Graeber, M. D. and Miller, U. (1992) Dystonia–parkinsonism syndrome (KDP) locus-flanking markers in Xq12-q21.1 *Am. J. Hum. Genet.*, **50**, 808–815.
12. Ahmad, F., Davis, M. B., Waddy, H. M., Oley, C. A., Marsden, C. D. and Harding, A. E. (1993) Evidence for locus heterogeneity in autosomal dominant torsion dystonia. *Genomics*, **15**, 9–12.

13. Bressman, S. B., deLeon, D., Brin, M.F., Risch, N. J., Burke, R. E., Greene, P. E., Shale, H. *et al.* (1989) Idiopathic torsion dystonia among Ashkenazi Jews: evidence for autosomal dominant inheritance. *Ann. Neurol.*, **26**, 612–620.
14. Greene, P. E., Kang, U. J. and Fahn, S. (1995) Spread of symptoms in idiopathic torsion dystonia. *Mov. Disord.*, **10**, 143–152.
15. Bernstein, S. (1912) Ein Fall von Torsionkrampf. *Wien. Klin. Wochenschr.*, **25**, 1567–1571.
16. Abrahamson, I. (1920) Presentation of cases of familial dystonia musculorum of Oppenheim. *J. Nerv. Ment. Dis.*, **51**, 451–454.
17. Mankowsky, B. N. and Czerny, L. I. (1929) Zur frage uber die Hereditat der Torsiodystonie. *Mschr. Psychiat. Neurol.*, **72**, 165–197.
18. Regensburg, J. (1930) Zur Klinik des hereditaren torsiondystonischen Symptomen komplexen. *Mschr. Psychiat. Neurol.*, **75**, 323–345.
19. Zeman, W., Kaelbling, R. and Pasamanick, B. (1959) Idiopathic dystonia musculorum deformans I. The hereditary pattern. *Am J. Hum. Genet.*, **II**, 188–202.
20. Johnson, W., Schwartz, G. and Barbeau, A. (1962) Studies on dystonia musculorum deformans. *Arch. Neurol.*, **7**, 301–313.
21. Larsson, T. and Sjogren, T. (1966) Dystonia musculorum deformans: a genetic and clinical population study of 121 cases. *Acta Neurol. Scand.*, **17** (Suppl), 1–232.
22. Zeman, W. and Dyken, P. (1967) Dystonia musculorum deformans; clinical, genetic and pathoanatomical studies. *Psychiatr. Neurol. Neurochir.*, **70**, 77–121.
23. Eldridge, R. (1970) The torsion dystonias: literature review: genetic and clinical studies. *Neurology*, **35**, 73–77.
24. Korczyn, A. D., Zilber, N., Kahana, E. and Alter, M. (1981) Inheritance of torsion dystonia. Reply. *Ann. Neurol.*, **10**, 204–205.
25. Burke, R. E., Brin, M. F., Fahn, S., Bressman, S. B. and Moskowitz, C. B. (1986) An analysis of the clinical course of non-Jewish autosomal dominant torsion dystonia. *Mov. Disord.*, **1**, 163–178.
26. Zilber, N., Korczyn, A. D., Kahana, E., Fried, K. and Alter, M. (1984) Inheritance of idiopathic torsion dystonia among Jews. *J. Med. Genet.*, **21**, 13–20.
27. Risch, N., Bressman, S. B., deLeon, D., Brin, M.F., Burke, R. E., Greene, P. E. *et al.* (1990) Segregation analysis of idiopathic torsion dystonia in Ashkenazi Jews suggest autosomal dominant inheritance. *Am. J. Hum. Genet.*, **46**, 533–538.
28. Pauls, D. L. and Korczyn, A. D. (1990) Complex segregation analysis of dystonia pedigrees suggest autosomal dominant inheritance. *Neurology*, **40**, 1107–1110.
29. Fletcher, N. A., Harding, A. E. and Marsden, C. D. (1990) A genetic study of idiopathic torsion dystonia in the United Kingdom. *Brain*, **113**, 379–395.
30. Defazio, G., Livrea, P., Guanti, G., Lepore, V. and Ferrari, E. (1993) Genetic contribution to idiopathic adult-onset blepharospasm and cranial–cervical dystonia. *Eur. Neurol.*, **33**, 345–350.
31. Waddy, H. M., Fletcher, N. A., Harding, A. E. and Marsden, C. D. (1991) A genetic study of idiopathic focal dystonias. *Ann. Neurol.*, **29**, 320–324.
32. Ozelius, L. J., Kramer, P. L., Moskowitz, G. B., Kwiatkowski, D. J., Brin, M. F., Bressman, S. B. *et al.* (1989) Human gene for torsion dystonia located on chromosome 9q32-34. *Neuron*, **2**, 1427–1434.
33. Kramer, P. L., deLeon, D., Ozelius, L. J., Risch, N. J., Bressman, S. B., Brin, M. F., Schuback, D. E., *et al.* (1990) Dystonia gene in Ashkenazi Jewish population is located on chromosome 9z32-34. *Ann. Neurol.*, **27**, 114–120.
34. Kwiatkowski, D. J., Ozelius, L., Kramer, P. L., Perman, S., Shuback, D. E., Gusella, J. F. *et al.* (1991) Torsion dystonia genes in two populations confined to a small region on chromosome 9q32-34. *Am. J. Hum. Genet.*, **49**, 366–371.

35. Schuback, D., Kramer, P., Ozelius, L., Holmgren, G., Forsgren, L., Kyllerman, M. *et al.* (1991) Dopamine beta-hydroxylase gene excluded in four subtypes of hereditary dystonia. *Hum. Genet.*, **87**, 311–316.
36. Warner, T. T., Fletcher, N. A., Davis, M. B., Ahmad, F., Conway, D., Feve, A. *et al.* (1993) Linkage analysis in British and French families with idiopathic torsion dystonia. *Brain*, **116**, 739–744.
37. Kramer, P. L., Heiman, G., Gasser, T., Ozelius, L., deLeon, D., Brin, M. F. *et al.* (1994) The DYT1 gene on 9q34 is responsible for most cases of early-onset idiopathic torsion dystonia in non-Jews. *Am. J. Hum. Genet.*, **55**, 468–475.
38. Ozelius, L. J., Kramer, P. L., deLeon, D., Risch, N., Bressman, S. B., Schuback, D. E. *et al.* (1992) Strong allelic association between the torsion dystonia gene (DYT1) and loci on chromosome 9q34 in Ashkenazi Jews. *Am. J. Hum. Genet.*, **50**, 619–628.
39. Bressman, S. B., deLeon, D., Kramer, P. L., Ozelius, L. J., Brin, M. F., Greene, P. E., *et al.* (1995) Dystonia in Ashkenazi Jews: clinical characterization of a unique mutation. *Ann. Neurol.*, **36**, 771–777.
40. Bressman, S. B., Heiman, G., Nygaard, T. G., Ozelius, L. J., Hunt, A. L., Brin, M. F. *et al.* (1994) A study of idiopathic torsion dystonia in a non-Jewish family: evidence for genetic heterogeneity. *Neurology*, **44**, 283–287.
41. Bressman, S. B., Hunt, A. L., Heiman, G. A., Brin, M. F., Burke, R. E., Fahn, S., *et al.* (1995) Exclusion of the DYT1 locus in a non-Jewish family with early-onset idiopathic dystonia. *Mov. Disord.*, **9**, 626–632.
42. LaBuda, M. C., Fletcher, N. A., Korczyn, A. D., Inzelberg, R., Harding, A. E. and Pauls, D. L. (1993) Genomic imprinting and anticipation in idiopathic torsion dystonia. *Neurology*, **43**, 2040–2043.
43. deLeon, D., Bressman, S., Brin, M. F., Risch, N. and Fahn, S. (1992) Torsion dystonia in Ashkenazi Jews: Is there evidence for an imprinted gene? *Mov. Disord.*, **7**, 297.
44. Fletcher, N. A., Harding, A. E. and Marsden, C. D. (1991) Intrafamilial correlation in idiopathic torsion dystonia. *Mov. Disord.*, **6**, 310–314.
45. Fletcher, N. A., Harding, A. E. and Marsden, C. D. (1991) The relationship between trauma and idiopathic torsion dystonia. *J. Neurol. Neurosurg. Psychiatry*, **54**, 713–717.
46. Risch, N., deLeon, D., Ozelius, L., Kramer, P., Almasy, L., Singer, B. *et al.* (1995) Genetic analysis of idiopathic torsion dystonia in Ashkenazi Jews: evidence for the recent descent of Ashkenazim from a small founder population. *Nature Genet.*, **9**, 152–159.
47. Nygaard, T. G., Marsden, C. D. and Fahn, S. (1991) Dopa-responsive dystonia; long-term treatment response and prognosis. *Neurology*, **41**, 174–181.
48. LeWitt, P. A., Miller, L. P., Levine, R. A., Lovenberg, W., Newman, R. P., Papavasiliou, A. *et al.* (1986) Tetrahydrobiopterin in dystonia: identification of abnormal metabolism and therapeutic trials. *Neurology*, **36**, 760–764.
49. Furukawa, Y., Nishi, K., Kondo, T., Mizuno, Y., Narabayashi, H., *et al.* (1993) CSF biopterin levels and clinical features of patients with juvenile parkinsonism. *Adv. Neurol.*, **60**, 562–567.
50. Snow, B. J., Nygaard, T. G., Takahashi, H. and Calne, D. B. (1993) Positron emission tomographic studies of dopa-responsive dystonia and early-onset idiopathic parkinsonism. *Ann. Neurol.*, **34**, 733–738.
51. Rajput, A. H., Gibb, W. R. G., Kish, S. J. and Hornykiewicz, O. (1992) Dopa-responsive dystonia—clinical, pathological and biochemical studies in one case. (Abstract). *Mov. Disord.*, **7**, 124.
52. Nygaard, T. G. (1993) An analysis of North American families with dopa-responsive dystonia. In *Hereditary Progressive Dystonia with Marked Diurnal*

Fluctuation (M. Segawa, Ed). Parthenon Publishing, Carnforth, pp. 97–104.
53. Nygaard, T. G., Takahashi, H., Heiman, G. A., Snow, B. J., Fahn, S. and Calne, D. B. (1992) Long-term treatment response and fluorodopa positron emission tomographic scanning of parkinsonism in a family with dopa-responsive dystonia. *Ann. Neurol.*, **32**, 603–608.
54. Nygaard, T. G., Wilhelmsen, K. C., Risch, N. J., Brown, D. L., Trugman, J. M., Gilliam, T. C. *et al.* (1993) Linkage mapping of dopa-responsive dystonia (DRD) to chromosome 14q. *Nature Genet.*, **5**, 386–391.
55. Ichinose, H., Ohye, T., Takahashi, E., Seki, N., Hori, T. Segawa, M. *et al.* (1994) Hereditary progressive dystonia with marked diurnal fluctuation caused by mutations in the GTP hydrolase 1 gene. *Nature Genet.*, **8**, 263–241.
56. Hayden, M. R. (1981) *Huntington's Chorea*. Springer, New York.
57. Harper, P. S. (1991) *Huntington's Disease*. W. B. Saunders, London.
58. Conneally, P. M. (1984) Huntington's disease: genetics and epidemiology. *Am. J. Hum. Genet.*, **36**, 506–526.
59. Telenius, H., Kremer, H. P. H., Theilmann, J., Andrew, S. E., Almqvist, E., Anvret, M., *et al.* (1993) Molecular analysis of juvenile Huntington disease: the major influence on $(CAG)^n$ repeat length is the sex of the affected parent. *Hum. Mol. Genet.*, **2**, 1535–1540.
60. Myers, R. H., Vonsattel, J. P., Stevens, T. J., Cupples, L. A., Richardson, E. P., Martin, J. B. and Brid, E. D. (1988) Clinical and neuropathologic assessment of severity in Huntington's disease. *Neurology*, **38**, 341–347.
61. Merritt, A. D., Conneally, P. M., Rahman, N. F. and Drew, A. L. (1973) Juvenile Huntington's chorea. In *Progress in Neurogenetics* (A. B. Barbeau and J. R. Brunett, Eds). Excerpta Medica, Amsterdam, pp. 645–650.
62. Newcombe, R. G., Walker, D. A. and Harper, P. S. (1981) Factors influencing age at onset and duration of survival in Huntington's chorea. *Ann. Hum. Genet.*, **45**, 387–396.
63. Gusella, J. F., Wexler, N. S., Conneally, P. M., Naylor, S., Anderson, M. A., Tanzi, R. E. *et al.* (1983) A polymorphic DNA marker genetically linked to Huntington's disease. *Nature*, **306**, 234–238.
64. Conneally, P. M., Haines, J. L., Tanzi, R. E., Wexler, N. S., Penchaszadeh, G. K., Harper, P. S. *et al.* (1989) Huntington disease: no evidence for locus heterogeneity. *Genomics*, **5**, 304–308.
65. MacDonald, M. E., Haines, J. L., Zimmer, M., Cheng, S. V., Youngman, S., Whaley, W. L. *et al.* (1989) Recombination events suggest potential sites for the Huntington's disease gene. *Neuron*, **3**, 183–190.
66. Macdonald, M. E., Lin, C., Srinidi, L., Bates, G., Altherr, M., Whaley, W. L. *et al.* (1991) Complex patterns of linkage disequilibrium in the Huntington's disease region. *Am. J. Hum. Genet.*, **49**, 723–734.
67. Huntington Disease Collaborative Research Group. (1993) A novel gene containing a trinucleotide repeat that is expanded and unstable on Huntington's disease chromosomes. *Cell*, **72**, 971–983.
68. Duyao, M., Ambrose, C., Myers, R., Novelletto, A., Persichetti, F., Frontali, M., *et al.* (1993) Trinucleotide repeat length instability and age of onset in Huntington's disease. *Nature Genet.*, **4** ,387–392.
69. Snell, R. G., MacMillan, J. C., Cheadle, J. P., Fenton, I., Lazarou, L. P., Davies, P., *et al.* (1993) Relationship between trinucleotide repeat expansion and phenotypic variation in Huntington's disease. *Nature Genet.*, **4**, 393–397.
70. Andrew, S. E., Goldberg, Y. P., Kremer, B., Telenius, H., Theilmann, J., Adams, S., *et al.* (1993) The relationship between trinucleotide ('CAG) repeat length and clinical features of Huntington's disease. *Nature Genet.*, **4**, 398–403.
71. Zuhlke, C., Riess, O., Schroder, K., Siedlazck, I., Epplen, J. T., Engel, W. and

Thies, U. (1993) Expansion of the $(CAG)^n$ repeat causing Huntington's disease in 352 patients of German origin. *Hum. Mol. Genet.*, **2**, 1467–1469.

72. Norremolle, A., Reiss, O., Epplen, J. T., Fenger, K., Hashold, L. and Sorensen, S. A. (1993) Trinucleotide repeat elongation in the Huntingtin gene in Huntington disease patients from 71 Danish families. *Hum. Mol. Genet.*, **2**, 1475–1476.
73. Stine, O. C., Pleasant, N., Franz, M. L., Abbott, M. H., Folstein, S. E. and Ross, C. A. (1993) Correlation between the onset age of Huntington's disease and length of the trinucleotide repeat in IT-15. *Hum. Mol. Genet.*, **2**, 1547–1549.
74. Rubinsztein, D. C., Barton, D. E., Davison, B. C. and Ferguson-Smith, M. A. (1993) Analysis of the huntingtin gene reveals a trinucleotide length polymorphism in the region of the gene that contains two CCG-rich stretches and a correlation between decreased age of onset of Huntington's disease and CAG repeat number. *Hum. Mol. Genet.*, **2** ,1713–1715.
75. De Rooij, K. E., De Koning Gans, P. A., Skraastad, M. I., Belfroid, R. D., Vegter Van Der Vlis, M., Roos, R. A. *et al.* (1993) Dynamic mutation in Dutch Huntington's disease patients: increased paternal repeat instability extending to within the normal size range. *J. Med. Genet.*, **30**, 996–1002.
76. Barron, L. H., Warner, J. P., Porteous, M., Holloway, S., Simpson, S., Davidson, R. and Brock, D. J. (1993) A study of the Huntington's disease associated trinucleotide repeat in the Scottish population. *J. Med. Genet.*, **30**, 1003–1007.
77. Craufurd, D. and Dodge, A. (1993) Mutation size and age at onset in Huntington's disease. *J. Med. Genet.*, **30**, 1008–1011.
78. Farrer, L. A., Cupples, L. A., Wiater, P., Conneally, P. M., Gusella, J. F. and Myers, R. H. (1993) The normal Huntington disease (HD) allele, or a closely linked gene, influences age at onset of HD. *Am. J. Hum. Genet.*, **53**, 125–130.

13 Functional Neuroanatomy of the Basal Ganglia

GARRETT E. ALEXANDER
Emory University School of Medicine, Atlanta, Georgia, USA

FUNCTIONAL ORGANIZATION OF THE BASAL GANGLIA

The basal ganglia comprise the striatum (including the neostriatum, composed of the putamen and caudate nucleus, and the ventral striatum), the globus pallidus, the substantia nigra and the subthalamic nucleus. All of these are functionally subdivided into skeletomotor, oculomotor, associative and limbic territories based on their physiological properties and on their interconnections with cortical and thalamic territories of the same functionalities[1]. As indicated in Fig. 13.1, the large-scale organization of the basal ganglia can be viewed as a family of re-entrant loops that are

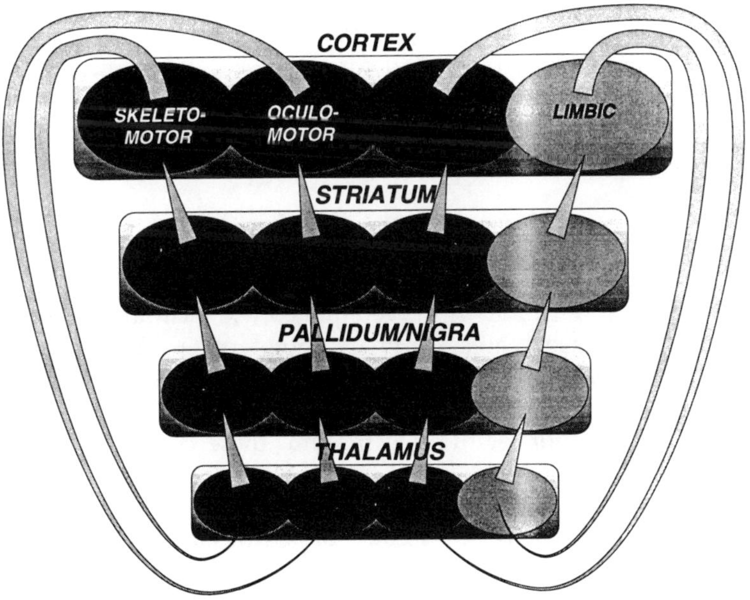

Figure 13.1. Parallel, functionally segregated, basal ganglia–thalamocortical loops. Information flow is from narrow to wide end of each pathway

Movement and Allied Disorders. Edited by M. M. Robertson and V. Eapen

organized in parallel, each taking its origin from a particular set of functionally related cortical fields (skeletomotor, oculomotor, etc.), passing through the functionally corresponding portions of the basal ganglia, and returning to parts of those same cortical fields by way of specific basal ganglia-recipient zones in the dorsal thalamus.

Due to maintained segregation along each of these cortico-basal ganglia-thalamocortical circuits, there is little direct communication among the separate functional domains. While virtually the entire cortical mantle is mapped topographically onto the striatum, often considered the 'input' portion of the basal ganglia, the cortically directed signals from the basal ganglia output nuclei (internal pallidum and substantia nigra pars reticulata) are returned exclusively to foci within the frontal lobe (after first passing through the corresponding portions of the thalamus). Because of their parallel organization, it is generally suspected that the operations performed at corresponding stations along each of these loops are quite similar. In this review, the focus will be on the organization and physiology of the skeletomotor loop.

MOTOR CIRCUITRY OF THE BASAL GANGLIA

The skeletomotor circuitry of the basal ganglia includes several noteworthy features, some of which may be important in shaping the specific contributions that these structures make to the control of movement. The broad outlines of basal ganglia motor circuitry are depicted in Fig. 13.2.

CORTICAL INPUTS

Like the cerebellum, the basal ganglia receive topographic inputs from most of the sensorimotor territories of the cerebral cortex, including primary and secondary somatosensory areas, primary motor cortex, and a variety of premotor areas including the supplementary motor area, the dorsal and ventral premotor areas, and the cingulate motor areas[2–11]. Directed toward the sensorimotor portion of the neostriatum, these co-ordinated cortico-striatal inputs impose a well-defined somatotopic organization upon their target nucleus which, in primates, coincides roughly with the putamen[12–14]. In addition to their respective corticostriatal neurons, most of the putamen-projecting sensorimotor areas also contain separate populations of neurons that project directly to the spinal cord[2,15,16]. Some evidence suggests that the cortical message conveyed to the striatum may differ from that projected directly to the spinal cord[17]. If so, the prevailing view that the basal ganglia

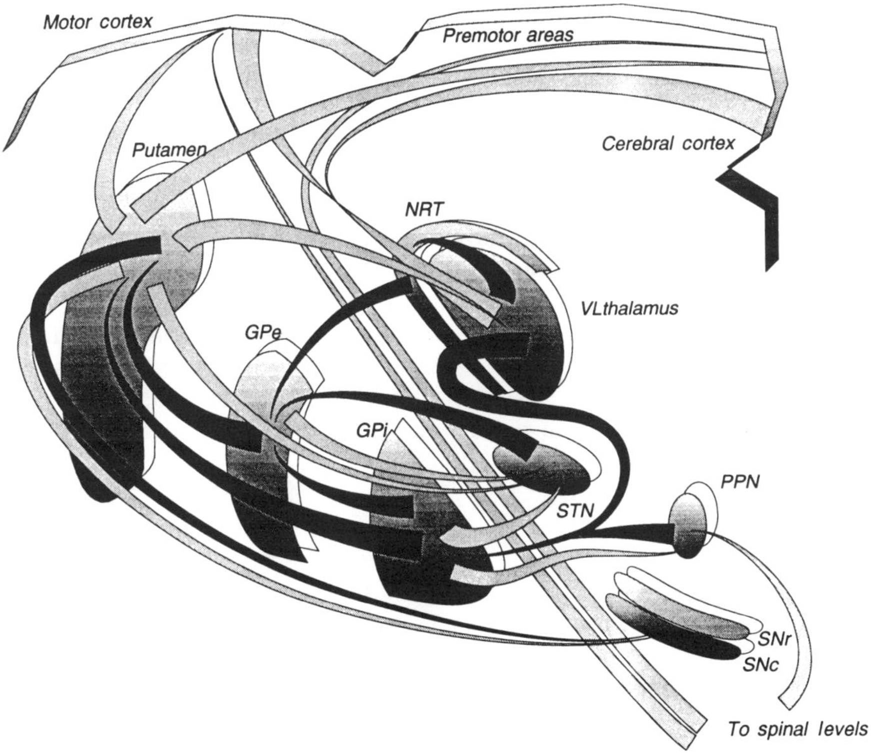

Figure 13.2. Basal ganglia skeletomotor circuitry. Major motor pathways involving the basal ganglia. Excitatory pathways are indicated by light shading, inhibitory by dark shading. Pathway origins and terminations are indicated by narrow and wide ends, respectively. Connections between thalamus and cortex are reciprocal. Not shown are connections to and from SNr, which parallel those of GPi. Abbreviations: GPe, external segment of globus pallidus; GPi, internal segment of globus pallidus; NRT, reticular nucleus of the thalamus; PPN, pedunculopontine nucleus; SNc, substantia nigra pars compacta; STN, subthalamic nucleus; VLthalamus, basal ganglia recipient zone in ventrolateral thalamus. To simplify the illustration, the thalamostriate projection from the centromedian nucleus is shown arising from VLthalamus

receive cortical signals that are faithful replicas of corticospinal commands, i.e. simple corollary discharges, may need to be revised.

The majority of the putamen-projecting sensorimotor areas also send topographic projections to the subthalamic nucleus[18]. Both the corticostriatal and the corticosubthalamic projections are excitatory and probably glutamatergic[19–22] (as are most of the corticospinal projections[23]), but the conduction velocities of these two pathways may differ significantly. Direct comparisons in the rat suggest that the corticostriatal projection may be substantially slower than the corticosubthalamic[24], which could have a significant influence on the way information is processed within the basal ganglia. Thus far, direct comparisons of these two pathways have not been made in the monkey, but it does seem clear from primate studies that conduction along the corticostriatal pathway is substantially slower than conduction along the pathways leading from cortex to brainstem and spinal levels[17].

Nevertheless, there are significant species differences in basal ganglia connectivity, so extrapolations must be made with caution. In rats, for example, the earliest cortically-induced excitatory postsynaptic potentials (EPSPs) in striatum appear to come from axon collaterals of large diameter, brainstem-projecting fibres[25], but in primates this collateral projection seems to be lacking, with the massive corticostriatal projection arising almost exclusively from a separate population of small-axoned, direct-projecting corticostriatal neurons[26].

STRIATUM

In the putamen, as in the rest of the striatum, the large majority of neurons (>75% in primates, up to 95% in rodents) are of the medium spiny type (MSN)[27]. MSNs are GABA(gamma-aminobutyric acid)-ergic projection neurons[28], and in primates they comprise two distinct populations, one projecting to the external segment of the globus pallidus (GPe) and the other projecting either to the internal segment of the globus pallidus (GPi) or to the substantia nigra pars reticulata (SNr)[29,30]. At rest, putamen projection neurons are nearly silent[31,32], but most have well-defined sensorimotor fields and discharge selectively in relation to specific parameters of movement or specific aspects of the preparation for movement[13, 33–36].

The other type of putamen neuron that has been well studied is the large, aspiny interneuron[37,38]. Converging evidence from anatomical studies as well as from extracellular and intracellular recording studies indicate that these neurons have the following properties. Unlike MSNs, the large interneurons are spontaneously active (with discharge rates of 3–7 Hz), and they do not discharge in relation to specific parameters of movement preparation or execution. Rather, they discharge briefly (only one or two spikes) and synchronously following the presentation of a conditioned sensory stimulus that signifies the imminent delivery of a reward[39]. These spontaneously active interneurons appear to be cholinergic[40], but their synaptic influence on neighbouring MSNs has not been directly determined. Electron microscopic studies have shown that cholinergic synapses on the somata and dendritic shafts and spines of MSNs are of the symmetrical type[41], which suggests that the aspiny interneurons may have an inhibitory effect on MSNs.

GLOBUS PALLIDUS AND SUBSTANTIA NIGRA

Those portions of GPi and SNr that receive input from the putamen constitute the sensorimotor output nuclei of the basal ganglia, sending GABA-ergic projections to their respective targets in both the ventrolateral thalamus (n. ventralis lateralis and n. ventralis anterior) and the centromedian nucleus of the thalamus[42–48]. Anatomically, GPi and SNr share many common features, and from a functional standpoint they can be viewed as two subdivisions of a single basal ganglia output nucleus[49,50]. In GPi/SNr, large projection neurons are by far the most abundant cell type, but a minute population of small cells that may represent interneurons has also been described[51,52]. Neurons in the sensorimotor territories of GPi/SNr have movement-related receptive fields that are similar to those of the putamen's MSNs, but GPi/SNr neurons differ from MSNs in having relatively high spontaneous discharge rates (60–80 Hz) that are modulated both upward and downward depending on their particular sensorimotor response fields[53–55]. Neurons in the sensorimotor territory of GPe have discharge properties and sensorimotor fields that are comparable to those in GPi/SNr[53].

DIRECT AND INDIRECT PATHWAYS

The basal ganglia output nuclei (GPi/SNr) receive not only *direct* inputs from the striatum via the GPi- and SNr-projecting MSNs, but also an important converging source of information via what has come to be termed the *indirect* pathway through the basal ganglia[56]. The direct and indirect pathways are illustrated in Figure 13.3. The indirect pathway takes its origin from the GPe-projecting MSNs. In turn, the GABA-ergic neurons of GPe project mainly to the subthalamic nucleus[57], whose excitatory, glutamatergic neurons send feedforward connections to GPi/SNr, completing one arm of the indirect pathway[58–60]. Subthalamic neurons also send glutamatergic feedback connections to GPe and to the putamen[59,61,62].

Recently, a second arm of the indirect pathway has been revealed. GPe projects not only to the subthalamic nucleus, but also to the output nuclei, GPi/SNr[63,64]. A remarkable consequence of this is that activation of MSNs associated with either arm of the indirect pathway should increase basal ganglia output by increasing neuronal activity at the level of GPi/SNr: in one case, by disinhibiting the subthalamic nucleus with its excitatory projections to GPi/SNr; in the other, by directly disinhibiting GPi/SNr. In contrast, activation of MSNs associated with the direct pathway should decrease basal ganglia output by directly suppressing activity at the level of GPi/SNr.

It has long been recognized that the large-scale organization of the basal ganglia constitutes a re-entrant system, with cortical influences passing

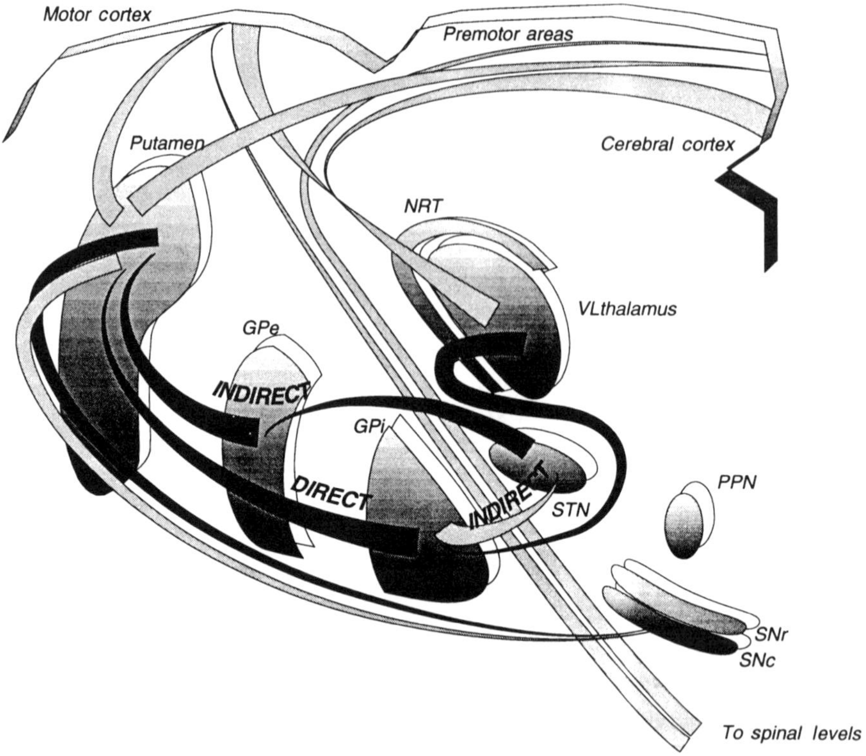

Figure 13.3. Direct and indirect pathways through basal ganglia. Conventions are the same as in Fig. 13.2

through the basal ganglia and being returned to cortical levels through specific portions of the thalamus[65]. Of some interest recently has been the question of how the direct and indirect pathways may differentially influence thalamocortical operations. Current evidence indicates that these two pathways have opposing effects on the output nuclei. Activation of the direct pathway should result in a corresponding suppression of GABA-ergic GPi/SNr output, thereby disinhibiting the basal ganglia-receiving portions of the thalamus, while activation of either arm of the indirect pathway should lead to an enhancement of GPi/SNr-mediated thalamic inhibition[56]. Given the re-entrant nature of basal ganglia-thalamocortical connections, cortically initiated activation of the direct pathway might therefore be expected to result in positive feedback at cortical levels, with corresponding activation of the indirect pathway giving rise, conversely, to negative feedback.

A detailed understanding of how the basal ganglia's motor circuitry operates is complicated by a variety of pathways that feed backwards or forwards across multiple nuclei. Two of the feedback pathways include excitatory projections returned to the putamen: already mentioned was the projection from the subthalamic nucleus[61], also noteworthy are the thalamostriatal projections that originate in the centromedian nucleus[66,67]. Both of these pathways appear to provide positive feedback to the putamen.

THALAMIC RETICULAR NUCLEUS

GPe sends an inhibitory, feedforward projection to the nucleus reticularis of the thalamus (NRT)[68], which in turn imposes a robust, GABA-ergic modulation upon the basal ganglia-recipient nuclei of the ventrolateral thalamus (as well as upon other thalamic nuclei)[69]. There appears to be a functional consistency among the various GPe projections, in that cortically induced activations of GPe-projecting MSNs should have the net effect of producing negative feedback at cortical levels, based on the functional effects of each of the known GPe projections—including both arms of the indirect pathway and the GPe projections to the NRT.

On the other hand, the role of the NRT in basal ganglia operations may be much more complicated. It is generally accepted that the NRT plays an important role in gating thalamocortical transmission from the dorsal thalamus, and that it does so in a roughly topographic manner that links specific portions of the NRT with specific thalamic nuclei and their cortical target zones[69]. The NRT receives collateral, excitatory inputs from corticothalamic as well as thalamocortical fibres that must pass through this nucleus *en route* to their respective termination zones in cortex and thalamus. In addition, the NRT may also receive collateral inputs[69] from both the inhibitory pallidothalamic pathway[42,70] and the excitatory thalamostriate projections[71].

PEDUNCULOPONTINE NUCLEUS

While the pedunculopontine nucleus (PPN) is not generally considered to be part of the basal ganglia, this structure has strong, reciprocal connections with the basal ganglia output nuclei and with the subthalamic nucleus, and it also sends unreciprocated projections to the dopaminergic neurons of the substantia nigra pars compacta (SNc; see below) as well as to the putamen and caudate nucleus[46,47,57,62,72–75]. In primates, the majority of pallidal inputs to the PPN are apparently collaterals of pallidothalamic projections[61,73,74]. The PPN contains two populations of neurons, one cholinergic and the other non-cholinergic[76]. It is mainly the non-cholinergic neurons that project back to GPi/SNr and the subthalamic nucleus[76,77], while the cholinergic neurons project primarily to the thalamus[78,79]. The non-cholinergic neurons have excitatory effects on their basal ganglia targets[80–82], and there is some evidence that they may use glutamate as their transmitter[83].

As with GPi/SNr, there is a convergence of inputs from both the direct and indirect pathways at the level of the PPN. In this case, however, activation of either pathway at the level of the MSNs leads to the same polarity of response within the PPN (that is, activation of PPN by disinhibited subthalamic inputs, or direct disinhibition of PPN by inputs from GPe or from GPi/SNr).

Until recently, descending projections of the basal ganglia output nuclei have received relatively little attention, it having been generally assumed that directly descending basal ganglia influences on the skeletomotor system extended no further caudally than the PPN. Recent studies in rats, however, have also revealed substantial PPN outflow to the reticulospinal system[84,85]. These findings have not yet been extended to primates.

FUNCTIONALLY SEGREGATED CIRCUITS

One of the remarkable features of basal ganglia circuitry is that functionally discrete channels of information processing are maintained throughout the various cortico-basal ganglia-thalamocortical pathways[86–88] in the face of layer-to-layer connectivity that is highly convergent[27,89]. In the case of the skeletomotor pathways, for example, basal ganglia neurons have been shown to have highly refined sensorimotor fields that are comparable in their somatotopic and behavioural specificity to the sensorimotor fields of neurons at cortical levels[34,90–92].

Recent anatomical studies using transneuronal tracers have revealed at least three separate channels of arm representation that extend continuously throughout the basal ganglia-thalamocortical pathways[3]. Each channel originates in a separate cortical motor area (motor cortex, ventral premotor area or supplementary motor area) and remains segregated from the others throughout the entire cortico-basal ganglia-thalamocortical loop.

On the other hand, at the cellular level there is considerable convergence of inputs along these same pathways. Based on electron microscopic analyses, it has been estimated that the convergence ratio along the corticostriatal pathways, which provide approximately one-half of the excitatory input to the neostriatum, may be in the order of 5000:1. Cell counts in the human striatum and globus pallidus[93,94] suggest minimum convergence ratios in the order of 300:1 and 100:1, respectively, for the striatal projections to GPe and GPi.

The mechanisms that underly the development and maintenance of functional specificity in basal ganglia networks (despite the abundant anatomical convergence) have yet to be identified. Much of this organization may be genetically determined, but experience-dependent synaptic modification may also play a role. If synaptic plasticity in basal ganglia network operates according to Hebb-like principles[95], and there is some evidence that this may be the case (see below), the correlative nature of Hebbian learning might well be expected to strengthen preferentially those connections which link neurons with similar functional properties[96].

ROLE OF DOPAMINE

Another important feature of basal ganglia organization is the pervasive role of dopamine. The functionality of dopamine in basal ganglia operations appears to be very complex. Dopaminergic input to the putamen consists of nigrostriatal projections that originate in the substantia nigra pars compacta (SNc)[61], and the cortical motor and premotor areas receive separate dopaminergic projections from the ventral tegmental area[97–99]. At the network level, dopamine appears to have differential effects on the direct and indirect pathways, tending to activate striatal MSNs that project directly to GPi while suppressing those that project to GPe[56]. Given the fact that there appear to be reciprocal re-entrant effects associated with differential activation of the direct versus indirect pathways (i.e. positive feedback to cortex via the direct pathway, and negative feedback via the indirect, see above), the differential effects of dopamine on these two pathways suggest that its overall impact on basal ganglia operations may include the enhancement of positive feedback, and suppression of negative feedback, returned to the various cortical areas that receive basal ganglia influences.

Dopamine has also been shown to have a role in synaptic plasticity within the striatum, being implicated in both long-term potentiation (LTP) and long-term depression (LTD)[100–102]. The nigrostriatal pathway provides an extraordinarily dense dopaminergic input to each MSN, which is comparable in magnitude to the 5000 or so corticostriatal synapses that individual MSNs receive[103]. The behavioural correlates of dopamine neurons have been studied in depth by Schultz and his colleagues[104,105]. Unlike nearly all the other basal ganglia motor circuit neurons, except perhaps the large, aspiny interneurons of the striatum[31,39], dopamine neurons do not show activity changes in relation to movement *per se*, but discharge instead in relation to conditions involving the probability and imminence of behavioural reinforcement[104,105].

The newly discovered facts that dopamine may play a crucial role in the cellular mechanisms of LTD and LTP within the striatum, and that dopamine neurons discharge selectively in relation to specific reward contingencies, combine to suggest the intriguing hypothesis that dopamine neurons may play an important role in determining when striatal synapses should be strengthened or weakened. In this respect, dopamine neurons might be seen as playing a role in striatal information processing analogous to that of an 'adaptive critic' in connectionist networks[106].

It is noteworthy, however, that the striatum is not the only basal ganglia structure for which there is evidence of adaptive synapses. With their combined voltage dependency and ligand specificity, N-methyl-D-aspartate (NMDA) receptors are widely assumed to play a role in at least one form of activity-dependent synaptic plasticity, namely LTP[107]. Evidence for the existence of NMDA receptors has been found in a number of basal ganglia nuclei that are believed to receive significant glutamatergic input, including the striatum (putamen and caudate nucleus)[20,37,108], the subthalamic nucleus[19,108], and the SNc[109]. NMDA receptors have also been demonstrated at cortical levels[108,110,111], where the phenomenon of LTP has been documented in many regions including some of the sensorimotor fields[112–115]. Taken together, these findings indicate that adaptive synapses may be distributed at multiple junctures along the basal ganglia-thalamocortical pathways.

FUNCTIONAL MODELS OF BASAL GANGLIA ORGANIZATION

Disinhibition plays an important role in many current models of basal ganglia operation[116]. In the case of the basal ganglia's oculomotor pathways, for example, there is compelling evidence that striatally induced, phasic inhibition of SNr neurons leads to the generation of saccadic eye movements through the release of command neurons in the superior colliculus from the tonic, GABA-ergic inhibition they receive via the nigrotectal pathway[117–119]. The elegant simplicity of this model has helped to motivate similar models of how the basal ganglia's skeletomotor circuitry may contribute to movement control, the chief difference being the emphasis in most skeletomotor models on disinhibition at the level of the thalamus rather than brainstem[56].

These models of the basal ganglia's skeletomotor circuitry assume that voluntary movements are facilitated in the context of focused disinhibition of the basal ganglia-recipient portions of the ventrolateral thalamus. This focused thalamic disinhibition is thought to be generated either by phasic enhancement of transmission through the direct pathway, by phasic suppression of transmission through the indirect pathway, or by a combination of these two processes. Conversely, according to this same scheme, decreased transmission through the direct pathway, or increased transmission through the indirect, would have the effect of suppressing voluntary movements.

This relatively simplistic model raises questions of its own, however. It is not known, for example, whether a given corticostriatal neuron (or functional group of such neurons) engages both the direct and indirect pathways in a balanced manner. Nor is it known whether the convergence of inputs from the direct and indirect pathways onto individual GPi/SNr neurons[64] results in a functional interaction between the two pathways that is antagonistic or complementary. A possibility at one extreme would be a functionally antagonistic, push/pull system that could be used to scale and/or brake the intended movement (e.g. with flexion-activated inputs from the two pathways being superimposed and thereby tending to cancel one another out). At the other extreme would be a functionally complementary, centre-surround system that might serve to facilitate the intended movement pattern while suppressing potentially conflicting ones. Whether either of these alternative schemes applies, or whether instead there may be a purely random convergence of direct and indirect projections onto GPi/SNr neurons, has important implications for any functional model of basal ganglia organization.

HYPOKINETIC DISORDERS

Studies of various primate models of basal ganglia-induced movement disorders have tended to confirm many of the predictions of the thalamic disinhibition models[120]. These models predict that excessive basal ganglia outflow should be associated with hypokinetic states such as are seen in the various akinetic/rigid disorders of movement control. Because of dopamine's reciprocal effects on the direct and indirect pathways, experimental striatal dopamine deficiency should and does result in excessive discharge of neurons in the subthalamic nucleus as well as in GPi/SNr. In primates with parkinsonian akinesia induced experimentally by treatment with MPTP, the discharge rates of GPi neurons as well as of neurons in the subthalamic nucleus have been found to be abnormally high, consistent with predictions of the thalamic disinhibition models[121,122]. Voluntary movements can be restored in these akinetic animals by selective lesions of the subthalamic nucleus, which results in the return of GPi neurons to more normal rates of discharge[123]. Also consistent with thalamic disinhibition models is the fact that akinesia in humans with idiopathic Parkinson's disease can be relieved by selective stereotaxic lesions of GPi (especially when the lesions are centred in that nucleus' sensorimotor territory[124]).

HYPERKINETIC DISORDERS

Such models are also able to account for hyperkinetic disorders (e.g. involuntary ballistic or choreiform movements) on the basis of reduced basal ganglia outflow[120]. Such reduced outflow is thought to result in excessive disinhibition of the basal ganglia-receiving territories within the thalamus, with consequent release of involuntary movements. This explanation is consistent with various clinical and experimental data, including the fact that lesions of the subthalamic nucleus result in dyskinesias[125], and that such lesions are associated with reduced levels of spontaneous discharge in GPi[123].

LIMITS OF CURRENT MODELS

There are, however, a number of observations that are difficult to reconcile with simple models of basal ganglia function based primarily on the concept of thalamic disinhibition. One of the most serious such conflicts involves the fact that lesions of the basal ganglia output nuclei do not result in dyskinesias[126,127] as the models predict they should, although dyskinesias have been reported in association with muscimol-induced suppression of GPi output[128]. A possible explanation for this discrepancy may be that the voltage-dependent, bistable properties of thalamic neurons[129] may cause them to respond to downward modulations of inhibitory basal ganglia input in a non-monotonic manner. On the one hand, moderate reductions of GABA-ergic input from the basal ganglia, as would be expected with subthalamic lesions, may partially, but inappropriately, depolarize some thalamic relay neurons to the point that they enter a non-relay burst mode when they are supposed to be maximally hyperpolarized, leading to bursts of inappropriate thalamocortical activity and resultant dyskinesias. On the other hand, severe reductions in GABA-ergic input, as would be expected with GPi lesions, may actually restore some stability by increasing the level of depolarization of all basal ganglia-recipient thalamic relay cells to the point where they enter into a more or less permanent, non-bursting, relay mode. Or perhaps the reason that complete removal of inhibitory basal ganglia input to the thalamus is not associated with dyskinesias is that the emergence of dyskinesias may require that reduced tonic levels of thalamic inhibition be combined with the preservation of at least some degree of phasic modulation of these same inhibitory inputs (see Steriade and Llinas[129]).

A related difficulty for thalamic disinhibition theories is that lesions of the ventrolateral thalamus do not result in akinesia, and yet according to such theories parkinsonian akinesia is generally attributed to increased basal ganglia outflow that results in excessive inhibition at the level of the ventrolateral thalamus[120]. One possible explanation for this apparent discrepancy is that we may have underestimated the functional significance of descending basal ganglia outflow to the PPN (and from there to the reticulospinal system), in which case lesions of the thalamus that block only the re-entrant (cortically-projected) influences of the basal ganglia may leave intact those descending influences that are conveyed more directly to the segmental motor apparatus.

Further inconsistencies and unanswered questions continue to surface, making it difficult to accept any of the current theories of basal ganglia function as definitive. For example, why should striatal dopamine deficiency lead to severe akinesia whereas structural lesions of the striatum fail to do so? And if basal ganglia dysfunction can lead to akinesia at one extreme and involuntary movements at the other, which suggests that the basal ganglia may play some role in the generation of movement, why is it that movement-related neuronal activity in the basal ganglia begins relatively late with respect to movement onset, well after the beginnings of movement-related activity in cortical motor areas or in the cerebellum[13,130,131]? And perhaps most disconcerting of all, what sort of role can the basal ganglia be playing in normal motor control, and how significant might that role be, if lesions of the output nuclei result only in minor disturbances of motor output[126,127]?

SUMMARY AND CONCLUSIONS

Enormous progress has recently been made in characterizing the structure and the functional organization of the basal ganglia. We now know which parts of the basal ganglia are involved in movement control, how movement parameters are encoded in the discharge patterns of basal ganglia neurons, how the basal ganglia communicate with cortical and other subcortical structures involved in movement control, how abnormal activity within the basal ganglia can lead to a variety of movement disorders, and how therapeutic manipulations of these nuclei can restore motor function in certain types of basal ganglia disorders.

At the same time, much has yet to be learned. Although the anatomy and physiology—and to some extent even the pathophysiology—of these structures are now understood in some detail, we still do not understand precisely what functions the basal ganglia subserve in the course of their normal operations. In particular, we have yet to learn what specific contributions the basal ganglia may make to the generation and co-ordination of voluntary movements. Of course, it should also be noted that the same can be said of virtually every other brain structure now known to be involved in skeletomotor control. Based on the impressive pace of recent discoveries concerning the functional organization of the basal ganglia, there is reason to hope that new insights into the basal ganglia's role in movement control may soon be forthcoming.

ACKNOWLEDGEMENTS

This work was supported by grants NS-17678 from the National Institutes of Health and N00014-92-J-1132 from the Office of Naval Research.

REFERENCES

1. Alexander, G. E., Crutcher, M. D. and DeLong, M. R. (1990) Basal ganglia-thalamocortical circuits: parallel substrates for motor, oculomotor, 'prefrontal' and 'limbic' functions. *Prog. Brain Res.*, **85**, 119–146.
2. Drum, R. P. and Strick, P. L. (1991) The origin of corticospinal projections from premotor areas in the frontal lobe. *J. Neurosci,*. **11**, 667–689.
3. Hoover, J. E. and Strick, P. L. (1993) Multiple output channels in the basal ganglia. *Science*, **259**, 819–821.
4. Flaherty, A. W. and Graybiel, A. M. (1993) Two input systems for body representations in the primate striatal matrix: experimental evidence in the squirrel monkey. *J. Neurosci.*, **13**, 1120–1137.
5. Flaherty, A. W. and Graybiel, A. M. (1991) Corticostriatal transformations in the primate somatosensory system. Projections from physiologically mapped body-part representations. *J. Neurophysiol.*, **66**, 1249–1263.
6. Künzle, H. (1975) Bilateral projections from precentral motor cortex to the putamen and other parts of the basal ganglia. An autoradiographic study in Macaca fascicularis. *Brain Res.*, **88**, 195–209.
7. Künzle, H. (1977) Projections from the primary somatosensory cortex to basal ganglia and thalamus in the monkey. *Exp. Brain Res.*, **30**, 481–492.
8. Künzle, H. (1978) An autoradiographic analysis of the efferent connections from premotor and adjacent prefrontal regions (areas 6 and 9) in macaca fascicularis. *Brain Behav. Evol.*, **15**, 185–234.
9. Cavada, C. and Goldman-Rakic, P. S. (1991) Topographic segregation of corticostriatal projections from posterior parietal subdivisions in the macaque monkey. *Neuroscience*, **42**, 683–696.
10. Selemon, L. D. and Goldman-Rakic, P. S. (1985) Longitudinal topography and interdigitation of cortico-striatal projections in the rhesus monkey. *J. Neurosci.*, **5**, 776–794.
11. Yeterian, E. H. and Pandya, D. N. (1993) Striatal connections of the parietal association cortices in rhesus monkeys. *J. Comp. Neurol.*, **332**, 175–197.
12. Alexander, G. E. and DeLong, M. R. (1985) Microstimulation of the primate neostriatum. II. Somatotopic organization of striatal microexcitable zones and their relation to neuronal response properties. *J. Neurophysiol.*, **53**, 1417–1430.
13. Crutcher, M. D. and Alexander, G. E. (1990) Movement-related neuronal activity selectively coding either direction or muscle pattern in three motor areas of the monkey. *J. Neurophysiol.*, **64**, 151–163.
14. Crutcher, M. D. and DeLong, M. R. (1984) Single cell studies of the primate putamen. I. Functional organization. *Exp. Brain Res.*, **53**, 233–243.
15. Hutchins, K. D., Martino, A. M. and Strick, P. L. (1988) Corticospinal projections from the medial wall of the hemisphere. *Exp. Brain Res.*, **715**, 667–672.
16. Hummelsheim, H., Wiesendanger, M., Bianchetti, M., Wiesendanger, R. and Macpherson, J. (1986) Further investigations of the efferent linkage of the supplementary motor area (SMA) with the spinal cord of the monkey. *Exp. Brain Res.*, **65**, 75–82.
17. Bauswein, E., Fromm, C. and Preuss, A. (1989) Corticostriatal cells in comparison with pyramidal tract neurons: contrasting properties in the behaving monkey. *Brain Res.*, **493**, 198–203.
18. Hartmann-von Monakow, A., Akert, K. and Künzle, H. (1978) Projections of the precentral motor cortex and other cortical areas of the frontal lobe to the subthalamic nucleus in the monkey. *Exp. Brain Res.*, **33**, 395–403.
19. Nakanishi, H., Kita, H. and Kitai, S. T. (1988) An N-methyl-D-aspartate

receptor mediated excitatory postsynaptic potential evoked in subthalamic neurons in an *in vitro* slice preparation of the rat. *Neurosci. Lett.*, **95**, 130–134.
20. Cherubini, E., Herrling, P. L., Lanfumey, L. and Stanzione, P. (1988) Excitatory amino acids in synaptic excitation of rat striatal neurones in vitro. *J. Physiol. (Lond)*, **400**, 677–690.
21. Kawaguchi, Y., Wilson, C.J. and Emson, P. C. (1989) Intracellular recording of identified neostriatal patch and matrix spiny cells in a slice preparation preserving cortical inputs. *J. Neurophysiol.*, **62**, 1052–1068.
22. Wilson, C. J. (1986) Postsynaptic potentials evoked in spiny neostriatal projection neurons by stimulation of ipsilateral and contralateral neocortex. *Brain Res.*, **367**, 201–213.
23. Valtschanoff, J. G., Weinberg, R. J. and Rustioni, A. (1993) Amino acid immunoreactivity in corticospinal terminals. *Exp. Brain Res.*, **93**, 95–103.
24. Kitai, S. T. and Deniau, J. M. (1981) Cortical inputs to the subthalamus: an intracellular analysis. *Brain Res.*, **214**, 411–415.
25. Donoghue, J. P. and Kitai, S. T. (1981) A collateral pathway to the neostriatum from corticofugal neurons of the rat sensory-motor cortex: an intracellular HRP study. *J. Comp. Neurol.*, **20**, 1–13.
26. Jones, E. G., Coulter, J. D., Burton, H. and Porter, R. (1977) Cells of origin and terminal distribution of corticostriatal fibers arising in the sensory-motor cortex of monkeys. *J. Comp. Neurol.*, **173**, 53–80.
27. Wilson, C. J. and Groves, P. M. (1980) Fine structure and synaptic connections of the common spiny neuron of the rat neostriatum: a study employing intracellular injection of horseradish peroxidase. *J. Comp. Neurol.*, **194**, 599–615.
28. Kita, H. and Kitai, S. T. (1988) Glutamate decarboxylase immunoreactive neurons in rat neostriatum: their morphological types and populations. *Brain Res.*, **447**, 346–352.
29. Selemon, L. D. and Goldman-Rakic, P. S. (1990) Topographical intermingling of striatonigral and striatopallidal neurons in the rhesus monkey. *J. Comp. Neurol.*, **297**, 359–376.
30. Flaherty, A. W. and Graybiel, A. M. (1993) Output architecture of the primate putamen. *J. Neurosci.*, **13**, 3222–3237.
31. Kimura, M., Kato, M. and Shimazaki, H. (1990) Physiological properties of projection neurons in the monkey striatum to the globus pallidus. *Exp. Brain Res.*, **82**, 672–676.
32. Alexander, G. E. and DeLong, M. R. (1985) Microstimulation of the primate neostriatum. I. Physiological properties of striatal microexcitable zones. *J. Neurophysiol.*, **53**, 1401–1416.
33. Liles, S. L. (1985) Activity of neurons in putamen during active and passive movements of wrist. *J. Neurophysiol.*, **53**, 217–236.
34. Alexander, G. E. and Crutcher, M. D. (1990) Preparation for movement: neural representations of intended direction in three motor areas of the monkey. *J. Neurophysiol.*, **64**, 133–150.
35. Alexander, G. E. and Crutcher, M. D. (1990) Neural representations of the target (goal) of visually guided arm movements in three motor areas of the monkey. *J. Neurophysiol.*, **64**, 164–178.
36. Kimura, M., Aosaki, T., Hu, Y., Ishida, A. and Watanabe, K. (1992) Activity of primate putamen neurons is selective to the mode of voluntary movement: visually guided, self-initiated or memory guided. *Exp. Brain Res.*, **89**, 473–477.
37. Kawaguchi, Y. (1992) Large aspiny cells in the matrix of the rat neostriatum *in vitro*: physiological identification, relation to the compartments and excitatory postsynaptic currents. *J. Neurophysiol.*, **67**, 1669–1682.
38. Wilson, C. J., Chang, H. T. and Kitai, S. T. (1990) Firing patterns and synaptic

potentials of identified giant aspiny in the rat neostriatum. *J. Neurosci.*, **10**, 508–519.

39. Kimura, M. (1986) The role of primate putamen neurons in the association of sensory stimuli with movement. *Neurosci., Res.* **3**, 436–443.
40. Bolam, J. P., Wainer, B. H. and Smith, A. D. (1984) Characterization of cholinergic neurons in rat striatum. A combination of choline acetyltransferase immunocytochemistry, Golgi-impregnation and electron microscopy. *Neuroscience*, **12**, 711–718.
41. Phelps, P. E., Houser, C. R. and Vaughn, J. E. (1985) Immunocytochemical localization of choline acetyltransferase within the rat neostriatum: a correlated light and electron microscopic study of cholinergic neurons and synapses. *J. Comp. Neurol.*, **238**, 286–307.
42. Uno, M., Ozawa, N. and Yoshida, M. (1978) The mode of pallido-thalamic transmission investigated with intracellular recording from cat thalamus. *Exp. Brain. Res.*, **33**, 483–507.
43. Yamamoto, T., Samejima, A. and Oka, H. (1985) An intracellular analysis of the entopeduncular inputs on the centrum medianum-parafascicular nuclear complex in cats. *Brain Res.*, **348**, 343–347.
44. Penney, J. B. Jr. and Young, A. B. (1981) GABA as the pallidothalamic neurotransmitter: implications for basal ganglia function. *Brain Res.*, **207**, 195–199.
45. Carpenter, M. B., Nakano, K. and Kim, R. (1976) Nigrothalamic projections in the monkey demonstrated by autoradiographic technics. *J. Comp. Neurol.*, **165**, 401–416.
46. Kim, R., Nakano, K., Jayaraman, A. and Carpenter, M. B. (1976) Projections of the globus pallidus and adjacent structures: an autoradiographic study in the monkey. *J. Comp. Neurol.*, **169**, 263–290.
47. DeVito, J. L. and Anderson, M. E. (1982) An autoradiographic study of efferent connections of the globus pallidus. *Exp. Brain Res.*, **46**, 107–117.
48. Ueki, A., Uno, M., Anderson, A. and Yoshida, M. (1977) Monosynaptic inhibition of thalamic neurons produced by stimulation of the substantia nigra. *Experientia*, **33**, 1480–1482.
49. Nauta, H. J. W. (1979) A proposed conceptual reorganization of the basal ganglia and telencephalon. *Neuroscience* **4**, 1875–1881.
50. Parent, A. (1986) *Comparative Neurobiology of the Basal Ganglia*. John Wiley & Sons, New York.
51. Fox, C. A. and Rafols, J. A. (1976) The striatal efferents in the globus pallidus and in the substantia nigra. In *The Basal Ganglia* (M. D. Yahr, Ed). Raven Press, New York, pp. 37–55.
52. Difiglia, M. and Rafols, J. A. (1988) Synaptic organization of the globus pallidus. *J. Electron Microsc. Tech.*, **10**, 247–263.
53. Mitchell, S. J., Richardson, R. T., Baker, F. H. and Delong, M. R. (1987) The primate globus pallidus: Neuronal activity related to direction of movement. *Exp. Brain Res.*, **68**, 491–505.
54. DeLong, M. R., Crutcher, M. D. and Georgopoulos, A. P. (1983) Relations between movement and single cell discharge in the substantia nigra of the behaving monkey. *J. Neurosci.*, **3**, 1599–1606.
55. Hamada, I., DeLong, M. R. and Mano, N-I. (1990) Activity of identified wrist-related pallidal neurons during step and ramp wrist movements in the monkey. *J. Neurophysiol.*, **64**, 1892–1906.
56. Alexander, G. E. and Crutcher, M. D. (1990) Functional architecture of basal ganglia circuits: neural substrates of parallel processing. *Trends Neurosci.*, **13**, 266–271.

57. Carpenter, M. B. and Jayaraman, A. (1990) Subthalamic nucleus of the monkey: connections and immunocytochemical features of afferents. *J. Hirnforsch.*, **31**, 653–668.
58. Smith, Y. and Parent, A. (1988) Neurons of the subthalamic nucleus in primates display glutamate but not GABA immunoreactivity. *Brain Res.*, **453**, 353–356.
59. Robledo, P. and Feger, J. (1990) Excitatory influence of rat subthalamic nucleus to the substantia nigra pars reticulata and the pallidal complex: electrophysiological data. *Brain Res.*, **518**, 47–54.
60. Kita, H. and Kitai, S. T. (1987) Efferent projections of the subthalamic nucleus in the rat: light and electron microscopic analysis with the PHA-L method. *J. Comp. Neurol.*, **260**, 435–452.
61. Parent, A. (1990) Extrinsic connections of the basal ganglia. *Trends Neurosci.*, **13**, 254–258.
62. Nakano, K., Hasegawa, Y., Tokushige, A., Nakagawa, S., Kayahara, T. and Mizuno, N. (1990) Topographical projections from the thalamus, subthalamic nucleus and pedunculopontine tegmental nucleus to the striatum in the Japanese monkey, Macaca fuscata. *Brain Res.*, **537**, 54–68.
63. Hazrati, L-N., Parent, A., Mitchell, S. and Haber, S. N. (1990) Evidence for interconnections between the two segments of the globus pallidus in primates: a PHA-L anterograde tracing study. *Brain Res.*, **533**, 171–175.
64. Bolam, J. P. and Smith, Y. (1992) The striatum and the globus pallidus send convergent synaptic inputs onto single cells in the entopeduncular nucleus of the rat: a double anterograde labelling study combined with postembedding immunocytochemistry for GABA. *J. Comp. Neurol.*, **321**, 456–476.
65. DeLong, M. R. and Georgopoulos, A. P. (1981) Motor functions of the basal ganglia. In *Handbook of Physiology. The Nervous System. Motor Control.* (J. M. Brookhart, V. B. Mountcastle, V. B. Brooks and S. R. Geiger, Eds). Sect. 1, Vol. II, Pt. 2. American Physiological Society, Bethesda, pp. 1017–1061.
66. Parent, A. (1983) The subcortical afferents to caudate nucleus and putamen in primate: a fluorescence retrograde double labeling study. *Neuroscience* **10**, 1137–1150.
67. Francois, C., Percheron, G., Parent, A., Sadikot, A. F., Fenelon, G. and Yelnik, J. (1991) Topography of the projection from the central complex of the thalamus to the sensorimotor striatal territory in monkeys. *J. Comp. Neurol.*, **305**, 17–34.
68. Hazrati, L-N. and Parent, A. (1991) Projection from the external pallidum to the reticular thalamic nucleus in the squirrel monkey. *Brain Res.*, **550**, 142–146.
69. Jones, E. G. (1985) *The Thalamus*. Plenum Press, New York.
70. Uno, M. and Yoshida, M. (1975) Monosynaptic inhibition of thalamic neurons produced by stimulation of the pallidal nucleus in cats. *Brain Res.*, **99**, 377–380.
71. Wilson, C. J., Chang, H. T. and Kitai, S. T. (1983) Disfacilitation and long-lasting inhibition of neostriatal neurons in the rat. *Exp. Brain Res.*, **51**, 227–235.
72. DeVito, J. L., Anderson, M. E. and Walsh, K. E. (1980) A horseradish peroxidase study of afferent connections of the globus pallidus in Macaca mulatta. *Exp. Brain Res.*, **38**, 65–73.
73. Harnois, C. and Filion, M. (1982) Pallidofugal projections to thalamus and midbrain: a quantitative antidromic activation study in monkeys and cats. *Exp. Brain Res.*, **47**, 277–285.
74. Hazrati, L-N. and Parent, A. (1991) Contralateral pallidothalamic and pallidotegmental projections in primates: an anterograde and retrograde labeling study. *Brain Res.*, **567**, 212–223.
75. Smith, Y., Hazrati, L-N. and Parent, A. (1990) Efferent projections of the subthalamic nucleus in the squirrel monkey as studied by PHA-L anterograde tracing method. *J. Comp. Neurol.*, **294**, 306–323.

76. Lee, H. J., Rye, D. B., Hallanger, A. E., Levey, A. I. and Wainer, B. H. (1988) Cholinergic vs. noncholinergic efferents from the mesopontine tegmentum to the extrapyramidal motor system nuclei. *J. Comp. Neurol.*, **275**, 469–492.
77. Rye, D. B., Saper, C. B., Lee, H. J. and Wainer, B. H. (1987) Pedunculopontine tegmental nucleus of the rat: cytoarchitecture, cytochemistry and some extrapyramidal connections of the mesopontine tegmentum. *J. Comp. Neurol.*, **259**, 483–528.
78. Hallanger, A. E., Levey, A. I., Lee, H. J., Rye, D. B. and Wainer, B. H. (1987) The origins of cholinergic and other 'nonspecific' afferents to the thalamus in the rat. *J. Comp. Neurol.*, **262**, 105–124.
79. Hallanger, A. E. and Wainer, B. H. (1988) Ascending projections from the pedunculopontine tegmental nucleus and the adjacent mesopontine tegmentum in the rat. *J. Comp. Neurol.*, **274**, 483–518.
80. Gonya-Magee, T. and Anderson, M. E. (1983) An electrophysiological characterization of projections from the pedunculopontine area to entopeduncular nucleus and globus pallidus in the cat. *Exp. Brain Res.*, **49**, 269–279.
81. Hammond, C., Rouzaire-Dubois, B., Feger, J., Jackson, A. and Crossman, A. (1983) Anatomical and electrophysiological studies on the reciprocal projections between the subthalamic nucleus and nucleus tegmenti pendunculopontinus in the rat. *Neuroscience*, **9**, 41–52.
82. Scarnati, E., Prioa, A., DeLoreto, S. and Pacitii, C. (1987) The reciprocal electrophysiological influence between the nucleus tegmenti pedunculopontinus and the substantia nigra in normal and decorticated rats. *Brain Res.*, **423**, 116–124.
83. Scarnati, E., Prioa, A., Campana, E. and Pacitii, C. (1986) A microiontophoretic study on the nature of the putative synaptic neurotransmitter in the pedunculopontine-substantia nigra pars compacta excitatory pathway in the rat. *Exp. Brain Res.*, **62**, 470–478.
84. Nakamura, Y., Kudo, M. and Tokuno, H. (1990) Monosynaptic projection from the pedunculopontine tegmental region to the reticulospinal neurons of the medulla oblongata: an electron microscopic study in the cat. *Brain Res.*, **524**, 353–356.
85. Nakamura, Y., Tokuno, H., Moriizumi, T., Kitao, Y. and Kudo, M. (1989) Monosynaptic nigral inputs to the pedunculopontine tegmental nucleus neurons which send their axons to the medial reticular formation in the medulla oblongata. An electron microscopic study in the cat. *Neurosci. Lett.*, **103**, 145–150.
86. Nambu, A., Yoshida, S. and Jinnai, K. (1988) Projection on the motor cortex of thalamic neurons with pallidal input in the monkey. *Exp. Brain Res.*, **71**, 658–662.
87. Nambu, A., Yoshida, S. and Jinnai, K. (1990) Discharge patterns of pallidal neurons with input from various cortical areas during movement in the monkey. *Brain Res.*, **519**, 183–191.
88. Nambu, A., Yoshida, S. and Jinnai, K. (1991) Movement-related activity of thalamic neurons with input from the globus pallidus and projection to the motor cortex of the monkey. *Exp. Brain Res.*, **84**, 279–284.
89. Yelnick, J., Percheron, G. and Francois, C. (1984) A golgi analysis of the primate globus pallidus. II. Quantitative morphology and spatial orientation of dendritic aborizations. *J. Comp. Neurol.*, **227**, 200–213.
90. Crutcher, M. D. and DeLong, M. R. (1984) Single cell studies of the primate putamen. II. Relations to direction of movement and pattern of muscular activity. *Exp. Brain Res.*, **53**, 244–258.

91. Georgopoulos, A. P., DeLong, M. R. and Crutcher, M. D. (1983) Relations between parameters of step-tracking movements and single cell discharge in the globus pallidus and subthalamic nucleus of the behaving monkey. *J. Neurosci.*, **3**, 1586–1598.
92. DeLong, M. R., Crutcher, M. D. and Georgopoulos, A. P. (1985) Primate globus pallidus and subthalamic nucleus: functional organization. *J. Neurophysiol.*, **53**, 530–543.
93. Schroder, K. E., Hopf, A., Lange, H. and Thorner, G. (1975) Morphemetrisch-statistche Strukturanalysen des Striatum, Pallidum und Nucleus Subthalamicus beim Menschen. I. Striatum. *J. Hirnforsch.*, **16**, 333–350.
94. Thorner, G., Lange, H. and Hopf, A. (1975) Morphometrisch-statische Strukturanalysen des Striatum, Pallidum und Nucleus Subthalamicus beim Menschen. II. Pallidum. *J. Hirnforsch.*, **16**, 401–413.
95. Brown, T. H., Kairiss, E. W. and Keenan, C. L. (1990) Hebbian synapses: biophysical mechanisms and algorithms. *Annu. Rev. Neurosci.*, **13**, 475–511.
96. Linsker, R. (1990) Perceptual neural organization: some approaches based on network models and information theory. *Annu. Rev. Neurosci.*, **13**, 257–281.
97. Smiley, J. F., Williams, S. M., Szigeti, K. and Goldman-Rakic, P. S. (1992) Light and electron microscopic characterization of dopamine-immunoreactive axons in human cerebral cortex. *J. Comp. Neurol.*, **321**, 325–335.
98. DeKeyser, J., Herregodts, P. and Ebinger, G. (1990) The mesoneocortical dopamine neuron system. *Neurology*, **40**, 1660–1662.
99. Gaspar, P., Berger, B., Febvret, A., Vigny, A. and Henry, J. P. (1989) Catecholamine innervation of the human cerebral cortex as revealed by comparative immunohistochemistry of tyrosine hydroxylase and dopamine-beta-hydroxylase. *J. Comp. Neurol.*, **279**, 249–271.
100. Calabresi, P., Maj, R., Pisani, A., Mercuri, N. B. and Bernardi, G. (1992) Long-term synaptic depression in the striatum: physiological and pharmacological characterization. *J. Neurosci.*, **12**, 4224–4233.
101 Calabresi, P., Pisani, A., Mercuri, N. B. and Bernardi, G. (1992) Long-term potentiation in the striatum is unmasked by removing the voltage-dependent magnesium block of NMDA receptor channels. *Eur. J. Neurosci.*, **4**, 929–935.
102. Walsh, J. P. (1993) Depression of excitatory synaptic input in rat striatal neurons. *Brain Res.*, **608**, 123–128.
103. Doucet, G., Descarries, L. and Garcia, S. (1986) Quantification of the dopamine innervation in adult rat neostriatum. *Neuroscience*, **19**, 427–445.
104. Schultz, W. and Romo, R. (1990) Dopamine neurons of the monkey midbrain: contingencies of responses to stimuli eliciting immediate behavioral reactions. *J. Neurophysiol.*, **63**, 607–624.
105. Romo, R. and Schultz, W. (1990) Dopamine neurons of the monkey midbrain: contingencies of responses to active touch during self-initiated arm movements. *J. Neurophysiol.*, **63**, 592–606.
106. Barto, A. G. (1992) Reinforcement learning and adaptive critic methods. In *Handbook of Intelligent Control: Neural, Fuzzy, and Adaptive Approaches* (D. A. White and D. A. Sofge, Eds). Van Nostrand Reinhold, New York, pp. 469–491.
107. Rauschecker, J. P. (1991) Mechanisms of visual plasticity: Hebb synapses. NMDA receptors, and beyond. *Physiol. Rev.*, **71**, 587–615.
108. Young, A. B., Dauth, G. W., Hollingsworth, Z., Penney, J. B., Kaatz, K. and Gilman, S. (1990) Quisqualate- and NMDA-sensitive [3H]glutamate binding in primate brain. *J. Neurosci. Res.*, **27**, 512–521.
109. Mercuri, N. B., Stratta, F., Calabresi, P. and Bernardi, G. (1992) A voltage-clamp analysis of NMDA-induced responses on dopaminergic neurons of the rat substantia nigra zona compacta and ventral tegmental area. *Brain Res.*, **593**, 51–56.

110. Kobayashi, T., Nagao, T., Fukuda, H., Hicks, T. P. and Oka, J. I. (1993) NMDA receptors mediate neuronal burst firing in rat somatosensory cortex *in vivo*. *Neuroreport*, **4**, 735–738.
111. Armstrong, J. M., Welker, E. and Callahan, C. A. (1993) The contribution of NMDA and non-NMDA receptors to fast and slow transmission of sensory information in the rat SI barrel cortex. *J. Neurosci.*, **13**, 2149–2160.
112. Iriki, A., Pavlides, C., Keller, A. and Asanuma, H. (1989) Long-term potentiation in the motor cortex. *Science*, **245**, 1385–1387.
113. Iriki, A., Pavlides, C., Keller, A. and Asanuma, H. (1991) Long-term potentiation of thalamic input to the motor cortex induced by coactivation of thalamocortical and corticocortical afferents. *J. Neurophysiol.*, **65**, 1435–1441.
114. Bindman, L. J., Murphy, K. P. S. J. and Pockett, S. (1988) Postsynaptic control of the induction of long-term changes in efficacy of transmission at neocortical synapses in slices of rat brain. *J. Neurophysiol.*, **60**, 1053–1065.
115. Baranyi, A. and Szente, M. B. (1987) Long-lasting potentiation of synaptic transmission requires postsynaptic modifications in the neocortex. *Brain Res.*, **423**, 378–384.
116. Chevalier, G. and Deniau, J. M. (1990) Disinhibition as a basic process in the expression of striatal functions. *Trends Neurosci.*, **13**, 277–280.
117. Hikosaka, O. and Wurtz, R. H. (1983) Visual and oculomotor functions of monkey substantia nigra pars reticulata. IV. Relation of substantia nigra to superior colliculus. *J. Neurophysiol.*, **49**, 1285–1301.
118. Hikosaka, O. and Wurtz, R. H. (1985) Modification of saccadic eye movements by GABA-related substances. I. Effect of muscimol and bicuculline in monkey superior colliculus. *J. Neurophysiol.*, **53**, 266–291.
119. Hikosaka, O., Sakamoto, M. and Usui, S. (1989) Functional properties of monkey caudate neurons. I. Activities related to saccadic eye movements. *J. Neurophysiol.*, **61**, 780–798.
120. DeLong, M. R. (1990) Primate models of movement disorders of basal ganglia origin. *Trends Neurosci.*, **13**, 281–285.
121. Miller, W. C. and DeLong, M. R. (1988) Parkinsonian symptomatology: an anatomical and physiological analysis. *Ann. NY Acad. Sci.*, **515**, 287–302.
122. Filion, M., Tremblay, L. and Bedard, P. J. (1988) Abnormal influences of passive limb movement on the activity of globus pallidus neurons in parkinsonian monkeys. *Brain Res.*, **444**, 165–176.
123. Bergman, H., Wichmann, T. and DeLong, M. R. (1990) Reversal of experimental parkinsonism by lesions of the subthalamic nucleus. *Science* **249**, 1436–1438.
124. Laitinen, L. V., Bergenheim, A. T. and Hariz, M. I. (1992) Leksell's posteroventral pallidotomy in the treatment of Parkinson's disease. *J. Neurosurg.*, **76**, 53–61.
125. Carpenter, M. B., Whittier, J. R. and Mettler, F. A. (1950) Analysis of choreoid hyperkinesia in the rhesus monkey: surgical and pharmacological analysis of hyperkinesia resulting from lesions in the subthalamic nucleus of Luys. *J. Comp. Neurol.*, **92**, 293–332.
126. Horak, F. B. and Anderson, M. E. (1984) Influence of globus pallidus on arm movements in monkeys. I. Effects of kainic-induced lesions. *J. Neurophysiol.*, **52**, 290–304.
127. Mink, J. W. and Thach, W. T. (1991) Basal ganglia motor control. III. Pallidal ablation: normal reaction time, muscle cocontraction, and slow movement. *J. Neurophysiol.*, **65**, 330–351.
128. Kato, M. and Kimura, M. (1992) Effects of reversible blockade of basal ganglia on a voluntary arm movement. *J. Neurophysiol.*, **68**, 1516–1534.
129. Steriade, M. and Llinas, R. R. (1988) The functional states of the thalamus and the associated neuronal interplay. *Physiol. Rev.*, **68**, 649–742.

130. Anderson, M. E. and Horak, F. B. (1985) Influence of the globus pallidus on arm movements in monkeys. III. Timing of movement-related information. *J. Neurophysiol.*, **54**, 433–448.
131. Thach, W. T. (1978) Correlation of neural discharge with pattern and force of muscular activity, joint position, and direction of intended next movement in motor cortex and cerebellum. *J. Neurophysiol.*, **41**, 654–676.

14 Structural Neuroimaging: Magnetic Resonance

ALINA GRECO
Centre Hospitalier Princesse Grace, Principality of Monaco

INTRODUCTION

The advent of magnetic resonance imaging (MRI) in clinical practice during the mid-1980s has had an enormous impact on paediatric neuroradiology. MRI is a non-invasive modality which employs radiofrequency radiation in the presence of a strong magnetic field. Multiplanar (coronal, axial and sagittal) pictures of the body, mapping the distribution of hydrogen nuclei and parameters related to their motion in cellular water and lipids are produced. Variation in the timing of the radiofrequency pulse produces changes in the contrast between different tissues, and pathological processes are highlighted. MRI is safe and provides unique information about brain anatomy.

The bony calvarium, inducing streak artefacts on computed tomography (CT) scans, and limiting the window for ultrasound (US) examinations, poses no difficulty for MRI studies.

The multiplanar imaging capabilities of MRI, combined with the differential contrast of the variety of pulse sequences available, allow improved detection of the morphostructural changes associated with neurological and/or developmental impairment[1].

Proton MRI spectroscopy, which can be integrated with conventional MRI equipment, allows a means of measuring the levels of various biochemical changes within the brain[2].

TECHNICAL CONSIDERATIONS

A detailed consideration of the technical aspects of MRI is beyond the scope of this chapter. As mentioned above, several inherent tissue parameters influence the MRI signal intensity, namely proton density, T1 and T2 relaxation times and flow. T1 and T2 relaxation times can be considered a type of measure of molecular motion.

Movement and Allied Disorders. Edited by M. M. Robertson and V. Eapen

MRI contrast depends on an interplay between the inherent tissue parameters and imaging parameters (pulse sequence, interpulse delay times, etc.) which are appropriately chosen by the operator at the time of the examination, according to the clinical problem.

The screening protocol for intracranial pathology includes first sagittal T1-weighted images. These serve as a localizer for axial as well as coronal T2-weighted and T1-weighted images, but also display the morphology of the corpus callosum, cerebellum, cortex, sellar and suprasellar regions, as well as of the craniocervical junction. The high level of grey–white matter contrast achieved with both T2- and T1-weighted images allows depiction of normal anatomy and improved detection of structural abnormalities which is unrivalled by the other available imaging modalities.

All MRI systems have the same basic components: a magnet, radiofrequency transmitter and receiver coil, gradient coils and sophisticated software to analyse the data.

MRI time varies according to the equipment used and the pulse sequence parameters chosen. In general, an adequate study requires between 20 and 30 min.

Inherent difficulties of examining very young, uncooperative patients are easily overcome by using appropriate sedation.

NORMAL PAEDIATRIC MRI ANATOMY

Due to the higher water content of the infant brain, both T1 and T2 relaxation times of the white matter are longer than the T1 and T2 of the grey matter. Therefore, during the first 6 months of life, the signal intensity of the white matter is lower than that of the grey matter on T1-weighted images, and higher than that of the grey matter on T2-weighted images.

Normal infants after the age of 12 months show a progressive increase in the signal intensity of myelinated white matter on T1-weighted images. Myelinated white matter is hypointense relative to grey matter on T2-weighted images (see Fig. 14.1).

Early in childhood, normal basal ganglia are isointense relative to the cortex on T2-weighted images (Fig. 14.1). With normal maturation, progressive darkening of the signal intensity of the deep grey nuclei is seen on T2-weighted images. In the mature brain, the extrapyramidal nuclei contain a relatively high concentration of iron, which is relatively more prominent in the globus pallidus, followed by the red nucleus, substantia nigra and putamen[3]. The deposition of iron in the extrapyramidal system is responsible for the T2 effect, that is a local inhomogeneity in the magnetic field, responsible for spin dephasing and, consequently, signal loss on T2-weighted images.

Depending on the pathological process underlying the movement disorder, T2-weighted images may show either an increase or a decrease in the signal intensity of the basal ganglia or a combination of the two.

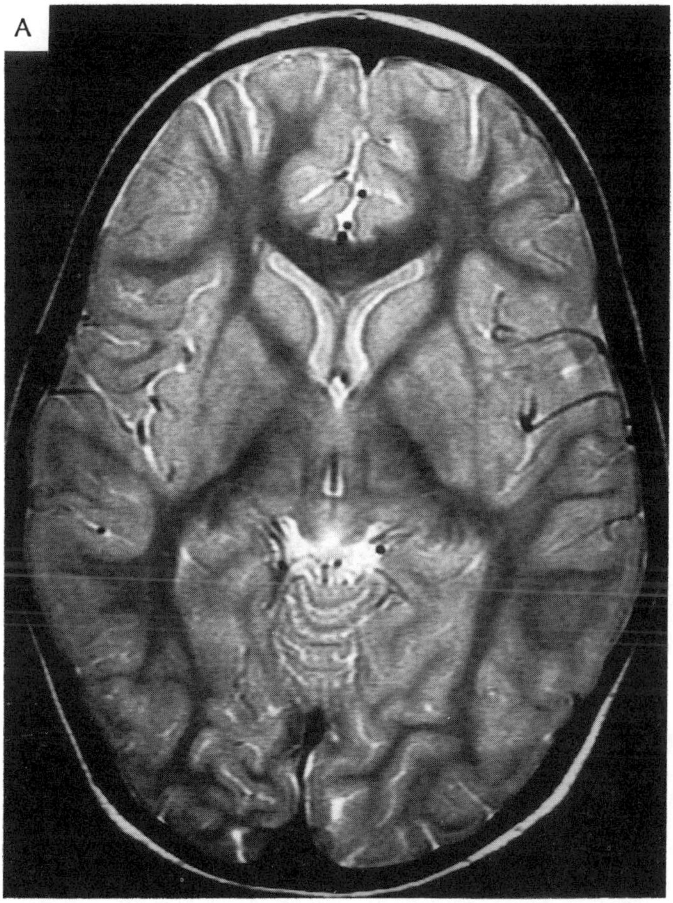

Figure 14.1.(A) Normal 4-year-old boy. Axial proton density (A), and axial T2-weighted image (B) images. Basal ganglia, white matter and grey matter. Myelinated white matter is hypointense relative to the grey matter due to the relatively short T2 of myelin. Cerebrospinal fluid is hyperintense, due to its very long T2 relaxation time

Figure 14.1. *continued overleaf*

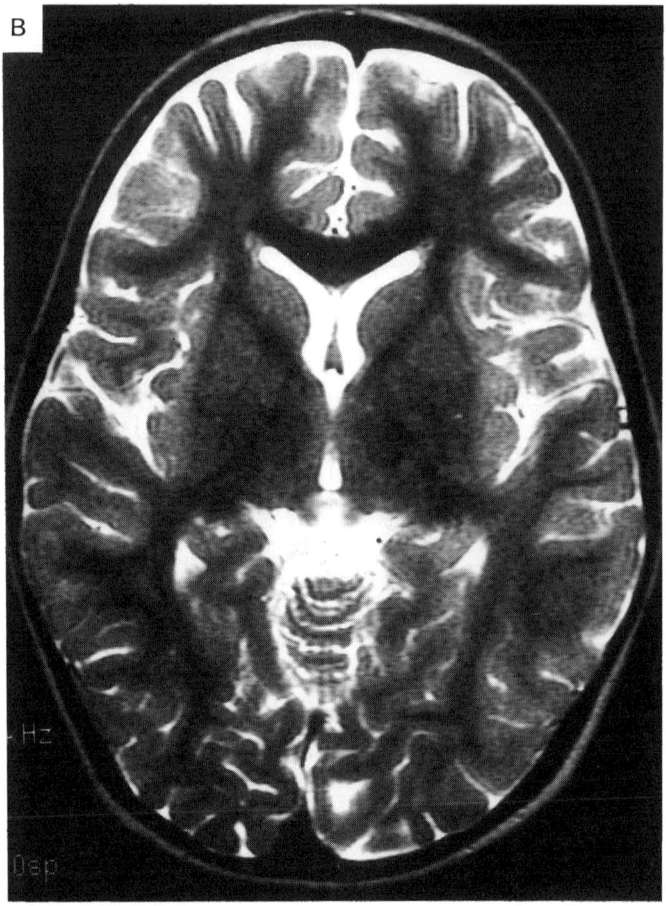

Figure 14.1.(B)

ABNORMAL CONDITIONS

The ability of MRI to display the nuclei of the extrapyramidal motor system helps the physician to correlate the neurological impairment with structural abnormalities involving the basal ganglia, which are revealed as signal changes (increased or decreased) as well as focal atrophy.

CHOREA

An increased signal in the corpus striatum contralateral to the patient's symptomatic side has been reported on T2-weighted images in children with acute onset of Sydenham's chorea[4]. In Huntington's disease and in

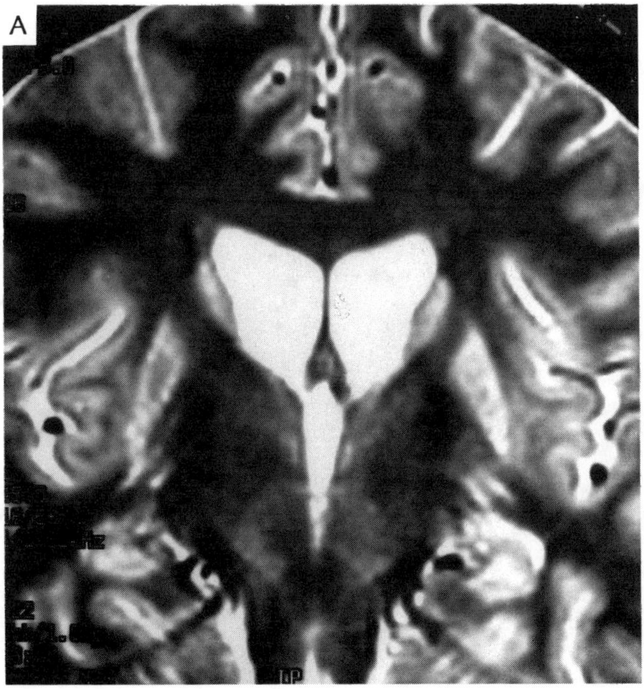

Figure 14.2.(A) Huntington disease. Coronal proton density (A) and coronal T2-weighted (B) images. Caudate nuclei and putamina display abnormal signal increase. On the coronal heavily T1-weighted (inversion recovery) image, (C), atrophy of the caudate nuclei and putamina is demonstrated, with signal reduction relative to normal globi pallidi

Figure 14.2. *continued overeleaf*

chorea-acanthocytosis, there is an abnormal signal involving the caudate and putamen (see Fig. 14.2). Atrophy of the caudate nuclei and, to a lesser extent, of the putamina, is also shown, with quantitative assessment of the frontal horn bicaudate ratio on coronal T1-weighted images (Fig. 14.2).

DYSTONIA

Dystonic conditions are also characterized by either an increase or a decrease in the signal intensity of the neostriatum. In patients with Hallervorden–Spatz disease[5], T2-weighted MRI shows hypo-intensity of the globus pallidus, reflecting excessive iron deposition at this level. There is no focal atrophy (Fig. 14.3).

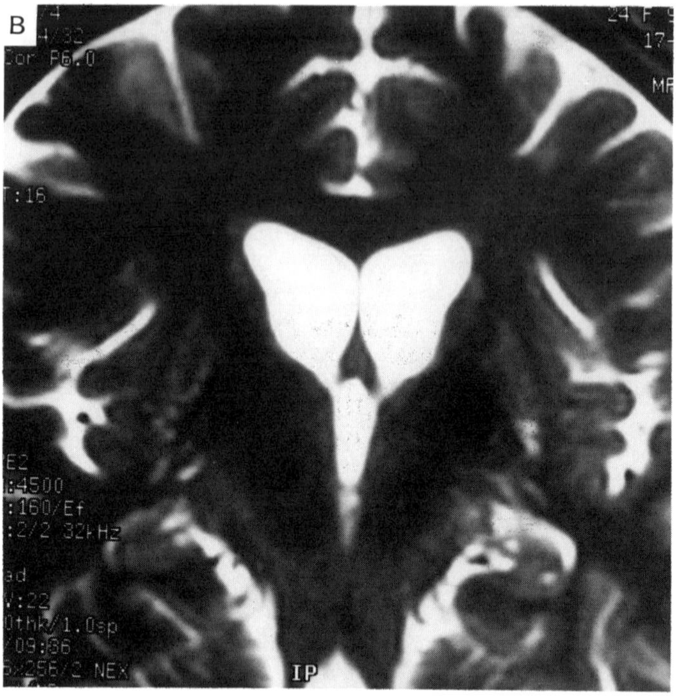

Figure 14.2.(B)

In Leigh's disease, symmetrical bilateral putaminal necrosis induces increased signal intensity on T2-weighted images[6] (Fig. 14.4).

MRI findings in Wilson's disease in children[7] include increased signal in the globus pallidus on T1-weighted images, presumably due to the accumulation of paramagnetic substances of some sort secondary to liver failure (Fig. 14.5). T2-weighted images are, in the early stages, normal or show signal reduction. Signal changes also occur in the thalamus as well as in the midbrain. In the advanced stages, necrosis and cystic changes account for T1 and T2 prolongation and, consequently, decreased signal on T1-weighted images and increased signal on T2-weighted images.

In phenylketonuria (Fig. 14.6), MRI signal abnormalities correlate with the described histopathological changes of cerebral white matter tracts, which vary from nonspecific vacuolization to frank demyelination and consist of white matter increased signal intensity on T2-weighted images.

Patchy to confluent areas of increased signal, most prominent in the periatrial regions, optic radiations and extending into the corona radiata, have been described[8–10]. However, none of the series published has shown clear correlation between the severity of the MRI white matter signal changes and IQ or diet.

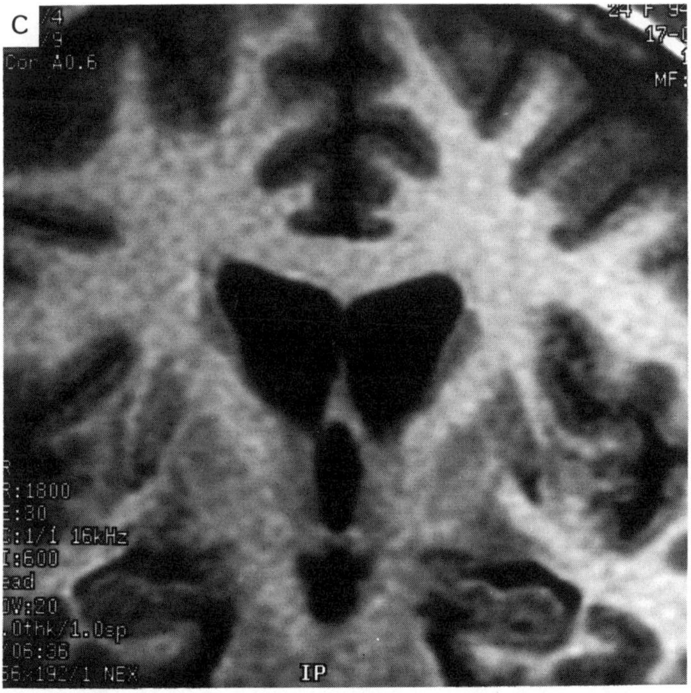

Figure 14.2(C)

HYPOXIA

MRI appears to be a powerful tool in assessing brain damage resulting from perinatal or prenatal asphyxia. Whatever the aetiology, hypoxia can result in diffuse basal ganglia injury[11] (Fig. 14.7).

RETT SYNDROME

Children with Rett syndrome have global brain hypoplasia and progressive cerebellar atrophy. MRI allows a quantitative assessment by measuring various dimensions of cerebral, cerebellar and brainstem structures on axial, sagittal and coronal images[12].

AUTISM

High resolution, three-dimensional volumetric MRI allows demonstration of cerebral volume loss in autistic children. Courchesne[13] has reported bilateral parietal cortical volume loss, extending to the adjacent superior

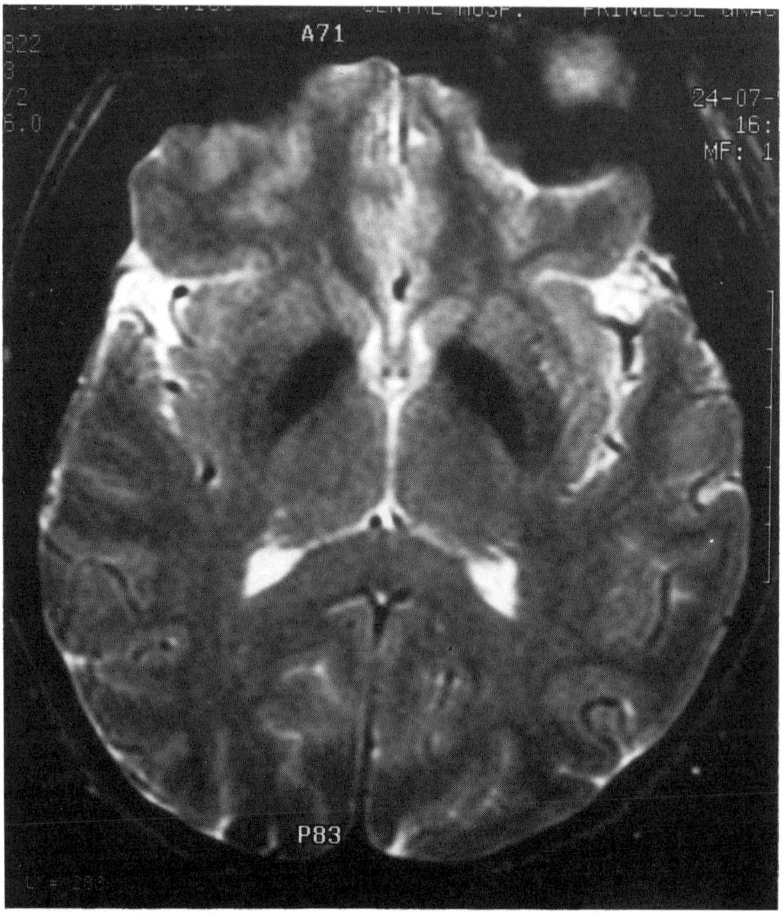

Figure 14.3. Hallervorden–Spatz disease. Axial T2-weighted image. There is a uniformly decreased signal of globus pallidus bilaterally, due to excessive iron deposition

frontal and occipital lobes. Thinning of the posterior corpus callosum and hypoplasia of the cerebellar vermis can also be demonstrated on sagittal MRI.

EPILEPSY

When an organic lesion needs to be ruled out in a young patient with a seizure disorder, MRI is the examination of first choice. In patients in whom no brain lesion is found on MRI or when EEG and MRI findings are

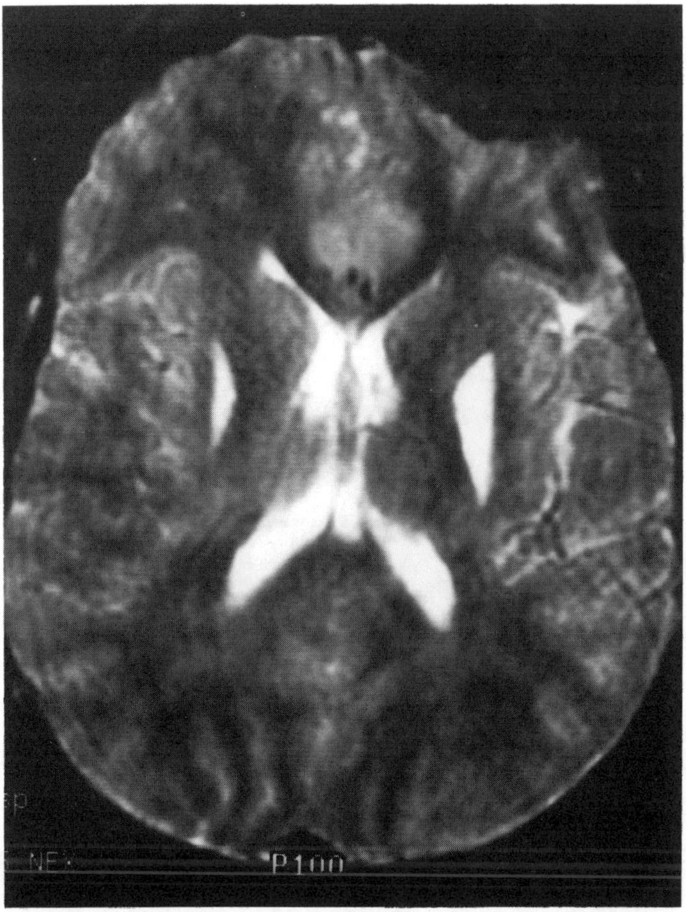

Figure 14.4. Leigh disease. Axial T2-weighted image. There is asymmetry of the putamina with associated marked signal increase. A pattern of hyperintense signal involving both putaminal regions is highly specific for Leigh disease. Head motion of the young, uncooperative patient has induced slight image degradation

discordant, then functional studies, such as single photon emission tomography (SPET) and positron emission tomography (PET) are needed.

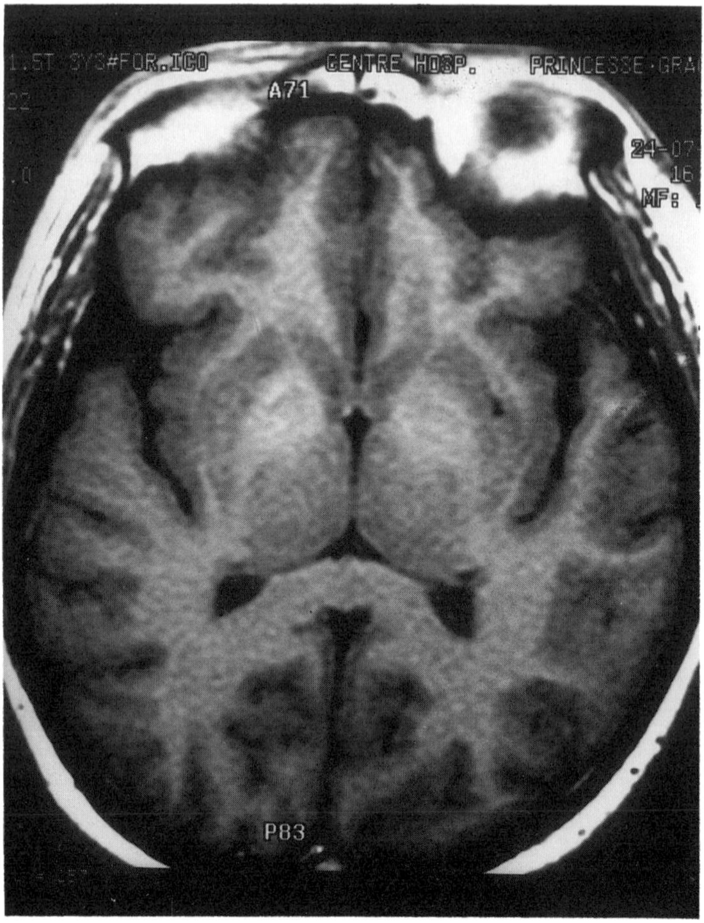

Figure 14.5. Wilson's disease. T1-weighted image. The signal intensity of the global pallidi is abnormally high. This is thought to be secondary to the accumulation of paramagnetic substances at this level secondary to liver failure

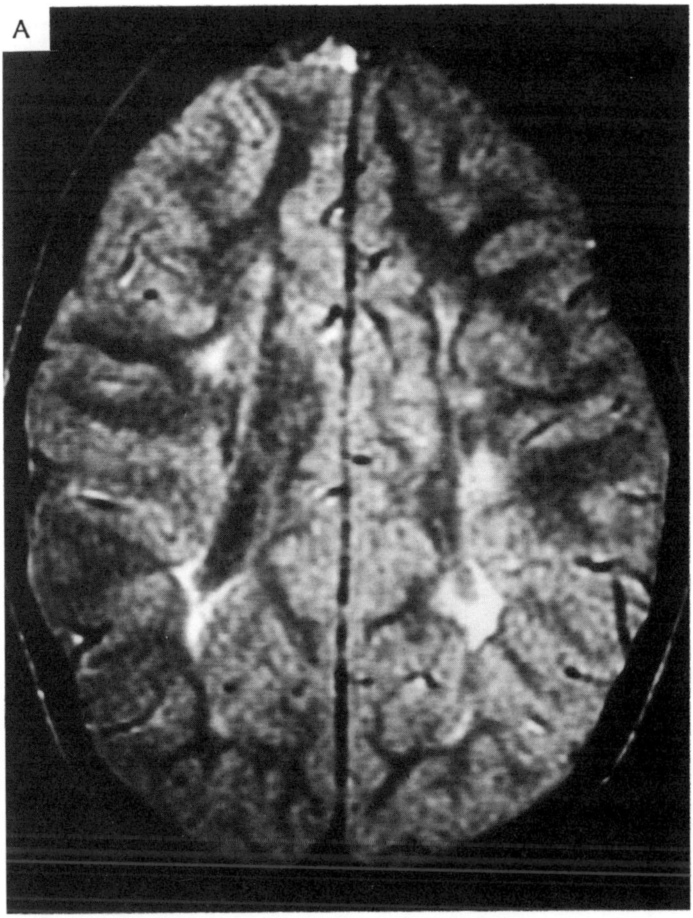

Figure 14.6.(A) Phenylketonuria. Axial proton density (A) and T2-weighted (B) images. There are patchy areas of abnormally high signal following the white matter distribution, with associated widening of the ventricular system

Figure 14.6. *continued overeleaf*

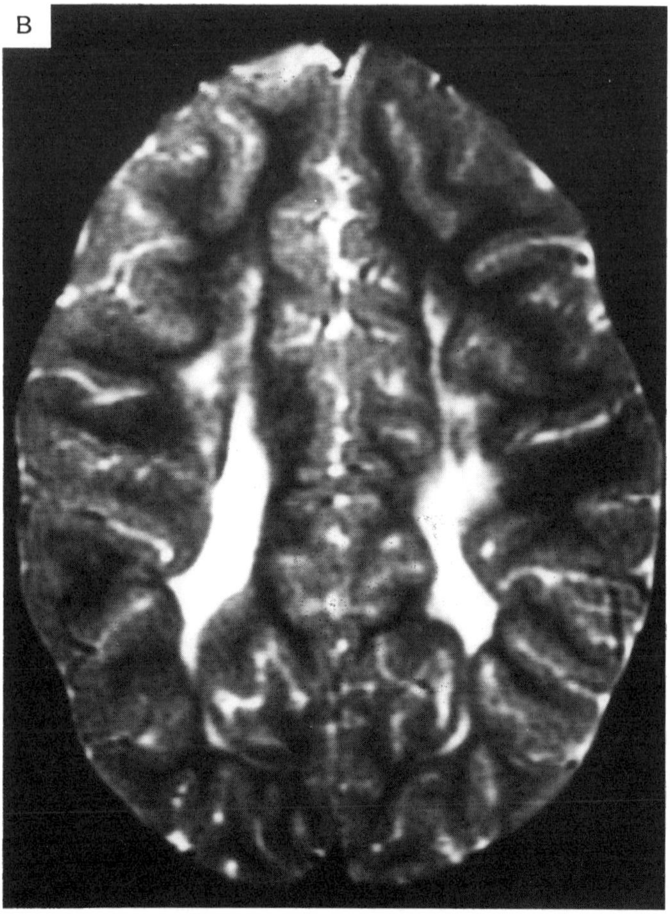

Figure 14.6.(B)

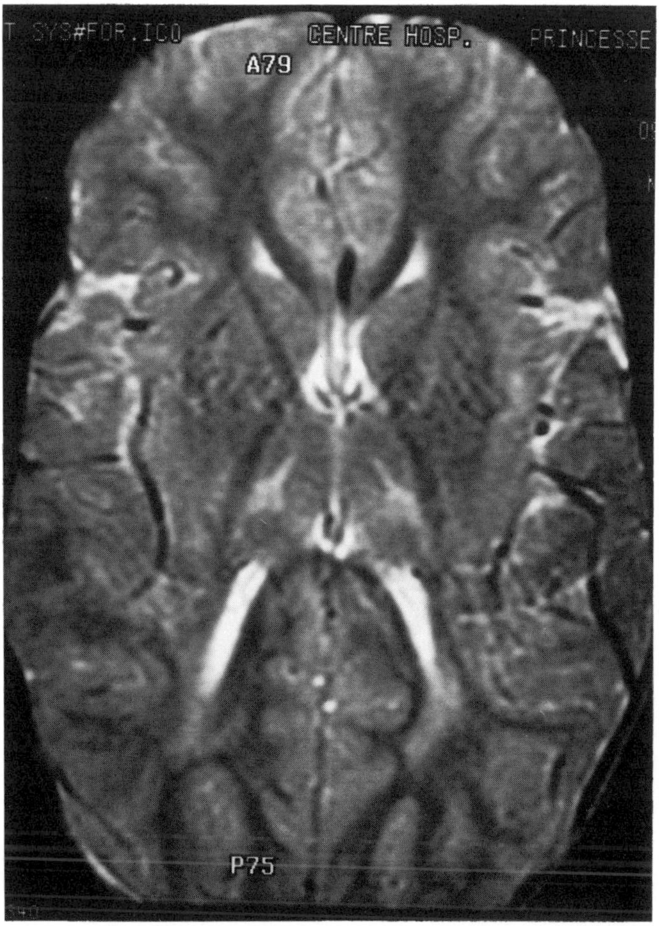

Figure 14.7. Perinatal asphyxia. Axial T2-weighted image. Both thalami are atrophic and display increased signal intensity

REFERENCES

1. Mirowitz Scott, A., Sartor, K., Prensky, A. J., Gado, M. and Hodges, F. (1991) Neurodegenerative diseases of childhood: MR and CT evaluation. *J. Comput. Assist. Tomogr.*, **15**, 210–220.
2. Cirodd, W., Krageloh-Mann, I., Klose, V. and Sauter, R. (1991) Metabolic and destructive brain disorders in children: findings with localized MR spectroscopy. *Radiology*, **181**, 173–181.
3. Aoki, S., Okada, Y., Nishimura, K., Barkovich, A. J., Kjos, B. O., Brasch, R. C. and Norman, D. (1989) Normal deposition of brain iron in childhood and adolescence: MR imaging at 1.5 Tesla. *Radiology*, **172**, 381–385.

4. Kienzle, G. D., Breger, R. K., Chun, R. W. M., Zupanc, M. L. and Sacket, J. F. (1991) Sydenham chorea: MR manifestations in two cases. *Am. J. Neuroradiol.*, **12**, 73–76.
5. Savoiardo, M., Halliday, W. C., Nardocci, N., Strada, L., D'Incerti, L., Angelini, L., Rumi, V. and Tesoro-Tess, J. D. (1993), Hallervorden–Spatz disease: MR and pathologic findings. *Am. J. Neuroradiol.*, **14**, 155–162.
6. Medina, L., Chi, T. L., Devivo, D. C. and Hilal, S. K. (1990) MR findings in patients with subacute necrotizing encephalomyelopathy (Leigh syndrome): correlation with biochemical defect. *Am. J. Neuroradiol.*, **11**, 379–384.
7. Kim, I., Yeon, K. M., Kin, W. S., Seo, J. K. and Han, M. C. (1993) MR imaging of the brain in Wilson disease in childhood. *Radiology*, **189**, 195.
8. Pearsen, K. D., Geant-Marton, A. D., Levy, H. L. and Davis, K. R. (1990) Phenylketonuria: MR imaging of the brain with clinical correlation, *Radiology*, **177**, 437–440.
9. Shaw, W. W. D., Weinberger, E. D. and Maravilla, K. (1990) Cranial MR in phenylketonuria. *J. Comput. Assist. Tomogr.*, **14**, 458–460.
10. Shaw, D. W. W., Maravilla, K. R., Weinberger, E. D., Garretson, J., Trahms, C. M. and Scott, C. R. (1991) MR imaging of phenylketonuria. *Am. J. Neuroradiol.*, **12**, 403–406.
11. Barkovich, A. J. and Truwit, C. L. (1990) Brain damage from perinatal asphyxia: correlation of MR findings with gestational age. *Am. J. Neuroradiol.*, **11**, 1087–1096.
12. Murakani, J. W., Courchesne, E., Haas, R. H., Press, G. A. and Yeung-Courchesne, R. (1992) Cerebellar and cerebral abnormalities in Rett syndrome: a quantitative MR analysis. *Am. J. Roentgenol.*, **159**, 177–183.
13. Courchesne, E., Press, G. A. and Yeung-Courchesne, R. (1993) Parietal lobe abnormalities in patients with infantile autism. *Am. J. Roentgenol.*, **160**, 387–393.

15 Radionuclide Neuroimaging

DURVAL CAMPOS COSTA
University College London Medical School, London UK

INTRODUCTION

Currently there is a wide variety of radiopharmaceuticals available to study brain functions. These drugs may be labelled with two types of radioactive elements (radionuclides): some emit positrons (positively charged electrons) and others decay into other elements by the emission of single photons from their nucleus. The former are the basic principle of positron emission tomography (PET), whilst the latter are used to carry out single photon emission tomography (SPET) also known as single photon emission computed tomography (SPECT). Both tomographic methodologies have been used to investigate, with success, a wide range of neuropsychiatric disorders in adults and children. A large body of literature demonstrating their research and clinical applications, particularly in adults, is already available.

Due to the recent development of new radiopharmaceuticals, both PET and SPET seem to be ideally suited to study the fundamental networks that become deranged during the evolution of movement disorders in general. In conjunction with high resolution structural imaging, particularly magnetic resonance imaging (MRI) (chapter 14), radionuclide neuroimaging techniques help to understand the physiology and biochemistry of both the pyramidal and extrapyramidal components of the motor system. In addition, there are PET and SPET radiotracers specifically designed to study crucial neurotransmission pathways implicated in the neuropathology of movement and allied disorders, thought to be based in the nigrostriatal system, particularly the basal ganglia[1,2]. In order to understand the clinical features and radionuclide neuroimaging modalities employed to study movement disorders, it is imperative to understand the fundamental neurochemistry of the interconnections between pyramidal, extrapyramidal and nigrostriatal systems. Thus the neurotransmitter implicated in the excitatory corticostriatal pathways is glutamate. The inhibitory striatonigral and striatopallidal pathways are both GABA-ergic and peptidergic (e.g. enkephalin, substance P, somatostatin and neuropeptide Y). The neurotransmitter of the nigrostriatal pathway is dopamine. The inhibitory transmission between the globus pallidus and the thalamus is made via GABA-ergic synapses. Taking

Movement and Allied Disorders. Edited by M. M. Robertson and V. Eapen

advantage of this knowledge, PET and SPET will play an increasing role in the management of patients with movement disorders, enabling the study of neuropharmacology *'in vivo'*.

RADIONUCLIDE NEUROIMAGING METHODOLOGIES

The first studies of brain function were carried out with the nitrous oxide method described by Kety and Schmidt[3]. Global cerebral blood flow (CBF) and oxygen utilization were measured *'in vivo'* in the developing brain. In nine normal children with age range of 3–11 years, the average global CBF was demonstrated to be approximately 1.8 times that of normal young adults[4]. It was also demonstrated that average cerebral oxygen utilization was higher in children than in adults. Later, larger series of patients were studied with radionuclide methods derived from the initial Kety–Schmidt technique. Initially Krypton-85 (^{85}Kr)[5] and later Xenon-133 (^{133}Xe)[6] were employed instead of nitrous oxide. However, these techniques lacked depth resolution, and no regional information on CBF values of deep structures could be obtained. The advent of tomography[7] made this a real possibility[8].

Tomography relies on the automatic acquisition of several equally spaced views around the brain (360° rotation is preferential). The number of views required is, to some extent, inversely proportional to the time per view—the more views around the brain are taken, the less time per view is needed. All the data acquired is then combined and 'reconstructed' using one of several algorithms according to the type of instrument. The reconstructed data is displayed as transaxial cross-sections of the brain. Nowadays, the majority of PET and SPET instruments have the ability to reorientate the reconstructed data in order to obtain oblique sections (transverse—parallel to the orbitomeatal or anterior commissure-posterior commissure lines, coronal and sagittal) as desired by the operator and the conditions of each particular study.

There are three main theoretical advantages of tomography. First, data is truly three-dimensional and volume measurements are relatively easy and only limited by the system resolution. Second, contrast resolution is much higher, allowing for the differentiation between grey and white matter in functional studies of the brain. Moreover, it enables the distinction between areas of grey matter or mixed brain substance with distinct tracer uptake. Finally, differences in uptake may be easily quantified. Theoretically, absolute quantification of the tracer uptake is possible if calibration with realistic phantoms and other corrections, particularly for radiation absorption, are performed.

RADIOPHARMACEUTICALS

The blood brain barrier (BBB) is the limiting step for the uptake of all radiopharmaceuticals in the brain tissue. Two main types of radiotracers are used to perform brain neuroimaging. The first is composed of tracers that cannot pass through the intact BBB and are thus referred to as the conventional BBB imaging radiopharmaceuticals. They are technetium-99m (^{99m}Tc) pertechnetate, ^{99m}Tc-diethylenetriamine penta-acetic acid (DTPA), ^{99m}Tc-glucoheptonate (GH) and thallium-201 (^{201}Tl) as thallous chloride. The other type of radiotracers consists of those with relatively high (although variable) lipophilicity, neutral charge and therefore able to cross the intact BBB[9]. PET and SPET involve the administration of one of these radiopharmaceuticals, made of an appropriate radionuclide labelling a specific drug or pharmaceutical. Tables 15.1 and 15.2 show the most common radionuclides used for PET and SPET respectively.

Each radiopharmaceutical is used to study a particular property of the central nervous system (CNS). It is possible to obtain information on regional cerebral blood flow (rCBF), nutrient utilisation (e.g. glucose), neurotransmitter physiology (at both pre- and postsynaptic levels), amino acid metabolism (e.g. methionine), etc. Although a large number of radiopharmaceuticals has been developed for use with PET and SPET, the most frequently used, to study patients with movement disorders, are shown in Table 15.3.

Table 15.1 Radionuclides commonly used for PET

Radionuclide	Photon energy (KeV)	Physical half-life (min)
^{82}Rb	511	1.25
^{15}O	511	2.0
^{13}N	511	10.0
^{11}C	511	20.0
^{68}Ga	511	68.0

Table 15.2 Radionuclides commonly used for SPET

Radionuclide	Photon energy (KeV)	Physical half-life (h)
^{99m}Tc	140	6.0
^{123}I	159	13.2
^{111}In	171, 245	67.3
^{201}TI	68–82	73.1
^{133}Xe	81	126.0

Table 15.3 Radiopharmaceuticals most commonly used in PET and SPET

	PET	SPET
Brain perfusion/rCBF	^{15}O-Water ^{13}N-Ammonia	^{133}Xe ^{99}Tc^{m}-HMPAO ^{99}Tc^{m}-ECD
Substrate utilization	^{18}F-FDG ^{11}C-Methylmethionine	–
Post-synaptic receptor imaging	^{18}F-Spiperone analogs ^{11}C-Flumazenil	^{123}I-IBZM ^{123}I-Iomazenil
Pre-synaptic receptor imaging	^{18}F-DOPA	^{123}I-βCIT

THE NORMAL BRAIN

Due to ethical considerations the study of normal brain function with radionuclide imaging is difficult, if not almost impossible. Radiation exposure, and particularly multiple venous and arterial sampling for quantitative PET studies are the major negative factors. Although several effective measures to reduce radiation exposure to children have been developed, it is still not morally and scientifically justifiable to perform radionuclide investigations in normal children. To obtain normal data it is necessary to use one of several strategies, passing through the use of children with transient neurological events that do not significantly interfere with normal neurological development, or other subjects in whom neurological diseases have been ruled out 'a posteriori'. It was by using similar strategies that the group from UCLA[10,11] defined so elegantly the maturation changes in cerebral function in infants with PET and ^{18}F-FDG. They included in their studies a group of 29 children with ages ranging from 5 days to 15 years, consisting of 16 males and 13 females. It was determined that the regional cerebral metabolic utilization rate of glucose in the first month of postnatal life was highest in the sensorimotor cortex, thalamus, brainstem and cerebellum, particularly the vermis. During the second and third months of extrauterine life, the glucose utilization increased in the basal ganglia, parietal, temporal, visual cortices (primary) and in the cerebellar hemispheres. The frontal cortex remained hypoactive until around the eighth month when together with the various associative cortical regions, the frontal cortices started to show significant increase in glucose metabolism. By the end of the first year of extrauterine life the anatomical distribution pattern of the regional cerebral glucose utilization rates was similar to the ones found in young healthy adults. The very low values of glucose utilization at birth rapidly rose to reach adult values by 2 years, and continued to rise until the third and fourth years when they were the highest. These high values were constant until 9–10 years of age, when they began to fall steadily to reach the values found in the latter part of the second decade.

It has been even more difficult to obtain data from SPET studies of rCBF using more widely available techniques. The same ethical considerations have played an important role in the lack of normative data in childhood. However, in some centres it has been possible to investigate, as in the UCLA studies, maturation changes in mature neonates with perinatal asphyxia and other neurological conditions, and who had no detectable clinical signs of neurological deficits by the end of their first year of extrauterine life[12]. They studied 11 babies and performed follow-up studies in four with ages ranging from 10 to 24 days. The follow-up studies were carried out in the first, fourth, seventh and twelfth months of life. Low rCBF values were found in the frontal and parietal cortices with strikingly high cerebellar and brainstem tracer uptake. The rCBF in the cortical regions increased significantly towards the end of the first year when the frontal hypoactivity was significantly less marked.

These reported measurements of glucose metabolism and rCBF represent only a small part of the functional changes in the developing brain during childhood that can be investigated with the aid of radionuclide imaging techniques. However, they are a fair and good representation of the wealth of information potentially gained by the utilization of these techniques. It is believed that in the foreseeable future, mapping of changes in other chemical maturation changes in the brain will be possible by using other already available methodologies which include neurotransmission imaging (dopamine D_2, benzodiazepine, presynaptic catecholaminergic system), protein synthesis, amino acid utilization (e.g. methionine), and other neuroreceptor imaging systems.

Plate 15.1 shows the distribution of rCBF in the brain of a healthy young adult obtained with SPET. It is similar to what can be seen in childhood as from age 3 or 4 years. The top row displays four transverse slices, the middle row four coronal slices and the bottom row four sagittal slices. The colour scale ranges from green (background) to white (the maximum in the study) with increasing steps through blue, orange and yellow. Brain structures with different rCBF values can be identified, particularly the cerebellar hemispheres, brainstem, frontal, parietal, visual cortices, basal ganglia (caudate nuclei and putamen), and thalamus in the transverse slices. The temporal cortices are particularly well seen in the coronal slices where they are displayed as small rings underneath the posterior frontal and parietal cortices. A direct comparison between frontal, parietal, temporal cortices and ipsilateral cerebellar hemispheres is possible with the sagittal slices.

Plate 15.2 shows the distribution of the ^{123}I-IBZM distribution in the brain of a healthy young adult obtained with SPET. Three transverse slices are shown. The one on the left (A) at the level of the cerebellum, the one in the middle (B) at the level of the basal ganglia, and the one on the right (C) at higher level through the periventricular white matter. The majority of the tracer uptake is seen in the striatum (middle slice), particularly the basal ganglia and, more intensely, in the caudate nuclei. The caudate nucleus/cortex (frontal or occipital) radioactivity ratio is 2.33 on the right and 2.30 on the left. The right over left radioactivity ratios for caudate and putamen are respectively 1.02 and 0.98, not significantly different from the unity. The caudate/putamen radioactivity ratios are 1.85 and 1.89 respectively on the right and left hemispheres.

ABNORMAL PATTERNS IN MOVEMENT DISORDERS

The basal ganglia have been considered the crucial set of structures implicated in the development of movement disorders, due to either their degeneration[1] or malfunction[2] and participation in the signs and symptoms manifested by patients. Amongst the wide range of movement and allied disorders, Gilles de la Tourette syndrome (GTS), epilepsy, cerebellar degeneration, Huntington's disease, Wilson's disease, obsessive–compulsive disorder and autism are the ones more frequently studied with radionuclide imaging techniques. Because different imaging methodologies and population samples have been used in different studies, the findings are sometimes conflicting and deserve further research with better design. However, some very important data have already been acquired. These data form important sources of reference and explain some of the clinical disturbances presented by each group of patients.

GILLES DE LA TOURETTE SYNDROME (GTS)

In GTS patients rCBF abnormalities are found in the basal ganglia and multiple cortical areas[13], particularly the frontal cortex[14] and its relationship with the striatum. Using PET to study the glucose metabolism, contradictory findings were reported by the same group of authors. An initial description of five GTS subjects showed increased glucose metabolism in the frontal cortex[15], whilst a later study of 12 untreated patients demonstrated reduction of the quantified glucose utilization rates in the frontal, cingulate and insular cortices, with an inverse correlation between the severity of both vocal and motor tics and glucose metabolic rates[16]. More recently, our group[17] has demonstrated statistically significant reductions of brain perfusion (rCBF) to the left caudate nucleus and anterior cingulate compared to normal controls. In addition, mildly affected patients were different from those moderately affected. The latter had worse perfusion ratios in the left anterior temporal cortex. Because the most significant abnormality was found in the striatum, dopamine D_2-receptor availability studies were carried out and showed a trend to lower binding of the ^{123}I-IBZM in the basal ganglia of GTS patients when compared to normals, particularly on the right hemisphere. However, the difference was not statistically significant and deserves further investigation with more homogeneous and better defined patient samples.

EPILEPSY

During the interictal, and particularly the postictal periods, both PET with FDG and SPET with rCBF/perfusion tracers there is reduction of the tracer uptake in the region of the epileptic focus. The opposite, increased tracer uptake in the region of the epileptic focus, is seen during the ictal phase.

Plate 15.3 shows two examples of interictal brain perfusion scans. The images display horizontal slices through the long axis of the temporal lobe in two cases of temporal lobe epilepsy on the left and right hemispheres, respectively on the top and bottom rows, compared to a normal control on the middle row.

It is well accepted that the sensitivity of brain perfusion (rCBF) SPET studies is at its best when the tracer is injected within a few seconds of the ictal period, reaching around 90% compared to EEG. Wide variations of sensitivity values (45–75%) have been reported in studies of the interictal period. Interestingly, patients with epilepsy and psychosis show reduced specific binding of IBZM to the dopamine D_2-receptor of the striatum compared to a control group of epileptic patients without psychosis[20]. This may be explained by a greater seizure-provoked release of dopamine, as previously suggested[21]. Indeed, epileptic patients treated with vigabatrin sporadically develop psychosis[22]. IBZM SPET studies before and after vigabatrin treatment in a group of six patients showed reduction of the IBZM binding to the striatum in the post-therapy compared to the pre-treatment study[23].

CEREBELLAR DEGENERATION

The characteristic pattern is seen in Plate 15.4 which demonstrates marked reduction in the rCBF to both cerebellar hemispheres and several cortical regions (left frontal and right temporal) probably due to deafferentation.

HUNTINGTON'S DISEASE

Although no systematic investigations of patients with Huntington's disease with either PET or SPET are available, there is increasing evidence of marked bilateral basal ganglia glucose hypometabolism[24], hypoperfusion and reduction of the dopamine D_2-receptor availability[25,26]. Presynaptic dopamine integrity seems to be intact in PET studies with ^{18}F-fluoro-L-DOPA[27].

WILSON'S DISEASE

Cerebral involvement in Wilson's disease (WD) is due to the deposition of copper throughout different brain structures with particular involvement of cerebellum, brainstem and basal ganglia, including the caudate nucleus and putamen. SPET studies of brain perfusion demonstrate reduction of the rCBF to the caudate and putamen, as well as other cortical regions[28]. IBZM SPET depicts reduction of the dopamine D_2-receptor availability[28,29] as shown in Plate 15.5. SPET studies of brain perfusion (HMPAO) and dopamine D_2-receptor availability (IBZM) of two sisters are shown. The slices are at similar basal ganglia level. The top row shows the studies of the asymptomatic carrier and the bottom row displays the studies of the sister with symptomatic WD. There is reduction of the perfusion and dopamine D_2-receptor availability in the right basal ganglia of the carrier—caudate/cortex = 1.92, caudate/putamen = 1.10. The symptomatic sister has marked bilateral reduction of the basal ganglia perfusion and availability of the dopamine D_2-receptors—caudate/cortex is equal to 1.45 (right) and 1.27 (left), caudate/putamen is 1.04 (right) and 0.99 (left). These images and unpublished data from our group indicate that ^{123}I-IBZM SPET will be able to detect very early abnormalities of the dopamine D_2-receptor availability in asymptomatic carriers of WD.

OBSESSIVE–COMPULSIVE DISORDER

Findings of PET and SPET studies in this heterogeneous syndrome are conflicting and sometimes contradictory. However, there is reported evidence of frontal hypometabolism with FDG PET[30]. rCBF SPET studies demonstrate elevated medial frontal cerebral blood flow[31].

AUTISM

This is another clinical area of conflicting evidence in different studies. Multiple explanations are available, mainly regarding patients' definition, in terms of intellectual performance and age of onset, and type of study, in particular, different methodologies employed to investigate similar cerebral functions. Frontal glucose hypermetabolism has been described, whilst more widespread reductions of regional perfusion were found more consistently[32].

OTHER DISEASES

A number of studies have reported abnormalities of brain perfusion, availability of dopamine D_2-receptors in the striatum and glucose metabolism changes in a wide variety of other movement disorders and related syndromes, particularly Rett syndrome[33,34], developmental stutterers[35], echolalia and palilalia[36].

Finally, it is important to mention that radionuclide imaging still plays an important role in the evaluation of patients with intracerebral space-occupying lesions, particularly in the differential diagnosis between postirradiation necrosis and tumour recurrence. ^{201}Tl as thallous chloride has demonstrated great potential in this area. Plate 15.6 shows an example of this tracer uptake in an intracerebral lymphoma in the left temporoparietal region.

REFERENCES

1. Penney, J. B. and Young, A. B. (1983) Speculations on the functional anatomy of basal ganglia disorders. *Ann. Rev. Neurosci.*, **6**, 73–94.
2. Penney, J. B. and Young, A. B. (1986) Striatal inhomogeneities and basal ganglia function. *Mov. Disord.*, **1**, 3–15.
3. Kety, S. S. and Schmidt, C. F. (1945) The determination of cerebral blood flow in man by the use of nitrous oxide in low concentrations. *Am. J. Physiol.*, **143**, 53–66.
4. Kennedy, C. and Sokoloff, L. (1957) An adaptation of the nitrous oxide method to the study of the cerebral circulation in children: Normal values for cerebral blood flow and cerebral metabolic rate in childhood. *J. Clin. Invest.*, **36**, 1130–1137.
5. Lassen, N. A. and Munck, O. (1955) The cerebral blood flow in man determined by the use of radioactive Krypton. *Acta. Physiol. Scand.*, **33**, 30–49.
6. Mallet, B. L. and Veall, N. (1963) Investigation of cerebral blood flow in hypertension, using radioactive-Xenon inhalation and extracranial recording. *Lancet*, **i**, 1081–1082.
7. Oldendorf, W. H. (1961) Isolated flying spot detection of radiodensity discontinuities—displaying the internal structural patterns of a complex object. *IRE Trans. Bio-Med. Elect. BME*, **8**, 68–72.
8. Kuhl, D. E. and Edwards, R. Q. (1970) The Mark III scanner. A compact device for multiple-view and section scanning of the brain. *Radiology* **96**, 563–570.
9. George, M. S., Ring, H. A., Costa D. C. *et al.* (Eds) (1991) *Neuroactivation and Neuroimaging with SPET.*, Springer-Verlag, London, pp. 3–28.
10. Chugani, H. T. and Phelps, M. E. (1986) Maturational changes in cerebral function in infants determined by [18]FDG positron emission tomography. *Science*, **231**, 840–843.
11. Chugani, H. T., Phelps, M. E. and Mazziotta, J. C. (1987) Positron emission tomography study of human brain functional development. *Ann. Neurol.*, **22**, 487–497.
12. Buga, K., Pávics, L., Sztriha, L., Kóbor, J. and Csernay, L. (1994) Relationship between human brain maturation and regional cerebral blood flow study in asphyxial neonates. *Eur. J. Nucl. Med.*, **21**, 734 (Abstract).

13. Hall, M., Costa, D. C., Shields, J., Heavens, J., Robertson, M. M. and Ell, P. J. (1991) Brain perfusion patterns with $^{99}Tc^{m}$-HMPAO/SPET in patients with Gilles de la Tourette syndrome—short report. *Nucl. Med.*, **27** (Suppl), 243–245.
14. George, M. S., Trimble, M. R., Costa, D. C., Robertson, M. M., Ring, H. A. and Ell, P. J. (1992) Elevated frontal cerebral blood flow in Gilles de la Tourette syndrome (GTS): A Tc-99m-HMPAO study. *Psychiatry Res.*, **45**, 143–151.
15. Chase, T. N., Foster, N. L., Fedio, P., *et al.* (1994) Gilles de la Tourette syndrome: studies with the fluorine-18-labelled fluorodeoxyglucose positron emission tomographic method. *Ann. Neurol.*, **15S**, S175 (Abstract).
16. Chase, T. N., Geoffrey, V., Gillespie, M., *et al.* (1984) Structural and functional studies of Gilles de la Tourette syndrome. *Rev. Neurol.*, **142**, 851–855.
17. Moriarty, J., Costa, D. C., Schmitz, B., Trimble, M. R., Ell, P. J. and Robertson, M. M. (1995) Brain Perfusion Abnormalities in Gilles de la Tourette's Syndrome. *Br. J. Psychiatry* (in press).
18. Costa, D. C., George, M. S., Ell, P. J., Pilowsky, L., Verhoeff, N. P. L. G. and Robertson, M. M. (1992) Dopamine D_2-receptor availability in patients with Gilles de la Tourette syndrome studied with SPET. *Nucl. Med.* **28** (Suppl), 414–417.
19. George, M. S., Robertson, M.M., Costa, D. C., Ell, P. J., Trimble, M. R., Pilowsky, L. and Verhoeff, N. P. L. G. (1994) Dopamine receptor availability in Tourette's syndrome. *Psychiatry Res.: Neuroimaging*, **55**, 193–203.
20. Ring, H. A., Trimble, M. R., Costa, D. C., Moriarty, J., Verhoeff, N. P. L. G. and Ell, P. J. (1994) Striatal dopamine receptor binding in epileptic psychosis. *Biol. Psychiatry*, **35**, 375–380.
21. Stevens, J. R. (1991) Psychosis and the temporal lobe. In *Adv. Neurol.* **55**, 79–96.
22. Sander, J. W. A. S., Hart, Y. M., Trimble, M. R. and Shorvon, S. D. (1991) Vigabatrin and psychosis. *J. Neurol. Neurosurg. Psychiatry*, **54**, 435–439.
23. Ring, H. A., Trimble, M. R., Costa, D. C., George, M. S., Verhoeff, N. P. L. G. and Ell, P. J. (1992) Effect of vigabatrin on striatal dopamine receptors: evidence in humans for interactions of GABA and dopamine systems. *J. Neurol. Neurosurg. Psychiatry*, **55**, 758–761.
24. Kuhl, D. E., Phelps, M. E., Markham, C. H., Metter, E. J., Riege, W. H. and Winter, J. (1982) Cerebral metabolism and atrophy in Huntington's disease determined by 18-FDG and computed tomographic scan. *Ann. Neurol.*, **12**, 425–434.
25. Boecker, H., Kuwert, T., Langen, K-J., Lange, H. W., Czech, N., Ziemons, K., Herzog, H., *et al.* (1994) SPECT with HMPAO compared to PET with FDG in Huntington's disease. *J. Comp. Assist. Tomogr.*, **18**, 542–548.
26. Ichise, M., Toyama, H., Fornazzari, L., Ballinger, J. R. and Kirsch, J. C. (1993) Iodine-123-IBZM dopamine D_2-receptor and technetium-99m-HMPAO brain perfusion SPECT in the evaluation of patients and subjects at risk for Huntington's disease. *J. Nucl. Med.*, **34**, 1274–1281.
27. Leenders, K. L., Frackowiak, R. S. J., Quinn, N. and Marsden, C. D. (1986) Brain energy metabolism and dopaminergic function in Huntington's disease measured *in vivo* using positron emission tomography. *Mov. Disord.*, **1**, 69–77.
28. Demetriadou, O., Costa, D. C., Gerasimou, G. P. and Walshe, J. (1994) Single photon emission tomography (SPET) in the assessment of patients with Wilson's disease. *Nucl. Med. Commun.*, **15**, 195 (Abstract).
29. Schwarz, J., Tatsch, K., Vogl, T., Kirsch, C. M., Trenkwalder, C., Arnold, G., Gasser, T. and Oertel, W. H. (1992) Marked reduction of striatal dopamine D_2-receptors as detected by ^{123}IBZM-SPECT in a Wilson's disease patient with generalized dystonia. *Mov. Disord.*, **7**, 58–61.
30. Martinot, J. L., Allilaire, J. F., Mazoyer, B. M., Hantouche, E., Huret, J. D.,

Legaut-Demare, F., Deslauriers, A. G., *et al.* (1990) Obsessive–compulsive disorder: a clinical, neuropsychological and positron emission tomography study. *Acta Psychiatr. Scand.*, **82**, 233–242.
31. Machlin, S. R., Harris, G. J., Pearlson, G. D., Hoehn-Saric, R., Jeffrey, P. and Camargo, E. E. (1991) Elevated medial-frontal cerebral blood flow in obsessive–compulsive patients: A SPECT study. *Am. J. Psychiatry*, **148**, 1240–1242.
32. George, M. S., Costa, D. C., Kouris, K., Ring, H. A. and Ell, P. J. (1992) Cerebral blood flow abnormalities in adults with infantile autism. *J. Nerv. Ment. Dis.*, **180**, 413–417.
33. Nielsen, J. B., Friberg, L., Lou, H., Lassen, N. A. and Sam, I. L. K. (1990) Immature pattern of brain activity in Rett syndrome. *Arch. Neurol.*, **47**, 982–986.
34. Yoshikawa, H., Fueki, N., Suzuki, H., Sakuragawa, N. and Masaaki, I. (1991) Cerebral blood flow and oxygen metabolism in Rett syndrome. *J. Child Neurol.*, **6**, 237–242.
35. Pool, K., Devous, M. D., Freeman, F. J., Watson, B. C. and Finitzo, T. (1991) Regional cerebral blood flow in developmental stutterers. *Arch. Neurol.*, **48**, 509–512.
36. Dierckx, R. A., Saerens, J., De Deyn, P. P. Verslegers, W., Marien, P. and Vandevivere, J. (1991) Evolution of technetium-99m-HMPAO SPECT and brain mapping in a patient presenting with echolalia and palilalia. *J. Nucl. Med.*, **32**, 1619–1621.

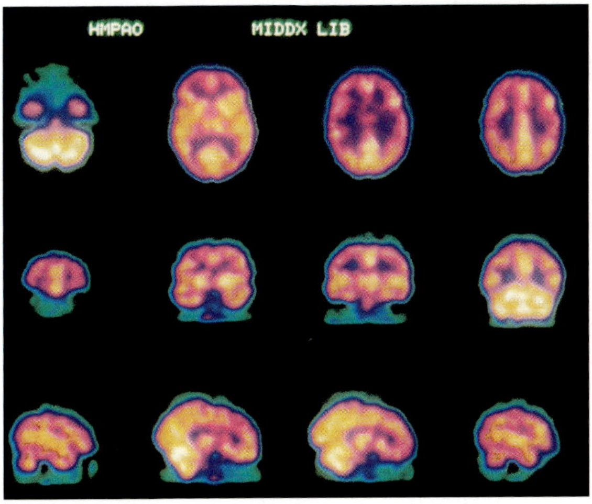

Plate 15.1 Brain perfusion SPET of a young healthy normal control

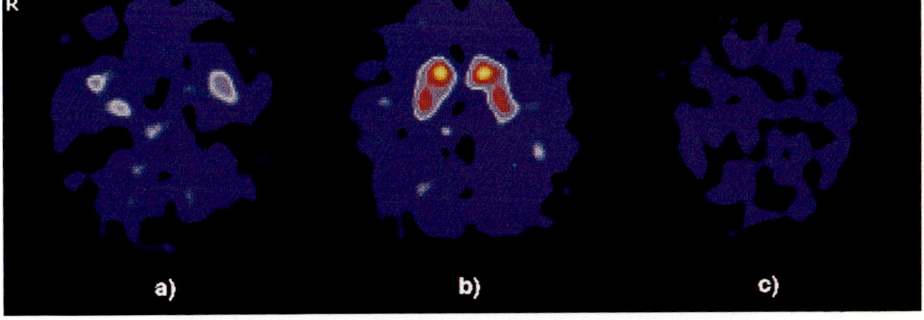

Plate 15.2 Three transverse slices of an IBZM SPET study of a normal control obtained at 2 hours post-injection are shown. R = right; a) level of cerebellum; b) level of basal ganglia; c) higher level through the periventricular white matter, frontal and parietal cortices

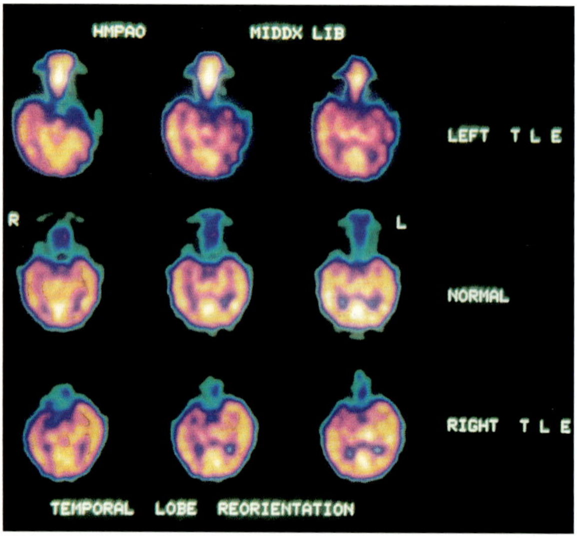

Plate 15.3 Horizontal long axis reorientation of the temporal lobes to show a case of left and a case of right temporal lobe epilepsy during the interictal period in comparison with a young healthy normal control

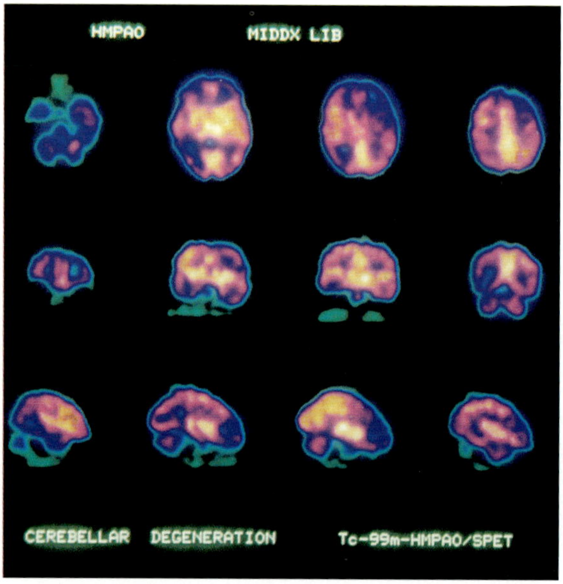

Plate 15.4 Cerebellar degeneration with very low perfusion to both cerebellar hemispheres and multiple cortical perfusion deficits

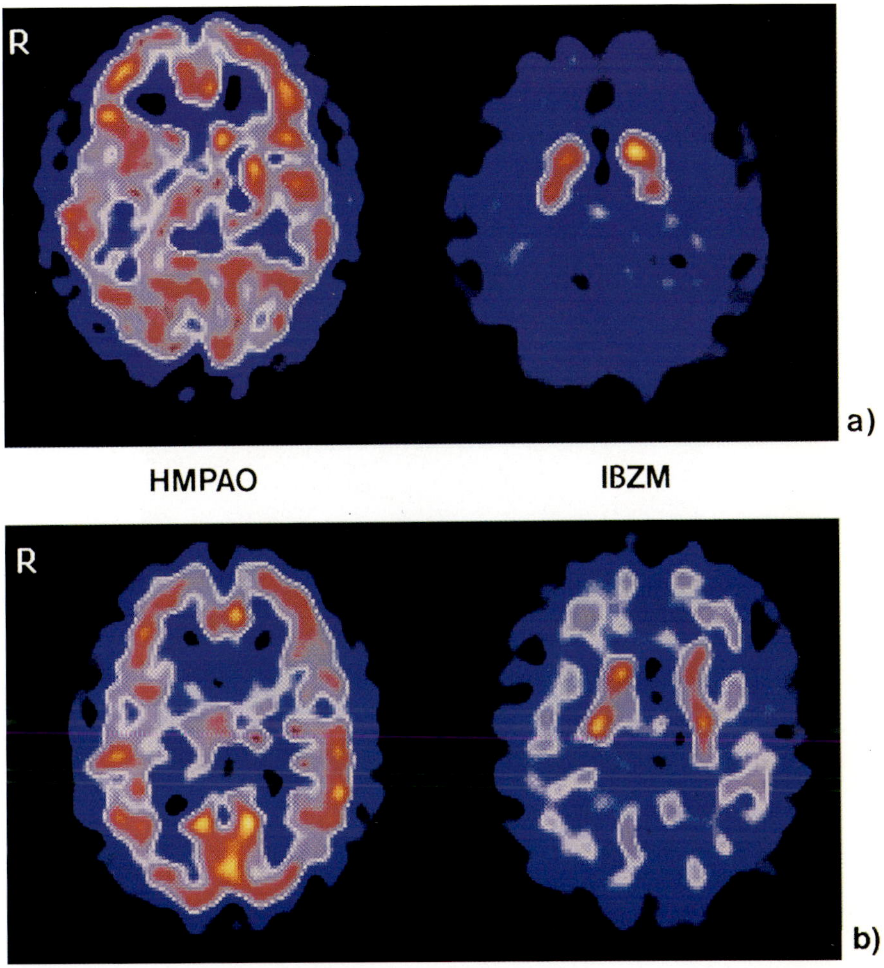

Plate 15.5 This figure shows the brain perfusion (HMPAO) and IBZM studies of two sisters. The studies on the top row a) are from an asymptomatic carrier of Wilson's disease, and the slices on the bottom row b) are from her Wilson's disease symptomatic sister. All the slices are at a similar level, through the basal ganglia. Perfusion is reduced in the right basal ganglia of the carrier and in both basal ganglia of the diseased sister. The abnormalities of the IBZM SPET are more marked

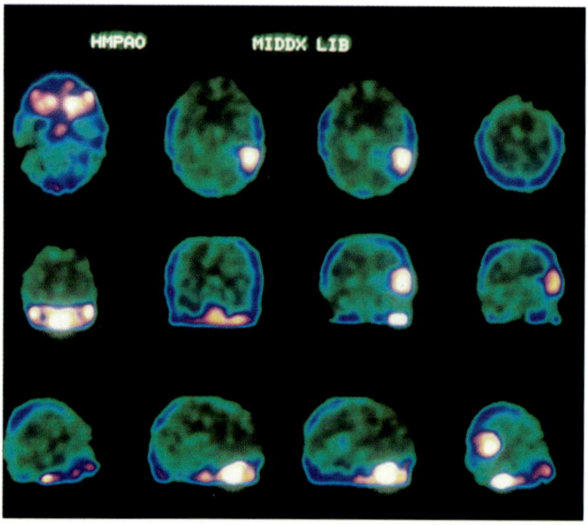

Plate 15.6 ^{201}Tl intracerebral focal uptake in a case of intracerebral lymphoma in the left temporo-parietal brain region

16 Developmental Dysexecutive Syndrome: Does it Exist? A Neuropsychological Perspective

SIMON BARON-COHEN
University of Cambridge, UK
and
JOHN MORIARTY
University of London, UK

ACTION CONTROL: NORMAN AND SHALLICE'S MODEL

In 1980, Norman and Shallice[1] proposed a general account of the control of action. The model was intended to account both for everyday slips of action (such as reaching for your keys at your front door, even when the door is not locked) to neurological disorders of action control (such as the perseverative behaviours of patients with frontal lobe damage). A schematic summary of their model is shown in Fig. 16.1.

Essentially, the model assumed that actions can be controlled in two

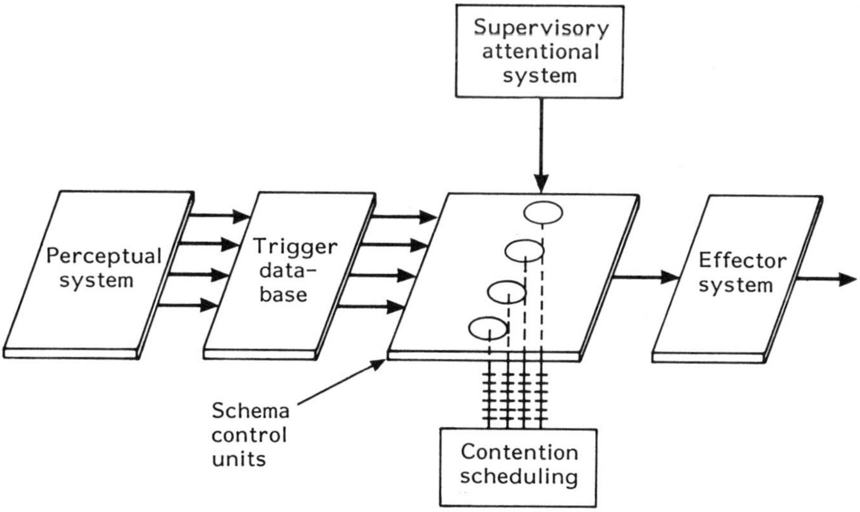

Figure 16.1. A schematic summary of Norman and Shallice's model of control of action

Movement and Allied Disorders. Edited by M. M. Robertson and V. Eapen

different ways. The first way is most clearly seen during well-learned, routine skills, in which strong learning effects allow actions to be performed relatively 'automatically'. An example that is often cited is driving a car. Experienced drivers can usually drive familiar routes whilst doing other things (having a conversation, thinking about a problem at work, etc.), even to the extent that when they stop to think about it, they may not be able to remember anything about the driving itself over the preceding 10 minutes or so. In such situations, action control is occurring in a complex and fluent fashion—the driver was breaking at the appropriate points during the journey, possibly overtaking other cars, changing gear appropriately, monitoring speed, and avoiding parked, obtruding vehicles, etc. Since the context for such driving is highly familiar, the 'automatic' action control system functions very successfully.

In Norman and Shallice's model, this automatic level of action control is explained as follows: well-learned actions are each represented by action-schemas, and built into each schema is information about their relative importance in given familiar contexts. It is the action-schemas which 'drive' the actions. As the contexts change, a process which the authors call 'contention scheduling' operates, whereby different possible schemas 'contend' with one another to determine which will be activated and executed.

However, the model also assumes that when the context becomes less familiar—for example, when novel events occur, then 'willed' action control can operate. This second action control system effectively allows the organism to act in a more 'deliberate' fashion, overriding the automatic activation of routine action schemas. This second system is called the 'supervisory attentional system' (or SAS). Thus, in the driving example above, on perceiving a less familiar event—e.g. a child who has fallen over in the street, the driver might stop the conversation s/he is engaged in, and 'decide' to stop the car and get out to help the child. It is the SAS that allows for such conscious decisions.

In Norman's subsequent work[2], this model was applied to the everyday *slips of action*, such as driving towards work on a weekend, when one really intended to drive to the supermarket. In this example, the routine action-schema for driving to work is activated by perceptual input but without any supervisory control, leading to the error. In contrast, Shallice[3] extended the theory in neuropsychological directions. He argued persuasively that patients with frontal lobe damage have a deficit in the SAS, leading to abnormalities in the planning, organizing and control of willed action. We turn to explore this neuropsychological direction in more detail next.

ACTION CONTROL AND FRONTAL LOBE DAMAGE

Three tasks on which patients with frontal lobe damage typically show difficulties are the Wisconsin card sorting test (WCST), the test of verbal fluency, and the Tower of London. These will now be briefly reviewed.

In the WCST, the subject is presented with a pack of cards with different numbers of shapes on each. Some shapes are circles, some triangles, some crosses or stars. The shapes vary in colour, number and form. The patient is asked to sort the cards into piles by following a rule. In the standard version the patient is not told the rule, but is given feedback as to whether s/he is correct or incorrect. In this way, the patient infers the rule the experimenter has in mind. (In modifications of this task, the patient is actually told the rule to sort the cards by.) The rule might be 'sorting by colour'. When it is clear that the patient is following this first rule, then the rule is changed without prior warning (e.g. sorting by number). The patient must now inhibit the 'learned' rule and discover the new rule. Again, once this has been followed clearly, the rule is again switched to a new one. Normal subjects find such rule-switching fairly easy and make few errors. In contrast, patients with frontal lobe damage typically persevere with the first rule they use, even when asked to try to switch to a new rule[4,5]. The brain region implicated in this rule switching is the left dorsolateral prefrontal cortex.

Similarly, on the verbal fluency task, patients are asked to come up with as many words as possible beginning with a specific letter (e.g. 'F'), in a one-minute period. Typically, patients with frontal lobe damage will produce relatively few new words (three or four), instead repeating the same few words that initially come to mind[6]. The normal person typically can produce at least a dozen, and usually as many as 30 or 40. The frontal lobe damaged patient may also break the rule and/or seek cues in the external environment. The brain region implicated in this verbal fluency task is the orbitofrontal cortex.

On the Tower of London problem (which is an adaptation of an older game, the Tower of Hanoi), the patient is shown a model of three pegs, with three differently coloured balls arranged on the pegs. This arrangement is called the 'initial position', and the patient is told to move the balls in order to reproduce a new pattern (the 'goal position'), in the fewest number of moves, and by only moving one ball at a time. Patients with left anterior frontal damage perform worse on this task[3].

Shallice's hypothesis is that such patients begin an activity, but then cannot interrupt it to change their behaviour flexibly, because they have an impairment in the SAS. The SAS in their case cannot interrupt ongoing actions to 'deliberately' switch to new actions. Thus, regarding the WCST, the patient with damage to the SAS continues to sort according to the previous rule, rather than changing to the new rule. Regarding the verbal fluency task, the idea is that because this is an unfamiliar task, there are no overlearned strategies for retrieving the information from memory, so the subject must produce novel retrieval strategies, normally a function of the SAS. Regarding the Tower of London task, the suggestion is that the task requires conscious planning, and inhibition of action prior to planning. Deficits in the SAS neatly explain four kinds of error: perseveration, poor generativity, impulsivity, and poor planning.

Shallice's hypothesis was also intended to account for a fifth symptom that such patients may show: distractibility. This is explained as follows: in the absence of an SAS, action-schemas can be triggered by any passing stimulus in the environment. Paradoxically, then, an impaired SAS can lead to two 'opposite' symptoms: perseveration and distractibility. The most extreme form of distractibility is seen in what L'Hermitte[7] described as 'utilization behaviour', where the patient grasps and uses any object that is presented to him or her, regardless of whether it is appropriate to do so. For example, seeing the clinician's spectacles lying on the table, the patient will pick them up and put them on his or her own face. Utilization behaviour has been reported in patients with frontal lobe damage (although many patients with frontal damage do not show utilization behaviour). Note that utilization behaviour has also been reported in patients with thalamic damage[8].

ACTION CONTROL AND WORKING MEMORY

Baddeley[9] makes an interesting link between the SAS from Norman and Shallice's model and the 'central executive' component in his own model of working memory. Here a small digression to summarize Baddeley's model of working memory will be made. Essentially, Baddeley's model proposes that short-term memory (STM) acts primarily as a working memory system, with three components (shown in Fig. 16.2). The first component is the central executive, which controls the allocation of attention and which coordinates the other two components, characterized as 'slave systems'. The two slave systems are summarized as follows:

1. The 'phonological loop'—this contains a phonological store, capable of holding phonological information-trace for about 1–2 s; and contains an articulatory control process, which reads such phonological traces and can rehearse them. It can also convert written information into a phonological code, and place it in the phonological store.
2. The 'visuo-spatial sketch pad'—this is held to be responsible for setting up and manipulating visuo-spatial images. Evidence from dual task paradigms suggest this is independent of the phonological loop.

In Baddeley's model, the central executive is held to allocate attention 'at will' to one or other of these two slave systems, enabling the subject to concentrate on phonological or visuo-spatial information processing. As mentioned above, Baddeley equates the central executive with the SAS. If this proposal is correct, then patients with frontal damage, who are held to

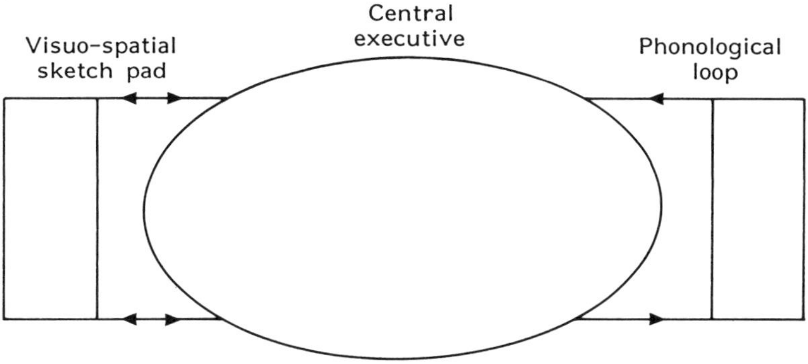

Figure 16.2. The three components of Baddeley's working memory system

have an impaired SAS, should also have problems in working memory. Shallice[5] and Baddeley and Wilson[10] summarize the evidence for 'frontal amnesia', and the evidence tying it to impairments in the SAS/central executive. On the basis of the evidence for SAS/central executive involvement in both attention-shifting, planning and working memory, Baddeley[11] coined the term *dysexecutive syndrome* to describe those patients with an impaired SAS/central executive.

DEVELOPMENTAL DYSEXECUTIVE SYNDROME

One obvious criticism of the SAS model is that it raises the 'homunculus' problem. That is, it implies that there is a system in the brain which controls all other systems, and which does so by exercising 'choice'. Whenever neural systems resemble homunculi, they pose problems, for the obvious reason that it is not clear what is controlling the homunculus. Another little homunculus inside the first one? An infinite regress looms large here. However, this argument can be levelled at many modular neurocognitive systems, and is not a fatal criticism. It simply means that the model needs greater specification in order to explain how the homunculus problem is to be avoided.

For the moment, let us accept both Shallice's and Baddeley's proposals about acquired frontal lobe damage in adulthood, and dysexecutive syndrome. Here we asked the question 'Is there a disorder which is a *developmental* instance of dysexecutive syndrome?' We aim to answer this question by briefly reviewing studies in which tests of the SAS have been used with clinical populations in childhood. In particular, we focus on autism, Gilles de la Tourette syndrome (GTS), attention deficit and hyperactivity disorder (ADHD), obsessive–compulsive disorder (OCD) and phenylketonuria (PKU). We approach this review highly selectively, by simply considering the use of the three tests above, as they have been applied to these five childhood neuropsychiatric samples.

AUTISM

Autism is a neurodevelopmental disorder characterized by abnormal social and communicative development, an absence of pretend play in childhood, and the presence of repetitive, perseverative, quasi-obsessional behaviour[12–14]. It is the latter symptoms that make it plausible that frontal lobe damage is involved in the disorder, given the resemblance to perseverative behaviour in adults with frontal damage. Adults with autism are significantly impaired on the WCST, relative to normal controls[15,16], and on the verbal fluency test, relative to dyslexic and normal controls[16]. In the latter study, the mean number of categories completed by the subjects with autism on the WCST was x = 1.7 (SD = 1.77), whereas for the dyslexic control subjects, the mean number of categories completed was x = 4.13 (SD = 1.19). Similarly, on the verbal fluency test, the mean number of words generated by the subjects with autism in 1 min was x = 30.8 (SD = 10.21), whereas for the subjects with dyslexia the mean number of words generated was x = 37.73 (SD = 9.8). Two studies[17,18] also reported a deficit on the WCST by subjects with autism, and the latter study[18] also found deficits on the other SAS test, the Tower of Hanoi.

Using a related measure (the Stockings of Cambridge, in which the subject has to move three balls from one 'billiard stocking' presented on a computer screen into another one, to match a new pattern of balls), Hughes and colleagues[19] also found deficits. Ozonoff and colleagues[20] also found that such executive function measures differentiated siblings of children with autism from siblings of children with mental handicap, suggesting that since autism has a genetic component[21], there may be a genetic abnormality in the development of executive function/the SAS in children with autism and their close relatives.

ATTENTION DEFICIT AND HYPERACTIVITY DISORDER (ADHD)

ADHD is a childhood disorder diagnosed when there are developmentally inappropriate degrees of inattention, impulsiveness and hyperactivity. The symptoms are usually present in a range of settings but can be confined to just one (e.g. at home). It is a common disorder, possibly occurring in as many as 3% of children, and is 5–10 times as common in males as in females in clinic populations (and three times as common in community samples). The disorder has its onset before the age of 7 years. The diagnosis is excluded in the presence of pervasive developmental disorder including autism. The diagnosis is only made if the behaviours are excessive for that child's mental age, and not only his or her chronological age. Thus, care must be taken in diagnosing ADHD in children with mental handicap. (For a full review of ADHD, see chapter 5.)

Chelune and colleagues[22] found that children with ADHD performed worse on the WCST than matched controls, and this was also reported by Gorenstein *et al.*[23]. This has not been consistently found, however (see Fischer *et al.*[24]; Loge *et al.*[25]). It may be that this impairment is more strongly linked to the conduct disorder that frequently co-occurs with ADHD, since the impairment has been found in children with conduct disorder[26]. Grodzinsky and Diamond[27] found boys with ADHD were impaired on the verbal fluency test, and this has also been reported by Felton *et al.*[28]. (Some failed replications of this have also been reported: see Grodzinsky and Diamond[27] for a discussion.)

PHENYLKETONURIA (PKU)

PKU is a classic inborn error of metabolism in which there is failure to metabolize phenylalanine (Phe) to tyrosine resulting in an accumulation of Phe in the blood, which becomes toxic[29]. (For a full review of PKU see chapter 7.) Early dietary treatment prevents the development of the severe mental handicap which is seen in this condition. However, even with dietary treatment, some mild deficits have been reported in executive function[30]. In this study, a variant of the verbal fluency test was used, namely a semantic fluency test, in which the subject has to name as many members of a specific semantic category as possible in 40 seconds. They also used the Tower of Hanoi. On the semantic fluency test, children with PKU produced a mean of $x = 14.09$ ($SD = 4.57$) words, whilst the control group produced a mean of $x = 20.82$ ($SD = 3.71$) words. On the Tower of Hanoi, the group with early-treated PKU were also significantly impaired. Pennington *et al.*[31] also reported that a group of older, early-treated children with PKU showed deficits on the WCST. Recently Diamond[32] has reported similar findings in very young children with early-treated PKU, using infancy measures of executive function.

GILLES DE LA TOURETTE SYNDROME (GTS)

GTS is a tic disorder characterized by the presence of multiple motor and one or more vocal tics. (For a full review see chapters 1, 2 and 3.)

Bornstein[33] found deficits on the WCST in children with GTS, and found that these correlated with obsessive–compulsive rather than the tic characteristics. Baron-Cohen *et al.*[34] found performance on a verbal fluency test task to be unimpaired in patients with GTS but they found impairments on the Tower of London task. In another study[35] they found a more specific deficit in what they term 'intention editing', as tested by the 'yes and no game', in which the subject has to answer a long series of closed questions without using the words 'yes' or 'no'. Subjects with GTS report more subjective difficulty in stopping themselves answering 'yes' or 'no', and made more errors on this task than normal children who were much younger.

OBSESSIVE–COMPULSIVE DISORDER (OCD)

OCD is a disorder with its onset typically in adolescence or early adulthood, although increasingly it is recognized that it may begin much earlier. The essential clinical feature is the presence of time-consuming obsessions and/or compulsions. Although the possible neurological basis of these symptoms was recognized in the last century, it has been regarded as a neurotic disorder of presumed psychological origin. (For a full review see chapter 4.) More recently, the presence of 'soft' neurological signs and impairments on traditional neuropsychological tests have been recognized.

Zielinski[36] reported that on the controlled oral word association (COWA) test (a word fluency test), and on the WCST, there were no group differences between patients with OCD and matched normal controls. Boone *et al.*[37] also report no group differences. However, Laplane *et al.*[38] reported that the majority of their patients with OCD were significantly impaired on a modified test of verbal fluency. This was also reported by Head *et al.*[39], who also found deficits in OCD patients on the WCST (short form). This was partially replicated by Christensen *et al.*[40].

NORMAL CHILDREN AND NEUROBIOLOGICAL FACTORS

It is worth pointing out that these tests are very sensitive to developmental factors. For example, Levin *et al.*[41] found that between the age groups of 7–8 years versus 9–12 years, major changes are seen on the WCST and on the verbal fluency test in normal children. On the latter test, the 7–8-year-old normal children generated a mean of $x = 15.9$ (SD = 6.3) words in 1 min, whilst the 9–12-year-olds generated a mean of $x = 26.3$ words (SD = 7.9). This implies that the 'growth' of executive function may be continuing until at least the end of childhood, possibly reflecting the maturation of the neural systems involved.

Regarding the neural basis to SAS, it has been reported that the WCST activates the dorsolateral prefrontal cortex (DLPFC) in normal subjects, as shown with single photon emission tomography (SPET)[42,43]. A position emission tomography (PET) study of word finding in four normal subjects[44] showed an increase in left dorsolateral prefrontal blood flow, consistent with an earlier study showing frontal activation[45]. Subjects with schizophrenia (who typically also have difficulty with the WCST) show reduced blood flow in the DLPFC during performance of this task[46]. Morris *et al.*[47] report DLPFC activation using SPET during a Tower of London task, with normal subjects. It is important to note that whilst frontal areas are implicated, it is likely that extrafrontal areas are also involved.

CONCLUSIONS

This review suggests that none of the five developmental disorders we have considered uniquely constitutes a developmental dysexecutive syndrome, in that, as measured by the three tests of WCST, Verbal Fluency, and/or the Tower of London/Hanoi, all five disorders have been reported to show deficits. Either this must mean that they *all* suffer from developmental dysexecutive syndrome—i.e. that it is a disorder that is so common that it is present in a wide range of neuropsychiatric syndromes—or it means that these tests are very sensitive to almost any kind of pathology. Either way, it throws doubt on the specificity of developmental dysexecutive syndrome.

We suggest that for theories of action control to have any explanatory power in relation to the range of disorders we have reviewed here, far more specific mechanisms will need to be postulated—possibly subcomponents of the SAS—each of which may be uniquely impaired in any specific neuropsychiatric disorder, thus accounting for the uniqueness of the symptoms observed. Our earlier proposal of an impaired intention editor in GTS is one example of this, which we suspect is indeed a subcomponent of the SAS[48]. In autism, the deficit in attributing mental states to themselves and others[49–51] appears to be unique to the syndrome (given an appropriate developmental level), and is therefore unlikely to be secondary to any SAS deficits. Future research needs to focus on demonstrating the specific links between such cognitive architecture, brain and behaviour.

ACKNOWLEDGEMENTS

During the preparation of this chapter, SBC was a member of the Institute of Psychiatry, University of London, and was supported by a grant from the Tourette Syndrome Association of the USA, and JM was supported by the Raymond Way Fund, Institute of Neurology. We are grateful to Mary Robertson, Donald Cohen, Michael Trimble, and Tim Shallice for discussions on this topic over the years. Catherine Mortimore also provided valuable feedback on this chapter.

REFERENCES

1. Norman, D. and Shallice, T. (1980) Attention to action: willed and automatic control of behaviour. In *Consciousness and Self-regulation*. Vol 4. (R. Davidson, G. Schwartz and D. Shapiro, Eds). Plenum Press, New York.

2. Norman, D. (1988) *The Psychology of Everyday Things*. Basic Books, New York.
3. Shallice, T. (1982) Specific impairments of planning. *Philos. Trans. R. Soc. Lond.*, **B 298**, 199–209.
4. Milner, B. (1964) Some effects of frontal lobectomy in man. In *The Frontal Granular Cortex and Behaviour*. (J. Warren and K. Akert, Eds). McGraw-Hill, New York.
5. Shallice, T. (1988) *From Neuropsychology to Mental Structure*. Cambridge University Press, Cambridge.
6. Perret, E. (1974) The left frontal lobe of man and the suppression of habitual responses in verbal categorical behaviour. *Neuropsychologia*, **16**, 527–537.
7. L'Hermitte, E. (1994) 'Utilization behaviour' and its relation to lesions of the frontal lobes. *Brain*, **106**, 237–255.
8. Eslinger, P., Warner, G., Grattan, L. and Easton, J. (1991) 'Frontal lobe' utilization behaviour associated with paramedian thalamic infarction. *Neurology*, **41**, 450–452.
9. Baddeley, A. (1991) *Human Memory: Theory and Practice*. Lawrence Erlbaum Associates, Hove.
10. Baddeley, A. and Wilson, B. (1988) Frontal amnesia and the dysexecutive syndrome. *Brain Cogn.*, **7**, 212–230.
11. Baddeley, A. (1986) *Working Memory*. Oxford University Press, Oxford.
12. Kanner, L. (1943) Autistic disturbance of affective contact. *Nervous Child* **2**, 217–250. Reprinted in Kanner, L. (1973) *Childhood Psychosis: Initial Studies and New Insights*. John Wiley and Sons, New York.
13. Wing, L. and Gould, J. (1979) Severe impairments of social interaction and associated abnormalities in children: epidemiology and classification. *J. Autism Dev. Disord.*, **9**, 11–29.
14. DSM-IV (1994) *Diagnostic and Statistical Manual of Mental Disorders*, 4th Edition, American Psychiatric Association, Washington, D.C.
15. Rumsey, J. and Hamburger, S. (1988) Neuropsychological findings in high functioning men with infantile autism, residual state. *J. Clin. Exp. Neuropsychology*, **10**, 201–221.
16. Rumsey, J. and Hamburger, S. (1990) Neuropsychological divergence of high-level autism and severe dyslexia. *J. Autism Dev. Disord.*, **20**, 155–168.
17. Prior, M. and Hoffman, W. (1990) Neuropsychological testing of autistic children through exploration with frontal lobe tests. *J. Autism Dev. Disord.*, **20**, 581–590.
18. Ozonoff, S., Pennington, B. and Rogers, S. (1991) Executive function deficits in high-functioning autistic children: relationship to theory of mind. *J. Child Psychol. Psychiatry*, **32**, 1081–1106.
19. Hughes, C., Russell, J. and Robbins, T. (1995) Evidence of a central executive dysfunction. *Neuropsychologia*, **32**, 477–492.
20. Ozonoff, S., Rogers, S., Farnham, J. and Pennington, B. (1995) Can standard measures identify subclinical markers of autism? *J. Autism Dev. Disord.* (in press).
21. Folstein, S. and Rutter, M. (1988) Autism: familial aggregation and genetic implications. *J. Autism Dev. Disord.*, **18**, 3–30.
22. Chelune, G., Ferguson, W., Koon, R. and Dickey, T. (1986) Frontal lobe disinhibition in attention deficit disorder. *Child Psychiatry Hum. Dev.*, **16**, 221–234.
23. Gorenstein, E., Mammato, C. and Sandy, J. (1989) Performance of inattentive-overactive children on selected measures of prefrontal type. *J. Clin. Psychol.*, **45**, 619–632.
24. Fischer, M., Barkeley, R., Edelbrock, C. and Smallish, L. (1990) The adolescent outcome of adolescent children diagnosed by research criteria. II: Academic,

attentional, and neuropsychological status. *J. Consult. Clin. Psychol.*, **58**, 580–588.

25. Loge, D., Staton, D. and Beatty, W. (1990) Performance of children with ADHD on tests sensitive to frontal lobe dysfunction. *J. Am. Acad. Child Adolesc. Psychiatry*, **29**, 540–545.
26. Taylor, E. (1994) Development and psychopathology of attention. In *Development through Life* (M. Rutter and D. Hay, Eds). Blackwell, Oxford.
27. Grodzinsky, G. and Diamond, A. (1992) Frontal lobe functioning in boys with attention deficit hyperactivity disorder. *Dev. Neuropsychol.*, **8**, 427–445.
28. Felton, R., Wood, F., Brown, I., Campbell, S. and Harter, M. (1987) Separate verbal naming deficits in attention deficit disorder and reading disability. *Brain Lang.*, **31**, 171–184.
29. Woo, S., Lidsky, A., Guttler, F., Chandra, T. and Robson, K. (1983) Cloned human phenylalanine hydroxylase gene allows prenatal diagnosis and carrier detection of classical phenylketonuria. *Nature*, **306**, 151–155.
30. Welsh, M., Pennington, B., Ozonoff, S., Rouse, B. and McCabe, E. (1990) Neuropsychology of early-treated phenylketonuria: specific executive function deficits. *Child Dev.*, **61**, 1679–1713.
31. Pennington, B., van Doorninck, W., McCabe, L. and McCabe, E. (1985) Neurological deficits in early treated phenylketonurics. *Am. J. Ment. Deficiency*, **89**, 467–474.
32. Diamond, A. (1994) Phenylalanine levels of 6–10 mg/dl may not be as benign as once thought. *Acta Paediatr.*, **83**, 89–91.
33. Bornstein, R. (1990) Neuropsychological correlates of obsessive characteristics in Tourette Syndrome. *J. Neuropsychiatry Clin. Neurosci.* **3**, 157–162.
34. Baron-Cohen, S., Moriarty, J., Mortimore, C. and Robertson, M. (1994) Executive function versus intention editing deficits in Gilles de la Tourette syndrome. Unpublished ms, Institute of Psychiatry, London.
35. Baron-Cohen, S., Cross, P., Crowson, M. and Robertson, M. (1994) Can children with Tourette's syndrome edit their intentions? *Psychol. Med.*, **24**, 29–40.
36. Zelinski, C., Taylor, M. and Juzwin, K. (1991) Neuropsychological deficits in obsessive–compulsive disorder. *Neuropsychiatry, Neuropsychol. Behav. Neurol.* **4**, 110–126.
37. Boone, K., Ananth, J., Philpott, L., Kaur, A. and Djenderedjian, A. (1991) Neuropsychological characteristics of non-depressed adults with obsessive–compulsive disorder. *Neuropsychiatry, Neuropsychol. Behav. Neurol.*, **4**, 96–109.
38. Laplane, D. Levasseur, M., Pillon, B., Dubois, B., Baulac, M., Mazoyer, B., Tran Dinh, S., Sette, G., Danze, F. and Baron, J. (1989) Obsessive compulsive and other behavioural changes with bilateral basal ganglia lesions. *Brain*, **112**, 699–725.
39. Head, D., Bolton, D. and Hymas, N. (1989) Deficit in cognitive shifting ability in patients with obsessive–compulsive disorder. *Biol. Psychiatry*, **25**, 929–937.
40. Christensen, K., Kim, S., Dysken, M. and Hoover, K. (1992) Neuropsychological performance in obsessive–compulsive disorder. *Biol. Psychiatry*, **31**, 4–18.
41. Levin, H., Culhane, K., Hartmann, J., Evankovich, K. and Mattson, A. (1991) Developmental changes in performance on tests of purported frontal lobe functioning. *Dev. Neuropsychol.*, **7**, 377–395.
42. Weinberger, D., Berman, K. and Zec, R. (1986) Physiologic dysfunction of dorsolateral prefrontal cortex in schizophrenia. I: Regional cerebral blood flow (rCBF) evidence. *Arch. Gen. Psychiatry*, **43**, 114–124.
43. Berman, K., Zec, R. and Weinberger, D. (1986) Physiologic dysfunction of dorsolateral prefrontal cortex in schizophrenia. II: The role of medication, attention, and mental effort. *Arch. Gen. Psychiatry*, **43**, 126–135.
44. Frith, C., Friston, K., Liddle, P. and Frackowiak, R. (1991) A PET study of word finding. *Neuropsychologia*, **29**, 1137–1148.

45. Parks, R., Lowenstein, D., Dodrill, K., Barker, W., Yoshii, F., Chang, J., Emran, A., Apicella, A., Sheramata, W. and Durar, R. (1988) Cerebral matabolic effects of a verbal fluency test: a PET scan study. *J. Clin. Exp. Neuropsychol.*, **10**, 565–575.
46. Berman, K., Illowsky, B. and Weinberger, D. (1988) Physiological dysfunction of dorsolateral prefrontal cortex in schizophrenia. IV: further evidence for regional and behavioural specificity. *Arch. Gen. Psychiatry*, **45**, 616–622.
47. Morris, R. *et al.* (1995) A SPECT study of the Tower of London task. *Neuropsychologia.*
48. Baron-Cohen, S., Robertson, M. and Moriarty, J. (1994) The development of the will: a neuropsychological analysis of Gilles de la Tourette's syndrome. In *The Self and its Dysfunction: Proceedings of the 4th Rochester Symposium* (D. Cicchetti and S. Toth, Eds). University of Rochester Press, New York.
49. Baron-Cohen, S., Leslie, A.M. and Frith, U. (1985) Does the autistic child have a 'theory of mind'? *Cognition*, **21**, 37–46.
50. Baron-Cohen, S. and Ring, H. (1994) A model of the mindreading system: neuropsychological and neurobiological perspectives. In *Origins of an Understanding of Mind* (P. Mitchell and C. Lewis, Eds). Lawrence Erlbaum Associates, Hove.
51. Baron-Cohen, S., Tager-Flusberg, H. and Cohen, D.J. (Eds) (1993) *Understanding Other Minds: Perspectives from Autism.* Oxford University Press, Oxford.

Index

action control
  frontal lobe damage, 306–8
  Norman and Shallice's model, 305–6
  working memory, 308–9
activity-dependent synaptic plasticity, N-methyl-D-aspartate receptors, 266
akathisia
  clinical features, 211–12
  combined scales, 229–30
  drug-related, 211–15
    as extrapyramidal disorder, 226
    course/outcome of, 213
    introduction to, 211
    pathophysiology, 213
    predisposing factors, 212–13
    prevalence/incidence of, 212
  single syndrome scales, 229
  tardive, 213
  treatment of, 214–15
ammonium tetrathiomolybdate, in Wilson's disease, 75
Angelman's syndrome, 191
anticholinergics
  acute dystonia, 206
  akathisia, 214
  drug-related parkinsonism, 210
anti-dopaminergic actions, 201
antiepileptic drugs, 201
antineuronal antibodies, and obsessive–compulsive disorder, 47–8
antipsychotics
  in acute dystonias, 204
  in tardive dyskinesia, 225
antistreptococcal antibodies, in obsessive–compulsive disorder, 48
anxiety, in obsessive–compulsive disorder, 48
Ashkenazi Jews
  idiopathic torsion dystonia, inheritance pattern of, 241
  9q markers, 244–5
Asperger's syndrome, 192–3
aspiny interneuron, basal ganglia motor circuitry, 260
ataxia
  and phenylketonuria, 88
  Friedreich's, 150
athetoid cerebral palsy, in developmental choreas, 107 (*table*)
athetosis, 180
atonic seizures, and drop attacks, 169–70
attention deficit disorder, 57–64
  behavioural approaches, 59
  gender difference in, 57
  and Gilles de la Tourette syndrome, 3–4, 20
  and movement disorders, 59–61
  operational definition of, 57–9
  and psychostimulants, 61–3
  and tic disorders, 61–3
  treatment of, 59
  treatment strategies, 63–4
autism, 310
  magnetic resonance imaging, 285–6
  radionuclide neuroimaging, 300
autosomal dominant inheritance
  cranial-cervical dystonia, 242
  Gilles de la Tourette syndrome, 18
  myoclonic dystonia, 123
autosomal recessive inheritance
  idiopathic torsion dystonia, 240
  phenylketonuria, 83, 84

ballismus, 180
  in chorea, 105
Baltic myoclonus, and progressive myoclonic epilepsies, 165
Barnes Akathisia Scale, 229
basal ganglia
  bilateral lucencies, 127–8
  calcification of, 127 (*table*)
    and dystonia, 126–7

basal ganglia *(cont.)*
  direct/indirect pathways, 262 *(fig.)*
  dysfunction
    in chorea, 106
    in hypoxia, 285
    in obsessive–compulsive disorder, 46
  functional models of, 266–9
  functional neuroanatomy of, 257–69
    role of dopamine, 265–6
  magnetic resonance imaging, 282
    thalamic reticular nucleus, 263
  motor circuitry of, 258–65
    direct/indirect pathways, 261–3
    functionally segregated circuits, 264–5
    globus pallidus, 261
    pedunculopontine nucleus, 263–4
    striatum, 260
    substantia nigra, 261
  organization
    current model limits, 268–9
    hyperkinetic disorders, 267–8
    hypokinetic disorders, 267
  output nuclei, 261, 263
  skeletomotor circuitry, 259 *(fig.)*
    movement control, 266
basal ganglia—thalamocortical loops, 257 *(fig.)*
  skeletomotor loop, 258
bedtime rituals, 48
benign familial chorea, in hereditary choreas, 109
benign idiopathic dystonia, in infancy, 123
benign myoclonic epilepsy, in infancy, 159
benzamides, in tardive dyskinesia, 225
benzhexol (Artane), in Wilson's disease, 76
bioamine neurotransmitter system, in dystonia, 115
blood brain barrier, radiopharmaceuticals, 295
bradykinesia, 200
  parkinsonism, 206–7
  single syndrome scales, 228
brain functions, radiopharmaceuticals and, 293
bucco-linguo-masticatory triad, in tardive dyskinesia, 216
bupropion and attention deficit disorder, 63
candidate gene approach, in tic disorders, 22–3
carbohydrate metabolism, disorders of, 183–4
central nervous system, and essential tremor, 134
cerebellar degeneration, radionuclide neuroimaging, 299
Children's Yale–Brown Obsessive–Compulsive Scale, 49
chlorpromazine, 199
chorea, 113
  aetiologies, 106–16
  athetosis, 105–13
  benign familial, 109
  developmental, 106–7
  and L-dopa therapy, 124
  drug-induced toxic, 111 *(table)*, 111–12
  hereditary, 107–10
  Huntington's, *see* Huntington's disease
  in hyperkinetic movement disorders, 180
  magnetic resonance imaging, 282–3
  metabolic/endocrine/nutritional, 112–13, 113 *(table)*
  and myoclonus, 150, 151
  paroxysmal, 109–10
  physiological, of infancy, 107 *(table)*
  Sydenham's, *see* Sydenham's chorea
choreiform syndrome, in developmental choreas, 107 *(table)*
choreoacanthocytosis, *see* neuroacanthocytosis
choreoathetosis, paroxysmal
  dystonic
    in hereditary choreas, 109
    treatment strategies, 116
  kinesiogenic, 116
clomipramine
  and attention deficit disorder, 63
  and obsessive–compulsive disorder, 52
clonazepam, in obsessive–compulsive disorder, 50
clonidine
  in attention deficit disorder, 62, 64
  in tardive dyskinesia, 225
clozapine, drug-related movement disorders, 201
compound heterozygotes, in phenylketonuria, 100
compulsive checking, 44

compulsive washing, 44
congenital rubella, and myoclonus, 157
contamination fears, 44
copper, in Wilson's disease, 70, 74
coprolalia, in Gilles de la Tourette syndrome, 2
copropraxia, in Gilles de la Tourette syndrome, 2
cortical atrophy, in Wilson's disease, 70
cortical inputs, basal ganglia motor circuitry, 258–60
cortico-basal ganglia-thalamocortical pathways, functionally segregated circuits, 264
corticostriatal neurons, basal ganglia motor circuitry, 258, 260
corticostriatal-thalamic-cortical circuits, in obsessive–compulsive disorder, 47
cranial-cervical dystonia, inheritance pattern, 242
cryptogenic myoclonic epilepsy, 158 *(fig.)*

dancing-eyes syndrome, and myoclonus, 157
defensive splitting, in Gilles de la Tourette syndrome, 33
degenerative disorders, rare, 178–9 *(table)*
dentatorubral-pallidoluysian atrophy, and dystonia, 125–6
deprenyl (monoamine oxidase inhibitor), and attention deficit disorder, 63
depression, parkinsonism and, 207
desipramine, and attention deficit disorder, 62
developmental dysexecutive syndrome, 305–13
  frontal lobe damage, 306–8
  Norman and Shallice's model, 305–6
  supervisory attentional system, 309
  working memory, 308–9
developmental delay, and phenylketonuria, 89, 90
dextroamphetamine, and attention deficit disorder, 59
dimercaprol, in advanced dystonic Wilson's disease, 75, 77
disinhibition, basal ganglia operation, 266
DNA-marker, in linkage analysis, 21–2
Doose syndrome, *see* myoclonic astatic epilepsy
dopa-responsive dystonia, 123–5
  childhood onset of, 124–5
  genetics of, 245–6
  pathophysiology of, 124
dopamine, in functional neuroanatomy of basal ganglia, 265–6
drop attacks, and complex partial seizures, 169
drug-related movement disorders, 199–231
  acute dystonias, 201–6
  akathisia, 211–15
  associated drugs, 200–1
  classification, 200
  parkinsonism, 206–11
  tardive dyskinesia, 215–26
  see also individual disorders
dysarthria, in Wilson's disease, 71
dyskinesia
  inhibitory basal ganglia output, 268
  tardive, *see* tardive dyskinesia
Dyskinesia Identification System Condensed User Scale, 230
dystonia, 114–29
  acute, 201–6
    aetiological category division, 237
  aetiologies of, 116, 117–18 *(table)*, 237
  age relationship, 203
    clinical features, 202–3
    course/outcome, 204
    drug-related movement disorders, 200
    mild, as extrapyramidal disorder, 226
    pathophysiology, 204
    predisposing factors, 203–4
    prevalence/incidence, 203
    treatment of, 205–6
    and myoclonus, 151, 156
  benign idiopathic, in infancy, 123
  causes of, 119 *(table)*
    adolescents, 122 *(table)*
    older children, 121 *(table)*
    preschool child, 120
  classification in Wilson's disease, 71
  clinical phenomenology, 114–15
  dopa-responsive, *see* dopa-responsive dystonia
  evaluation of, 116
  genetics of, 115–16

dystonia *(cont.)*
focal, 121, 242
hereditary progressive, 125
in hyperkinetic movement disorders, 181
idiopathic torsion, *see* idiopathic torsion dystonia
magnetic resonance imaging, 283–4
paroxysmal familial hypnogenic, 126
pathophysiology, 115
simulated disorders, 128–9, 129 *(table)*
tardive, 217
treatment strategies, 116, 120
dystonia musculorum deformans, *see* idiopathic torsion dystonia

eating dysfunction, in neuroacanthocytosis, 188
echolalia, in Gilles de la Tourette syndrome, 2
echopraxia, in Gilles de la Tourette syndrome, 2
electroencephalography, in attention deficit disorder, 58
epilepsia partialis continua, and myoclonus, 169
epilepsy
magnetic resonance imaging, 286–7
and myoclonus, 158–59, 163, 164
and phenylketonuria, 94
radionuclide neuroimaging, 299
essential myoclonus, 154–6
essential startle disease, and myoclonus, 156
essential tremor, 132–4
extraneous sensory stimuli, in tics, 32
extraocular dystonia, 202
extrapyramidal disorders, drug-related
assessment of, 226–31
examination for, 226–7
scale choice, 230–1
single syndrome scales, 228–9
standardized recording, 227
Extrapyramidal Symptoms Rating Scale, 229–30
eyelid myoclonus, absence epilepsy, 163

familial amyotrophic chorea with acanthocytosis, *see* neuroacanthocytosis
familial essential tremor, onset of, 133
familial paroxysmal kinesiogenic choreoathetosis, in hereditary choreas, 109
family studies, in obsessive–compulsive disorder, 45
fantasy, role of, in Gilles de la Tourette syndrome, 32–4
Friedreich's ataxia, and myoclonus, 150
frontal lobe damage, action control, in developmental dysexecutive syndrome, 306–8
functional neuroimaging, and obsessive–compulsive disorder, 47

GABA-ergic GPi/SNr output, direct/indirect pathways, 262
GABA-ergic treatment
in akathisia, 215
in tardive dyskinesia, 225
GABA-mediation, and tardive dyskinesia, 221
gallstones, pigment, in Wilson's disease, 75
genetics
of movement disorders, 237–52
of tic-related disorders, 19–21
Gilles de la Tourette syndrome, 1–7, 31–7, 311–12
adoption studies, 16–17
aetiology, 1–5
and akathisia, 214
assessment, in families, 39
and attention deficit disorder, 59–61
chemotherapy, 5
chromosomal abnormalities, 21–2
clinical characteristics, 2–3
defensive splitting, 33
demography, 1–2
and drug-induced/toxic choreas, 112
EEG findings, 5
electromyelogram patterns, 5
epidemiology, 1–2
family studies, 17–21, 37–9
genetics, 4, 15–19
identity issues, 37
in hyperkinetic movement disorders, 181
management of, 5–6
neuroimaging, 5
neurochemistry, 4–5
and obsessive–compulsive disorder, 45–6
onset, 38

pathophysiology, 5
psychopathology, 3–4
psychosocial interventions, 6
radionuclide neuroimaging, 298–9
self-regulation, 31–40
single-locus hypothesis, 17–18
tardive dyskinesia, 217
treatment, 40
twin studies, 16–17
globus pallidus, 261
Guthrie (heel prick) test, in phenylketonuria management, 86

haematuria, microscopic, in Wilson's disease, 76
haemolysis, in Wilson's disease, 71
Hallervorden–Spatz disease, 138–9, 189–90
and dystonia, 126
magnetic resonance imaging, 283, 286 *(fig.)*
pathophysiology of, 139
haplotypes, analyses, genetic linkage studies, 243
happy puppet, *see* Angelman's syndrome
hemiballismus, in chorea, 105
hepatolenticular degeneration, *see* Wilson's disease
Hillside Akathisia Scales, 229
horizontal nystagmus, and phenylketonuria, 88
huntingtin, identification of, 248–9
Huntington's disease
carrier testing, 251–2
current treatment, 108–9
gene mapping, 247–8
genetics of, 108, 246–52
huntingtin gene, 248–9
magnetic resonance imaging, 282–3, 283–5 *(fig.)*
and obsessive–compulsive disorder, 46
and parkinsonism, 136
and progressive myoclonic epilepsies, 165
radionuclide neuroimaging, 299–300
size/age correlation, 249–51
hyperekplexia, *see* essential startle disease
hyperkinetic disorders, 57, 200
basal ganglia organization, 267–8
evaluation, 180–1
long-term L-dopa use, 201
hyperphenylalaninaemia, in phenylketonuria, 86
hyperreflexia
and dopa-responsive dystonia, 245
generalized, and phenylketonuria, 90
hypersomnolence, and phenylketonuria, 89
hypersplenism, in Wilson's disease, 74
hyperthyroidism, in metabolic/endocrine/nutritional choreas, 113
hyperuricaemia, in Lesch–Nyhan syndrome, 186
hypokinetic disorders
basal ganglia organization, 267
evaluation, 180
hypomimia, and parkinsonism, 207
hypomyelination, in phenylketonuria, 85
hypoxanthine guanine phosphoribosyl transferase, in Lesch–Nyhan syndrome, 186–7
hypoxia, magnetic resonance imaging, 285
hypsarrhythmia, and infantile spasms, 167, 169

idiopathic torsion dystonia, 114, 120–3
and autosomal dominant gene, 115–16
clinical-genetic subtypes of, 238 *(table)*
counselling recommendations, 245
early onset, 239
genetics of, 237–45
linkage studies, 242–4
histopathological brain examination, 122
inheritance pattern of, 239–42
imipramine, and attention deficit disorder, 62
infantile spasms, 166–9
and phenylketonuria, 89, 90
distinct from myoclonus, 152
infectious/immunological choreas, 110 *(table)*
'intention editor' dysfunction, in Gilles de la Tourette syndrome, 4
intracerebral space-occupying lesions, radionuclide neuroimaging, 301
intracranial pathology, screening protocol, 280

Kayser–Fleischer rings, in Wilson's disease, 69–70, 79
kinetic and postural tremor, causes of, 131 *(table)*

L-dopa
in drug-related parkinsonism, 211
in dystonia, 116
in Wilson's disease, 76
Leigh's disease, 181–3
and dystonia, 128
magnetic resonance imaging, 284, 287 *(fig.)*
Lennox–Gastaut syndrome
and infantile spasms, 168
and myoclonus, 161–3
Lesch–Nyhan syndrome, 184–7
natural course of, 184 *(fig.)*
Levine–Critchley syndrome, *see* neuroacanthocytosis
limb contractures, in Wilson's disease, 74
limb-onset dystonia, genetic linkage studies, 243
linkage disequilibrium, idiopathic torsion dystonia, 244–5
liver cirrhosis, in Wilson's disease, 69–70

Machado–Joseph disease, 138
magnetic resonance imaging, 279
abnormal conditions, 282–91
and blood phenylalanine concentration, 96 *(fig.)*
group 1 subjects, 95 *(table)*
in Hallervorden–Spatz disease, 286 *(fig.)*
in Huntington's disease, 283–5 *(fig.)*
in Leigh's disease, 287 *(fig.)*
normal anatomy, 280–2
in perinatal asphyxia, 291 *(fig.)*
in phenylketonuria, 87–99, 92 *(table)*, 93 *(fig.)*, 289–90 *(fig.)*
technical aspects, 279–80
in Wilson's disease, 75, 288 *(fig.)*
measles, and myoclonus, 157
mental retardation (learning disability)
in Lennox–Gastaut syndrome, 162
in Lesch–Nyhan syndrome, 185–6
metabolic disorder, 177–93
and myoclonus, 156–7
methylphenidate, and attention deficit disorder, 59, 61, 62
microcephaly, in phenylketonuria, 85
milkmaid grasp, in chorea, 105
monoamine oxidase inhibitors, in attention deficit disorder, 64
myelin vulnerability, in phenylketonuria management, 86
myoclonus, 149–66
absence seizures in, 163
aetiology of, 155 *(table)*
dystonia and, 123
classification of, 152–4, 153–4 *(table)*
definition of, 150–2
encephalopathy, neonatal, 159
essential, 154–6
history of, 149–50
in hyperkinetic movement disorders, 181
investigation, 170–1
nocturnal, 155
non-epileptic, 169–70
progressive epilepsies, 164–6
diagnosis and classification, 165 *(table)*

N-acetyl aspartate, and phenylketonuria, 98 *(fig.)*, 99
narcissism, in Gilles de la Tourette syndrome, 36
National Phenylketonuria Register, 94
neonatal screening, phenylketonuria, 93 *(fig.)*
neuroacanthocytosis, 187–9
magnetic resonance imaging, 283
neuroblastoma, and myoclonus, 157
neurodegenerative diseases, 177–93
neurohormonal systems, and obsessive–compulsive disorder, 47
'neuroleptic' disorders, 199
neuropathic tremor, 134
neuropsychiatric disorders, radionuclide neuroimaging, 293
neuropsychological testing, in attention deficit disorder, 58
neurosecretory peptides, and obsessive–compulsive disorder, 47
neurotransmitter deficiency, and phenylketonuria, 85
nitrous oxide, radionuclide neuroimaging methodologies, 294
nocturnal myoclonus, 155

Norman and Shallice's model, action control, 305 (*fig.*)
nortriptyline, and attention deficit disorder, 62

objective dystonia, clinical features, 202
obsessive–compulsive disorder, 43–52
  aetiology, 45–8
  assessment and differential diagnosis, 48–50
  behavioural treatment, 51–2
  clinical phenomenology of, 44–5
  diagnostic criteria, 43
  epidemiology, 43
  in Gilles de la Tourette syndrome, 3–4, 19–22
  neurobiological factors, 46–7
  pharmacological treatment, 50–1
  prognosis, 52
  radionuclide neuroimaging, 300
Ohtahara syndrome, and myoclonic encephalopathy, 159
opsoclonus-myoclonus syndrome, 157
orofacial dyskinesia, 223
oxidative metabolic disorders, 11–13

palatal myoclonus, and rhythmic repetitive movements, 151
palilalia, in Gilles de la Tourette syndrome, 2
paramyoklonus multiplex, 150
parkinsonism, 180, 209–10
  akinetic–rigid syndromes, 136–9
  causes of, 137 (*table*)
  clinical features, 136, 207–8
  course/outcome, 208–9
  dystonia in, 125, 245
  pathophysiology of, 136, 209
  predisposing factors, 208
  prevalence/incidence of, 208
  single syndrome scales, 228
  and tardive movement, 220
  treatment of, 210–11
  tremor in, 135
paroxysmal choreas, 109–10
paroxysmal dystonic choreoathetosis
  in hereditary choreas, 109
  treatment strategies, 116
paroxysmal familial hypnogenic dystonia, 126
paroxysmal kinesiogenic choreoathetosis, 116
paroxysmal torticollis, in infancy, 129
pedunculopontine nucleus, basal ganglia motor circuitry, 263–4
pemoline, in attention deficit disorder, 63
penicillamine, in Wilson's disease, 74, 75, 77
  toxic reactions, 76
perinatal asphyxia, magnetic resonance imaging, 291
pertussis immunization, and infantile spasms, 167
phenylalanine
  in autosomal recessive disorder, 83
  excess in animals, 85
  low protein substitute, 94
  in phenylketonuria, 83–4, 86
phenylalanine/tyrosine conversion, 84 (*fig.*)
phenylketonuria, 83–100
  clinical manifestations, 84–5
  damage mechanism, 85
  future of, 100
  genetics of, 100
  history of, 83–4
  magnetic resonance imaging, 87–90, 284, 289–90 (*fig.*)
  management of, 86, 99
  neonatal screening, 93 (*fig.*)
  neurological abnormalities, 87–99
  neuropsychological impairments, 87 (*table*)
  pathology, 85
  psychological impairment, 86–7
phonological loop, and working memory, 308
pigment gallstones, in Wilson's disease, 75
polymorphic markers, linked with disease locus, 23
positional cloning, in linkage analysis, 21–2
positron emission tomography
  brain functions, 293
  radionuclides used in, 295 (*table*)
  radiopharmaceuticals used in, 296 (*table*)
postsynaptic receptor supersensitivity, 220
postural tremor, causes of, 130 (*table*)
Prader–Willi syndrome, 192
proteinuria, in Wilson's disease, 74
Proteus vulgaris, 84

proton magnetic resonance spectroscopy, 99
pseudosclerotic classification, in Wilson's disease, 71
psychostimulants, and attention deficit disorder, 59, 61–3
putamen-projecting sensorimotor areas, 258, 259
pyramidal tract signs, in phenylketonuria, 94

radionuclide neuroimaging, 293–301
 abnormal patterns, 298–301
 autism, 300
 cerebellar degeneration, 299
 epilepsy, 299
 Gilles de la Tourette syndrome, 298–9
 Huntington's disease, 299–300
 methodologies, 294
 normal brain, 296–8
 obsessive–compulsive disorder, 300
 Wilson's disease, 300
radiopharmaceuticals, 295–6
resting tremor, causes of, 130 *(table)*
restriction fragment length polymorphism, Huntington's disease, 248
Rett syndrome, 191
 hand movements/mouthing, 192 *(fig.)*
 magnetic resonance imaging, 285
rhythmical movements, and myoclonus, 151
rigidity, 207
risperidone, in tardive dyskinesia, 225
ritualistic behaviours, 48

St. Hans Scale, 230
Sandifer's syndrome, and dystonia, 129
schizophrenia, mimicked in Wilson's disease, 73
self-injurious behaviour
 in Gilles de la Tourette syndrome, 3–4
 in Lesch–Nyhan syndrome, 184–7, 185 *(fig.)*
sensory prodrome, in Gilles de la Tourette syndrome, 32
serotonin reuptake inhibitors, in obsessive–compulsive disorder, 46, 50
serum caeruloplasmin
 in Wilson's disease, 74
 screening test, Wilson's disease, 79
shuddering attacks, and tremor, 135
Simpson (Rockland) Dyskinesia Rating Scale, tardive dyskinesia, 229
Simpson–Angus Scale, parkinsonism, 228
single photon emission tomography
 brain functions, 293
 radionuclides used in, 295 *(table)*
 radiopharmaceuticals used in, 296 *(table)*
spasms, *see* infantile spasms
standardized recording, 227
startle disease, essential, 156
stereotypies, in hyperkinetic movement disorders, 181
streptococcal infections, and obsessive–compulsive disorder, 49
striatal dopamine deficiency, severe akinesia, 269
striatal postsynaptic dopamine receptor supersensitivity, and tardive dyskinesia, 221
structural neuroimaging, 279–91
substantia nigra, 261
subthalamic nucleus, 259, 263
supervisory attentional system
 action-schema triggering, 308
 Norman and Shallice's action control model, 306
 Tower of London test, 308
 utilization behaviour, 308
 verbal fluency test, 307–8
 Wisconsin card sorting test, 307
Sydenham's chorea, 105
 and infectious/immunological choreas, 110–11
 magnetic resonance imaging, 282
 and obsessive–compulsive disorder, 46, 47
synaptic plasticity, dopamine, role of, 265
systemic lupus erythematosus, 111

tardive akathisia, 213
tardive dyskinesia, 221–4, 222–3 *(table)*
 associated drugs, 200
 clinical features of, 216–17
 course/outcome, 219–20
 and drug-related movement disorders, 199, 215–26
 and drug-induced/toxic choreas, 112
 as epidemiological concept, 215
 non-drug-related variables, 219

pathophysiology, 220–1
persistent, estimated risk of, 218 *(table)*
predisposing factors, 218–19
prevalence/incidence of, 217–18
single syndrome scales, 228–9
treatment of, 224–6
tardive dystonia, and tardive dyskinesia, 217
Targeting Abnormal Kinetic Effects (TAKE), 228
tetrahydrobioptrin, and phenylketonuria, 84, 85
tetrarhiomolybdate, in Wilson's disease, 77
thalamic reticular nucleus, 263
thalamocortical operations, direct/indirect pathways, 262
tics, 61–3
extraneous sensory stimuli in, 32
family study data, 20–1
genetics of, 14–15
in Gilles de la Tourette syndrome, 17
in hyperkinetic movement disorders, 181
and myoclonus, 151
in obsessive–compulsive disorder, 49
tomography, radionuclide neuroimaging methodologies, 294
tonic seizures, and drop attacks, 169–70
torsion dystonia, idiopathic, *see* idiopathic torsion dystonia
torticollis, 202
paroxysmal, 129
Tower of London test, 307
transient obsessions, 48
tremor, 129–36
causes of, 131 *(table)*
classification of, 130
essential, 132–4
frequency of, 131
in hyperkinetic movement disorders, 181
pathophysiology of, 131–2
phenomenology of, 129–31
in phenylketonuria, 94
physiological, 132, 133 *(table)*
post-concussive, 135
postural, causes of, 130 *(table)*
trichotillomania, 45, 51, 52
tricyclic antidepressants, in attention deficit disorder, 62, 64
trientine, in Wilson's disease, 75, 76
triethylene tetramine dihydrochloride, in Wilson's disease, 75
tuberous sclerosis, and infantile spasms, 168
tyrosine, in phenylketonuria, 84

Unverricht–Lundborg disease, and progressive myoclonic epilepsies, 165

verbal fluency task, and frontal lobe damage, 307
viral infections, and myoclonus, 157
visuo-spatial sketch pad, and working memory, 308

Wechsler scales, in attention deficit disorder, 58
West syndrome
and infantile spasms, 167
and Lennox–Gastaut syndrome, 162
Whipple disease, and myoclonus, 157
Wilson's disease, 68–79
genetics of, 77–9, 78 *(fig.)*
historical background, 69–70
initial symptoms, 72 *(table)*
magnetic resonance imaging, 284, 288 *(fig.)*
movement disorders in, 71–4
patient management, 74–7
pseudosclerotic classification, 71, 72–3
radionuclide neuroimaging, 300
recorded initial signs, 73 *(table)*
Wisconsin card sorting test, 306–7
withdrawal emergent syndrome, 112

Yale–Brown obsessive–compulsive scale, 49

zinc salts, in Wilson's disease, 75, 76

Index compiled by A. Campbell Purton